FUNDAMENTALS OF PEDIATRIC CARDIOLOGY

FUNDAMENTALS OF PEDIATRIC CARDIOLOGY

David J. Driscoll, M.D.

Professor of Pediatrics
Consultant in Pediatric Cardiology
Mayo Clinic College of Medicine
Mayo Clinic and Foundation
Rochester, Minnesota

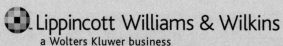. Lippincott Williams & Wilkins
a Wolters Kluwer business
Philadelphia · Baltimore · New York · London
Buenos Aires · Hong Kong · Sydney · Tokyo

Acquisitions Editor: Frances R. DeStefano
Managing Editor: Joanne Bersin
Developmental Editor: Lisa Consoli
Project Manager: Jennifer Harper
Senior Manufacturing Manager: Benjamin Rivera
Marketing Manager: Angela Panetta
Design Coordinator: Holly Reid McLaughlin
Production Services: Laserwords Private Limited
Printer: Edwards Brothers

Library of Congress Cataloging-in-Publication Data
Driscoll, David J.
  Fundamentals of pediatric cardiology / David J. Driscoll.
    p. ; cm.
  Includes bibliographical references and index.
  ISBN 0-7817-8500-6
  1. Pediatric cardiology. I. Title.
  [DNLM: 1. Heart Diseases. 2. Child. 3. Infant. WS 290 D781f 2006]
  RJ421.D75 2006
  618.92′12—dc22
                                        2006002395

Care has been taken to confirm the accuracy of the information presented and to describe generally accepted practices. However, the authors, editors, and publisher are not responsible for errors or omissions or for any consequences from application of the information in this book and make no warranty, expressed or implied, with respect to the currency, completeness, or accuracy of the contents of the publication. Application of this information in a particular situation remains the professional responsibility of the practitioner.

The authors, editors, and publisher have exerted every effort to ensure that drug selection and dosage set forth in this text are in accordance with current recommendations and practice at the time of publication. However, in view of ongoing research, changes in government regulations, and the constant flow of information relating to drug therapy and drug reactions, the reader is urged to check the package insert for each drug for any change in indications and dosage and for added warnings and precautions. This is particularly important when the recommended agent is a new or infrequently employed drug.

Some drugs and medical devices presented in this publication have Food and Drug Administration (FDA) clearance for limited use in restricted research settings. It is the responsibility of health care providers to ascertain the FDA status of each drug or device planned for use in their clinical practice.

The publisher has made every effort to trace copyright holders for borrowed material. If they have inadvertently overlooked any, they will be pleased to make the necessary arrangements at the first opportunity.

To purchase additional copies of this book, call our customer service department at (800) 638-3030 or fax orders to (301) 223-2320. International customers should call (301) 223-2300. Lippincott Williams & Wilkins customer service representatives are available from 8:30 am to 6:30 pm, EST, Monday through Friday, for telephone access. Visit Lippincott Williams & Wilkins on the Internet: http://www.lww.com.

10 9 8 7 6 5 4 3 2 1

To the women in my life:

My wife, Virginia V. Michels, M.D.
My daughter, Ginna Driscoll Wilson, J.D.
My mother, Dorothy Driscoll, M.O.M.

The Author

Dr. David Driscoll is Professor of Pediatrics, Division of Pediatric Cardiology, Mayo Clinic College of Medicine and the Mayo Clinic and Foundation. From 1985 to 2004, Dr. Driscoll was Chairman of the Division of Pediatric Cardiology. He has been the Chairman of the Council on Cardiovascular Disease in the Young of the American Heart Association and Chairman of the subboard of Pediatric Cardiology of the American Board of Pediatrics. Currently, he is the Editor of the subboard of Pediatric Cardiology.

Contents

Preface   xi

1   Cardiovascular Physiology   1

2   Clinical Evaluation   7

3   Basic Diagnostic Studies   17

4   Pediatric Exercise Testing   29

5   Innocent Murmurs   43

6   Chest Pain   49

7   Syncope and Sudden Death   55

8   Principles of Inheritance and Genetics of Congenital Heart Disease   61

9   Left-to-Right Shunts   73

10   Right-to-Left Shunts   89

11   Obstructive and Regurgitant Lesions   121

12   Acquired Heart Diseases   137

13   Cardiomyopathy   153

14   Coronary Artery Anomalies   161

Index   169

Preface

"Being a physician means living more lives than your own"

Many pediatricians and family practice physicians are intimidated by heart disease in infants, children, and adolescents. This may result from the perception that learning so many types of congenital heart defects and diseases may appear to be an insurmountable task. In addition becoming an expert in auscultation of the heart does require considerable experience, and it is easy to become frustrated when one is unable to make an anatomic diagnosis on the basis of physical examination. This is unfortunate because it is often difficult even for experts and frequently unnecessary to make an anatomical diagnosis on the basis of physical examination alone. Rather, it is important to determine whether the patient (i) does or does not have congenital heart disease, (ii) has cyanotic or acyanotic heart disease, (iii) has heart failure or pulmonary overcirculation (too much pulmonary blood flow), (iv) has reduced cardiac output, or (v) requires urgent detailed evaluation and treatment. I hope this book will facilitate all primary care physicians who care for infants and children to make these distinctions.

This book is intended for medical students with an interest in primary care, residents in pediatrics and family medicine, and first-year pediatric and adult cardiology trainees. I have tried to present information in a straightforward and organized manner. Excessive detail, unnecessary for initial evaluation and management of patients, has been avoided. This book was not intended to be encyclopedic. There are several excellent encyclopedic textbooks of pediatric cardiology, and the reader should refer to these textbooks, as well as the recent medical literature, if more detailed information is needed. The book also contains very little drug dosage data. Because there may be regional differences in drug use and dosage and because these may change over time, the reader should refer to current dosage recommendations for this information.

I have been fortunate in having had excellent teachers. It is impossible to recognize and thank all of them. However, I have included Drs. J. C. Peterson, William Gallen, Dan McNamara, Charles Mullins, Michael Nihill, Thomas Vargo, Paul Gillette, Howard Gutgesell, Robert Lewis, William Wiedman, Robert Feldt, Denton Cooley, Gordon Danielson, and Francisco Puga. I am grateful to all of them. In addition, I am grateful to Dr. William Edwards for providing the illustrations of pathologic materials, Dr. Patrick O'Leary for the echocardiographic images, and Mr. John Hagen for his excellent medical illustrations.

CHAPTER 1

Cardiovascular Physiology

"It is the physician's privilege
to cure sometimes,
to relieve often,
to comfort always"

BASIC CARDIOVASCULAR PHYSIOLOGY

It is essential to understand basic cardiovascular physiology to appreciate the pathophysiology of congenital and acquired heart problems. The primary function of the cardiovascular system is to pump blood. Cardiac output (liters per minute) is the basic measure of how much blood the heart pumps.

CARDIAC OUTPUT AND ITS DETERMINANTS

The determinants of cardiac output (CO) are heart rate (HR) and stroke volume (SV).

$$CO = HR \times SV$$

This relationship can be simplified using the determinants of SV—end-diastolic volume (EDV) and ejection fraction (EF).

$$CO = HR \times EDV \times EF$$

Therefore, the only way cardiac output can increase or decrease is if heart rate, end-diastolic volume, and/or ejection fraction increase(s) or decrease(s).

There are many factors that affect heart rate, end-diastolic volume, and ejection fraction. Hence, these factors change cardiac output. Heart rate may be affected by a variety of drugs and inherent conduction abnormalities. Factors that limit the increase in heart rate, such as β-blockers, atrioventricular block, and sick sinus syndrome, negatively affect the increase in cardiac output.

End-diastolic volume (preload) increases with an increase in intravascular volume and vice versa. Also, conditions such as restrictive cardiomyopathy, pericardial effusion, and constrictive pericarditis that limit ventricular filling decrease diastolic volume and hence cardiac output.

Ejection fraction decreases with decreased preload, increased afterload, and decreased contractility. Ejection fraction increases with increased preload, decreased afterload, increased contractility, and increased heart rate.

Contractility, by affecting ejection fraction, changes cardiac output. Contractility is easy to conceptualize but difficult to measure. Simplistically, ejection fraction would seem to be an excellent measure of contractility. However, because ejection fraction is affected by afterload, preload, heart rate, and contractility, it is not a pure measure of contractility. Contractility can change in response to either positive or negative inotropic agents.

As is apparent from this discussion, truly understanding a basic relationship such as $CO = HR \times EF \times EDV$ allows one to truly understand cardiovascular physiology and how diseases and different treatment strategies affect cardiac function.

There are several other relationships with which one should be acquainted. These are described in the following sections.

OHM'S LAW

$$Resistance\ (R) = \frac{Pressure\ (P)}{Flow\ (Q)}$$

Ohm's law describes the relationship between pressure, flow, and resistance. Understanding this relationship is essential to understand, for example, the difference between pulmonary hypertension and pulmonary vascular obstructive disease, the effect of left-to-right shunts on pulmonary artery pressure, and the effects of pulmonary artery and systemic vascular resistances on the volume of left-to-right and right-to-left shunts.

It is obvious from this relationship that increased pulmonary artery pressure could result from increased resistance in the pulmonary bed or increased flow into the pulmonary bed or both.

$$P = R \times Q$$

It also is clear from this relationship that flow decreases as resistance increases.

$$Q = \frac{P}{R}$$

This explains why a drug that decreases systemic vascular resistance (afterload reduction) increases cardiac output (Q).

POISEUILLE'S LAW

$$\Delta Pressure\ (P) = \frac{8LQ\ (Viscosity)}{\pi r^4}$$

or

$$Flow\ (Q) = \frac{\Delta P \pi r^4}{8L\ (Viscosity)}$$

or

$$Resistance\ (R) = \frac{8L\ (Viscosity)}{\pi r^4}$$

where $L =$ length and $r =$ radius.

This relationship helps understand the determinants of blood flow, pressure, and resistance.

By solving for each of these variables, it becomes apparent that *pressure* is directly related to the length of the tube through which a fluid flows, the volume of fluid flowing through the tube, and the viscosity of the fluid. Pressure is inversely related to the radius of the tube.

Flow is directly related to the driving pressure and the radius of the tube and indirectly to the viscosity of the fluid and the length of the tube through which flow occurs.

If one solves the equation for P/Q (which is resistance), it becomes apparent that *resistance* is related directly to viscosity and the length of the tube and inversely related to the radius of the tube. For example, as the viscosity of blood increases (as with polycythemia), pulmonary artery resistance and pressure increase.

FICK PRINCIPLE

In 1870, Fick conceived a method of determining cardiac output on the basis of oxygen consumption and mixed venous and arterial oxygen content. The Fick principle is described by the following formula:

$$CO = \dot{V}_{O_2}/[\text{Hemoglobin}] \times 1.36 \times (\text{Saturation}_{ART} - \text{Saturation}_{MV}) \times 10$$

where $\dot{V}_{O_2}$ = oxygen consumption, ART = arterial, and MV = mixed venous.

For oxygen to be consumed, it must be bound to the red blood cells entering the lungs and carried from the lungs to the tissues of the body. By knowing the amount of oxygen that is bound to the red blood cells entering the lungs, the amount that is bound to the red blood cells leaving the lungs, and the oxygen consumption, one can determine the rate of blood flow through the lungs. This is better understood if one considers this process as being analogous to coal being loaded onto a train (see Fig. 1.1). The coal represents oxygen, the train represents the pulmonary blood flow, and each car represents individual

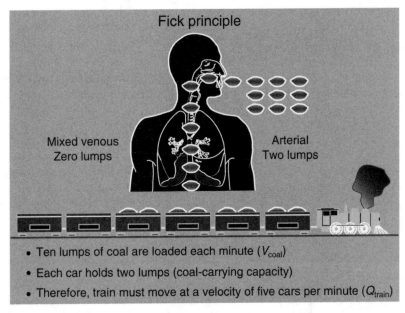

FIGURE 1.1 ● Schematic representation of the Fick principle. The coal represents oxygen. The train represents the pulmonary blood flow and each train car represents individual red blood cell. The coal-carrying capacity or each car (or the oxygen-carrying capacity of the red blood cells) is two lumps of coal. Knowing how many lumps of coal are in each car as it enters the lungs, how much coal is in each car as it exits the lung, and the rate of disappearance of lumps of coal from the environment, one can calculate the speed of the train (or the rate of pulmonary blood flow).

red blood cells. The formula describing the Fick principle allows a clear understanding of the relationship between oxygen consumption and cardiac output.

LAPLACE'S LAW

Laplace's law describes the relationship between pressure, wall tension, and radius.

$$\text{Pressure } (P) = \frac{\text{Wall tension}}{\text{Radius}}$$

Laplace's law is easily demonstrated by examining a partially inflated sausage-shaped balloon (see Fig. 1.2).

The cardiovascular implications of Laplace's law are important for at least two reasons. First, myocardial oxygen consumption increases as wall tension increases. Therefore, a heart with lower wall tension operates more efficiently than that with higher wall tension. One can appreciate that wall tension (tension = pressure × radius) will increase as the pressure and radius of the chamber increase. Hence, a dilated left ventricle pumping against a high afterload is at a disadvantage as compared to a small chamber pumping against a lower afterload. This makes it clear why lowering afterload is beneficial in treating patients with a dilated, poorly functioning ventricle.

Second, Laplace's law, when applied to a blood vessel wall, allows one to understand the determinants of vessel rupture. As wall tension increases, the chance of rupture increases, and as radius increases, wall tension increases. Hence, in a patient with Marfan syndrome whose aortic diameter is 5 cm, the aorta is more likely to rupture than in the case of a similar patient whose aortic diameter is 4 cm. Also, if the aortic diameter is the same in both patients, the one with higher blood pressure (and hence the higher wall tension) will be more likely to have an aortic rupture.

RESISTANCE AND COMPLIANCE

The term *resistance* is used to describe the ease or difficulty that a fluid encounters when flowing through a tube or blood vessel. *Compliance* is the term used to describe the difficulty or ease a fluid encounters when filling a chamber such as the left or right ventricle.

$$\text{Compliance} = \frac{\text{Change of volume}}{\text{Change of pressure}}$$

As described by Ohm's law, as resistance increases, flow in a blood vessel decreases and as compliance increases, flow into a chamber increases.

Two examples will illustrate these concepts and are useful in understanding cardiac pathophysiology.

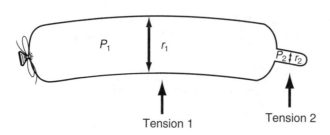

Tension 1   *Tension 2*

FIGURE 1.2 ● A partially inflated balloon is illustrative of the Laplace's law. If one squeezes the balloon where the radius is greater, the balloon feels "firmer" than when one squeezes it where the radius is lesser. Obviously, $P_1 = P_2$, but Tension 2 > Tension 1. This "firmness" is a result of greater wall tension.

Consider a patient with a very large ventricular septal defect (VSD). When ventricular contraction occurs, blood in the right ventricle could flow to the pulmonary artery or through the VSD to the aorta. Blood in the left ventricle could flow to the aorta or through the VSD to the pulmonary artery. The net flow of blood will be determined by the relative *resistances* to flow into the pulmonary bed and into the systemic bed. Normally, pulmonary resistance is lower than systemic resistance, so more blood will flow into the pulmonary artery than into the aorta.

Consider a patient with a large atrial septal defect (ASD). During diastole, blood in the left atrium could flow through the mitral valve or through the ASD and then through the tricuspid valve. Blood in the right atrium could flow through the tricuspid valve or through the ASD and then through the mitral valve. The net flow of blood will be determined by the relative *compliances* of the right and left ventricle during diastole. Because the right ventricle is a thin-walled structure, it is more "distensible" or "compliant" than the left ventricle, and hence more blood will flow through the tricuspid valve and into the right ventricle than through the mitral valve and into the left ventricle.

SELECTED REFERENCES

Katz A. *Physiology of the heart*. 3rd ed. Philadelphia, PA: Lippincott Williams & Wilkins; 2000.
Lilly L. *Pathophysiology of the heart*. 3rd ed. Philadelphia, PA: Lippincott Williams & Wilkins; 2003.

CHAPTER 2

Clinical Evaluation

*"Listen to what patients are saying
because they are telling you the diagnosis"*

In most cases, it is difficult to arrive at an accurate anatomic diagnosis of the specific congenital heart defect after only a history and physical examination. This is possible in some cases, such as for coarctation of the aorta and small ventricular septal defects (VSDs), but for more complex problems, sophisticated imaging studies, such as echocardiography, angiography, and magnetic resonance imaging (MRI), will be necessary.

However, it is extremely important to develop a differential diagnosis using the history, physical examination, chest x-ray, and electrocardiogram. To facilitate this, patients can be categorized on the following pathophysiologic bases. From this, one can plan the appropriate subsequent diagnostic and therapeutic steps.

A. Cyanotic heart disease with increased pulmonary blood flow

   Transposition of the great arteries
   Truncus arteriosus
   Totally anomalous pulmonary venous return
   Hypoplastic left heart syndrome
   Tricuspid atresia without pulmonary stenosis or atresia
   Tricuspid atresia with transposed great arteries

B. Cyanotic heart disease with decreased pulmonary blood flow

   Tetralogy of Fallot
   Pulmonary atresia and VSD
   Pulmonary atresia and intact ventricular septum
   Ebstein anomaly
   Tricuspid atresia with pulmonary stenosis or atresia
   Critical pulmonary stenosis (neonate)

C. Acyanotic heart disease with increased pulmonary blood flow and/or pulmonary congestion

   VSD
   Atrial septal defect (ASD)

Atrioventricular septal defect
Patent ductus arteriosus
Aorticopulmonary window
Systemic arteriovenous fistula
Pulmonary venous obstruction

Cor triatriatum
Obstructed total anomalous pulmonary venous return
Mitral stenosis

D. Acyanotic heart disease with ventricular outflow tract obstruction

Aortic stenosis
Pulmonic stenosis
Coarctation of the aorta
Obstructive hypertrophic cardiomyopathy

E. Acyanotic or cyanotic heart disease with poor systemic perfusion

Septic shock
Coarctation of the aorta (neonate)
Myocarditis
Cardiomyopathy
Critical aortic stenosis (neonate)
Critical pulmonary stenosis (neonate)

The presence of cyanosis is ascertained by observation or using a pulse oximeter. The presence of increased or decreased pulmonary blood flow is ascertained by the appearance of the pulmonary vasculature on chest x-ray. In addition, increased pulmonary blood flow is manifested by increased respiratory rate, poor feeding, failure to thrive, pallor, and intercostal, subcostal, and suprasternal notch retraction and head bobbing with breathing. The same signs and symptoms occur if there is an obstruction to pulmonary venous return such as in pulmonary vein stenosis, mitral valve stenosis, or decreased left ventricular compliance. Low cardiac output is manifested by fatigue, pallor, delayed capillary refill, tachycardia, peripheral cyanosis, syncope, and oliguria.

Unfortunately, with the proliferation of technology in the field of cardiology, trainees and practitioners are becoming less and less skilled in the art of history taking and physical examination. This is unfortunate because when the logical sequence of history, physical examination, chest radiogram, and electrocardiogram, followed by more technical tests such as echocardiography, cardiac catheterization, MRI, and magnetic resonance angiography (MRA) is not followed, mistakes in diagnosis and treatment will occur.

HISTORY AND PHYSICAL EXAMINATION

This chapter is not intended to supplant a detailed textbook of history taking and physical examination. Rather, useful suggestions about history taking and physical examination are presented.

HISTORY

The historical points of interest, of course, will vary considerably, depending upon the age of the patient and the presenting signs, symptoms, and complaints. When evaluating a newborn with cyanosis or congestive heart failure, the history will be rather brief. Obviously, one would want to know whether there is a family history of congenital heart disease or premature death and whether the baby was exposed to any teratogenic agents. It is very important to determine whether the baby is feeding well.

For older patients, one needs to ascertain the presence of cardiac symptoms such as dyspnea, shortness of breath, palpitations, and syncope. It is important to know that the patient, his/her family, and the physician are all using the same definition of terms. For example, patients often will state that they have "passed out." When asked what actually happened, it becomes clear that they did not really pass out but were just a bit light-headed. If patients respond that they are "short of breath," one must have them define and quantify what they mean by "short of breath."

Confusion frequently occurs when taking a family history of premature death. When asked about premature death, patients may respond that someone in the family died of a "heart attack." The term *heart attack* means different things to different individuals. Most physicians equate the term "heart attack" with "myocardial infarction." To the layperson, however, heart attack may include myocardial infarction, pulmonary embolism, sudden unexplained death (such as might occur with hypertrophic cardiomyopathy, prolonged QT-interval syndrome, or Brugada syndrome), and ruptured aortic aneurysm among many others. Hence, it is important to obtain accurate details to determine why a family member died.

Be aware of patients who do not answer the specific question or are imprecise in their answer.

For example,

SCENARIO A
Physician: "Have you ever fainted?"
Patient: "I had an aunt who fainted whenever she saw blood. . . and her sister died when she was 89 and the doctor thought that her heart had exploded."
Comment: When dealing with a patient such as this, who gives rambling, imprecise answers, it is important to redirect the patient's focus to the question.

SCENARIO B
Physician: "How many times have you fainted?"
Patient: "Lots of times."
Comment: Note that the patient has not answered the question. The follow-up question should be, "Well, have you fainted about 10 times or about 100 times?"

Subsequent questions should be aimed at refining the answer with more and more precision.

SCENARIO C
Physician: "When you faint, for how long are you unconscious?"
Patient: "A long time."
Comment: Follow-up question should be "Do you mean many seconds, minutes, hours, or days?"

Obtaining a family history is one of the pitfalls of good medical history taking. This is partly due to the patient's lack of knowledge of his/her complete family history and may also be due to the poor questions posed by the examiner.

PHYSICAL EXAMINATION

Inspection

> "Don't just look,
>   but see"

The following observations can be made by inspection:

Respiratory rate: Because infants have periodic respirations, it is important to count the respiratory rate for 1 entire minute (see Fig. 2.1).

Head bobbing: Infants with pulmonary edema, increased pulmonary blood flow, or pulmonary congestion demonstrate head bobbing with respiration.

Retractions

Pallor

Clubbing (see Fig. 2.2)

Cyanosis and differential cyanosis (see Fig. 2.3)

Sweating

Fat stores: Too little fat can result from chronic congestive heart failure and too much fat can be related to obesity, hypertension, and hyperlipidemia.

Dysmorphic features

Skin edema

Abnormal superficial vascular patterns

Palpation

> "Don't just touch,
>   but feel"

The following observations can be made by palpation:

Pulse volume (see Fig. 2.4): Increased pulse volume can be associated with patent ductus arteriosus, truncus arteriosus, anemia, arteriovenous fistula, fever, and aortic insufficiency. Reduced pulse volume can result from low cardiac output and arterial stenoses.

Precordial impulses (see Fig. 2.5): The quality of the right ventricular (RV) impulse is helpful in determining whether a significant cardiac defect exists, especially in infants. In general, in an infant, if the RV impulse is normal, it is unlikely that a potentially lethal

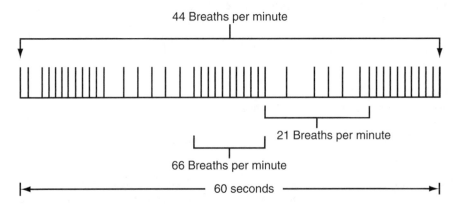

FIGURE 2.1 ● Illustration of periodic respiration. Note that if the respiratory rate is only counted for a short period, an incorrect respiratory rate could be calculated.

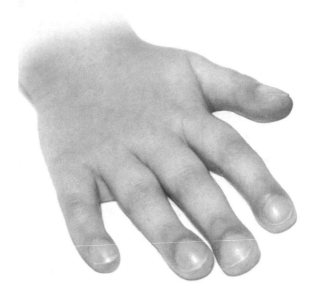

FIGURE 2.2 ● Digital clubbing.

congenital cardiac defect is present. The RV impulse is best felt at the lower left sternal border or below and behind the xiphoid process. Essentially, all important congenital cardiac defects that present in the newborn period are associated with an abnormally increased RV impulse. Patients with volume-overloaded ventricles will have a diffuse rocking precordial impulse. Thrills can alert the examiner to very turbulent blood flow patterns, as can occur with aortic and pulmonary stenosis and restrictive VSDs.

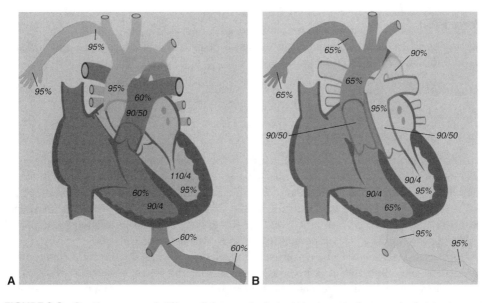

FIGURE 2.3 ● The causes of differential cyanosis. Patent ductus arteriosus and persistent pulmonary hypertension **(A)**. Transposition of the great arteries and coarctation of the aorta **(B)**.

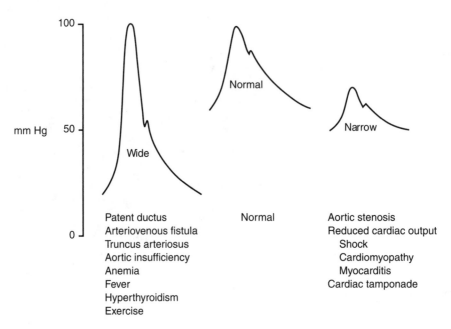

FIGURE 2.4 ● Illustration of the relationship of pulse pressure to specific cardiac conditions.

Temperature: One of the best indicators of survival or death after cardiac operation is toe temperature. The first thing that experienced clinicians do when evaluating a patient after cardiac operation is to feel the patient's toes.
Liver and spleen size
Peripheral edema
Ascites

Percussion

Percussion is useful in determining the presence of pleural effusion, ascites, and size and position of the liver and spleen.

Auscultation

> "Don't just listen,
>   but hear"

General principles. Cardiac auscultation involves more than just describing the presence of murmurs. It is used to describe the heart sounds, clicks, and rubs in addition to murmurs. To perform a complete and thorough auscultation of the heart, one must separate the auscultatory procedure into listening to the first heart sound, the second heart sound, occurs in systole, and lastly, occurs in diastole. Unless one listens carefully to each temporal portion of the cardiac cycle, important information will be missed.

Cardiac auscultation must be performed in a quiet room with a high-quality stethoscope. The patient must be quiet; it is a waste of time to auscult a crying baby. Therefore, the seasoned examiner employs techniques to keep infants and children quiet. Babies should be kept on the parent's lap and not undressed at the beginning of the examination (see Fig. 2.6). The examiner should first listen through the clothing and then gain further access

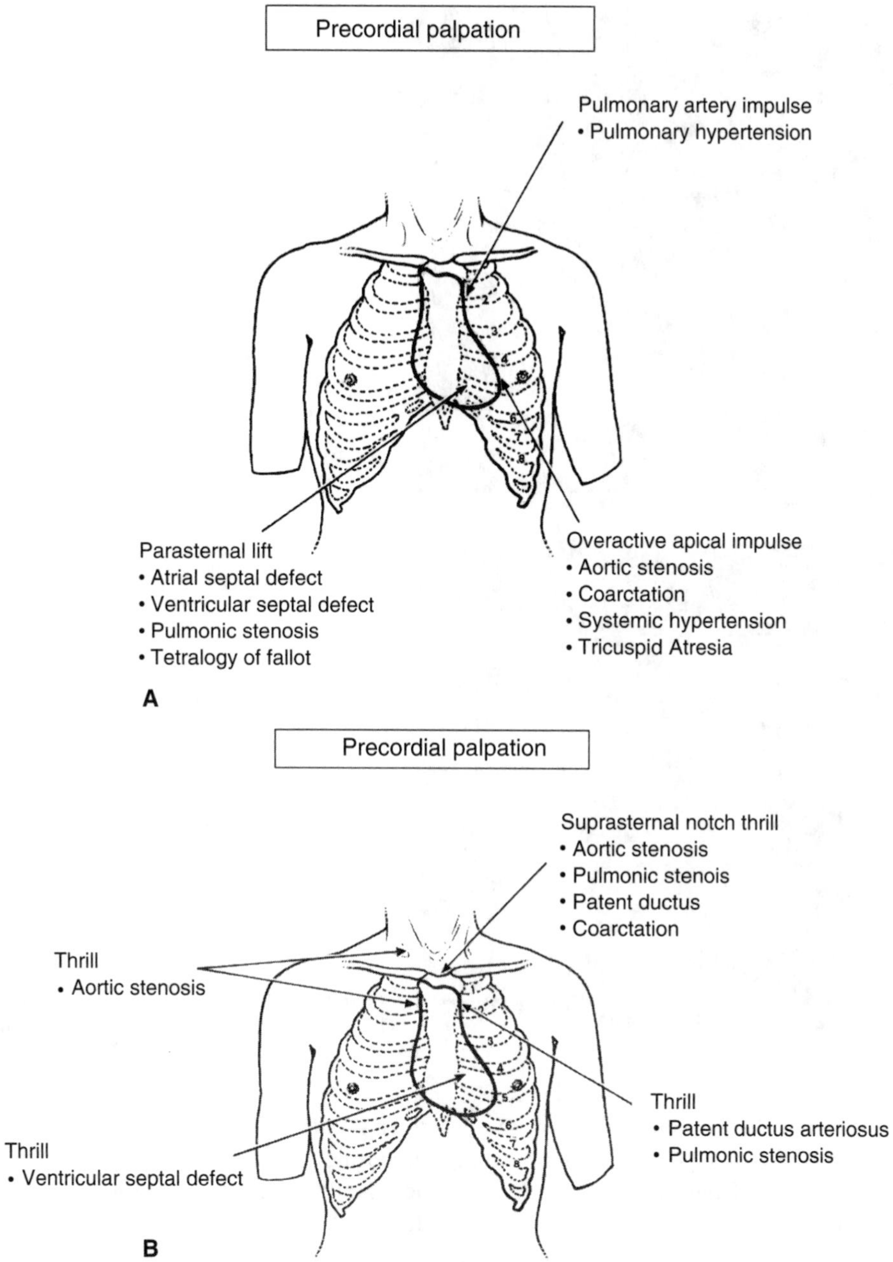

FIGURE 2.5 ● (A and B) Location of precordial impulses and thrills.

to the bare chest by carefully opening or removing pieces of clothing without disturbing the baby. As more access to the bare chest is obtained, the physician should continue to auscult the chest. If the baby is fussy and hungry, the examination should be continued after the baby has been fed.

Patients aged between 18 months and 3 years can be the most challenging to examine because they may be scared or uncooperative. When dealing with a child of this age-group,

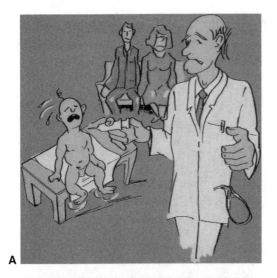

A

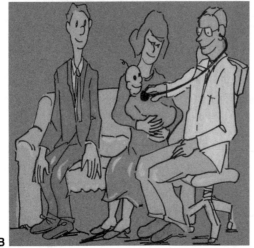

B   *FIGURE 2.6* ● When not to auscult the
                                heart **(A)**; when to auscult the heart **(B)**.

upon entering the examination room, the examiner should be seated as soon as possible so that he/she is not perceived as a towering, imposing figure to the child. For the first several minutes of the examination, the examiner should ignore the child and obtain the history from the parent. This will allow the child to "get used to" the presence of the examiner. After several minutes, the examiner can approach the child, but this should be done with the child on the parent's lap and with the examiner seated. All movements of the examiner should be slow. For example, reach out and ask to look at and touch the child's fingers. This allows initial contact to be made at a distance of several feet, thereby decreasing intimidation. While approaching the child, it is helpful to engage in some sort of banter to distract the child. It may be helpful to first listen with the stethoscope to the child's hand or arm before approaching the chest. Do not remove the child's clothing until one has established rapport with the child. Even then, remove only enough clothing to do a complete examination. With children of this age-group, it is generally better to exclude coarctation of the aorta by assessing the pedal pulses rather than the femoral pulses because the child may get upset if the examiner feels for the femoral pulses. Frequently, it is helpful to distract the child with some object of interest that the child *has not* seen before.

Heart sounds

S_1 *and* S_2. One needs to note whether the intensity of S_1 and S_2 is reduced or increased. Are they single or split? S_2 normally splits with inspiration and becomes single or nearly single with expiration. If S_2 is widely split and never becomes single, one must suspect the presence of an ASD or right bundle branch block. The intensity of S_2 will be increased if the chest wall is very thin, if there is pulmonary hypertension, or if the aorta is relatively anterior in the chest, as occurs with transposition of the great arteries, tetralogy of Fallot, and pulmonary atresia.

S_3 *and* S_4. The presence of an S_3 is normal in children. However, it must be distinguished from a mitral or tricuspid diastolic flow murmur. In general, mitral and tricuspid flow murmurs are of longer duration than an S_3. An S_4 is an abnormal sound and is associated with a stiff or noncompliant ventricle.

Heart murmurs. Heart murmurs should *not* be described in qualitative terms such as *rough, swishy, squeaky*, and *musical* because these terms mean different things to different individuals. Murmurs are described by the following characteristics.

Intensity or Loudness

For systolic murmurs, the standard convention is to describe the intensity and loudness in terms of grades 1/6 to 6/6. A grade 4/6 murmur is accompanied by a thrill. A 5/6 murmur can be heard with the stethoscope placed several centimeters away from the chest and a grade 6/6 murmur can be heard without a stethoscope.

The convention for diastolic murmurs is less well defined. Some suggest using the same convention as that for systolic murmurs (i.e., 1/6 to 6/6). But others use a range of 1/4 to 4/4.

The description of the change in the intensity of the murmur throughout its duration is important. A "crescendo–decrescendo" murmur is typical of the murmur produced by aortic or pulmonary stenosis. A "decrescendo" murmur is typical of aortic or pulmonary valve insufficiency. The term *holosystolic* is confusing because it refers to two different things. Obviously, it means that the murmur occurs throughout systole, but, by convention, it also means that the intensity of the murmur remains constant throughout its duration.

Frequency or Pitch

Frequency or pitch refers to the quality of the sound. Technically, frequency describes the physics of the sound wave in cycles per second. Pitch describes the quality of sound as heard by the listener and is usually directly related to the frequency. Pitch may also include the effect of harmonics on a person's perception of sound. Frequency and pitch are described as low, mid, or high. For example, the murmur of a VSD is a low-frequency murmur and that of mitral insufficiency is a high-frequency murmur. The murmurs of aortic and pulmonary stenosis are of the mid-frequency type.

Temporal Location Within the Cardiac Cycle

Temporal location refers to whether the murmur occurs in systole or diastole—early, mid, or late systole or diastole.

Location in the Chest

One must describe the position on the chest wall where the murmur is of maximum intensity and the position to which the murmur radiates. For example, the murmur of a VSD usually is best heard at the mid-left sternal border and may radiate toward the right sternal border or the base of the heart. The murmur of pulmonary stenosis is heard best at the left upper sternal border and radiates to the axillae and the back. The murmur of aortic stenosis is heard best along the mid-left sternal border and radiates to the right upper sternal border.

Effect of Maneuvers and Position Change

This is a topic that confuses many individuals, but some simple facts and concepts will be helpful. The innocent Still's murmur is one of the most common murmurs encountered in children. Hence, it is helpful to know that this murmur is louder in the supine than the sitting position.

The murmur of hypertrophic obstructive cardiomyopathy will become louder as left ventricular afterload decreases (essentially as blood pressure decreases) and softer as left ventricular afterload increases (essentially as blood pressure increases). Handgrip will increase afterload and make the murmur softer. Sublingual nitroglycerin reduces afterload and makes the murmur louder. Standing up will accentuate the murmur.

The murmur of mitral stenosis is best heard at the apex of the heart, with the patient in a left lateral decubitus position.

Much has been written about the effect of the Valsalva maneuver on murmurs, but this can be quite confusing because there are four phases to a Valsalva maneuver and the effect of Valsalva upon a murmur will depend on the phase of the Valsalva maneuver that exists when the murmur is assessed.

SELECTED REFERENCE

McKusick VA. *Cardiovascular sound in health and disease spectrograms*. Baltimore, MD: Lippincott Williams & Wilkins; 1958.

CHAPTER 3

Basic Diagnostic Studies

*"Absence of evidence
is not evidence of absence"*

ELECTROCARDIOGRAPHY

Numerous excellent textbooks on electrocardiography have been written, and this section is not intended to compete with or replace those textbooks. However, those textbooks may be a bit challenging for the medical student, family practice, or general pediatric resident. This chapter includes the essentials of cardiac rhythm analysis and treatment.

For each rhythm displayed, there is a brief comment about the treatment. One must recognize that the treatment of pediatric arrhythmias has become very complex. Indeed, pediatric electrophysiology is a specialty by itself. Therefore, the comments about treatment will be tailored to immediate rather than long-term treatment.

It is essential that all clinicians have the ability to determine the cardiac rhythm from an electrocardiographic tracing. Although it may be possible to determine the rhythm from a strip chart recording obtained from an electrocardiogram (ECG) monitor, one will make fewer errors if the interpretation is based upon a 12-lead surface ECG.

CARDIAC RHYTHM

1. The rhythm is *sinus* if there is a P wave in front of every QRS *and* if the P wave is upright in leads I and aVF (see Figure 3.1).

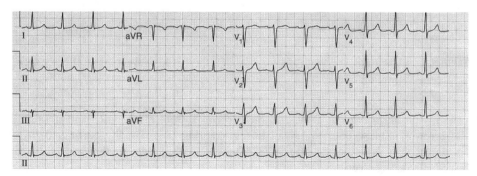

FIGURE 3.1 ● Sinus rhythm. This rhythm is indicated when there is a P wave in front of every QRS and if the P wave is upright in leads I and aVF.

2. The rhythm is *low right atrial* if there is a P wave in front of every QRS but if the P wave is upright in lead I and inverted in lead aVF (see Fig. 3.2). This is not an abnormal rhythm. It is a variant of normal and requires no special evaluation or treatment.

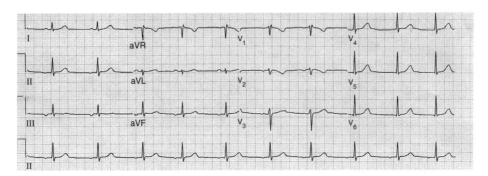

FIGURE 3.2 ● Low right atrial rhythm. This is indicated if there is a P wave in front of every QRS but the P wave is upright in lead I and inverted in lead aVF.

3. The rhythm is *left atrial* if there is a P wave in front of every QRS and the P wave is inverted in lead I (see Fig. 3.3). This rhythm can be associated with situs inversus totalis, in which the morphologic right atrium and the normal sinus node are to the left of the left atrium. In this case, the rhythm requires no treatment. A left atrial rhythm can also occur with normal situs when a left atrial electric focus supplants the normal sinus rhythm. In the absence of a left atrial ectopic focus tachycardia associated with this condition, no treatment is required.

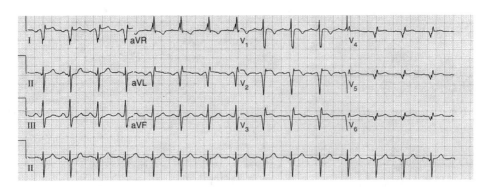

FIGURE 3.3 ● Left atrial rhythm. This is indicated if there is a P wave in front of every QRS and the P wave is inverted in lead I.

4. The rhythm is *junctional* if there is no P wave in front of the QRS and if the QRS is narrow (<80 msecond; two small boxes) (see Fig. 3.4). Usually, junctional rhythm is slower than the expected sinus rate. Intermittent junctional rhythm can be normal, especially during sleep.

    The treatment for junctional rhythm *in the absence of any sinus rhythm* may involves insertion of a pacemaker. However, it is difficult to identify patients who require a pacemaker.

When junctional rhythm is a complication of cardiac surgery, most experts recommend insertion of a pacemaker. If junctional rhythm is particularly slow or is associated with symptoms of lightheadedness or syncope, insertion of a pacemaker is indicated.

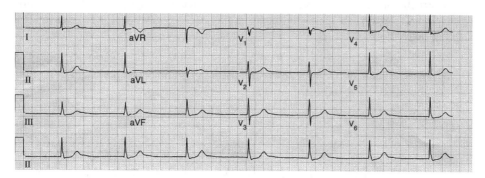

FIGURE 3.4 ● Junctional rhythm. This is indicated if there is not a P wave in front of the QRS and the QRS is narrow (<80 msecond; two small boxes).

5. If there is no P wave in front of the QRS and if the QRS is wide (>120 msecond), the rhythm likely is originating distal to the His bundle (see Fig. 3.5). The rhythm most likely is *ventricular* in origin. Alternatively, the rhythm could be originating from the *junction* if there is bundle branch block.

   The treatment of this condition depends upon many factors. Firstly, one must determine whether the rhythm is junctional with aberrant conduction or is ventricular or fascicular in origin. If a previous ECG is available when the patient was in sinus rhythm and if the morphology of the QRS complex in sinus rhythm is identical to that when there is no sinus rhythm, then the rhythm is junctional and treated accordingly (see preceding text).

   Secondly, if the rhythm is ventricular or fascicular, its cause must be determined. The causes of ventricular or fascicular rhythms include myocarditis, electrolyte imbalance, long–QT-interval syndrome, Brugada syndrome, and myocardial ischemia, among others. The treatment will depend upon the underlying cause but might include correction of metabolic abnormalities causing the arrhythmia, drugs to suppress the rhythm, and/or an implantable cardiac defibrillator (ICD).

   There is a condition of benign ventricular tachycardia (VT) of childhood that requires no treatment. However, before arriving at this diagnosis, all other causes of ventricular rhythms must be excluded.

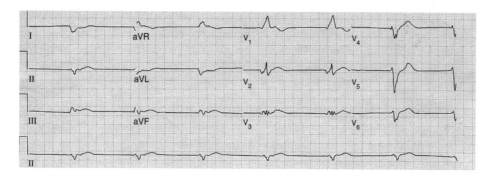

FIGURE 3.5 ● Rhythm likely originating distal to the His bundle. This is indicated if there is no P wave in front of the QRS and the QRS is wide (>120 msecond).

6. *Tachyarrhythmias* exist if the heart rate is faster than it should be on the basis of the patient's activity. For example, a heart rate of 180 beats per minute is normal for a 14-year-old engaged in vigorous exercise but is abnormal if the child is resting. Tachyarrhythmias can be classified into supraventricular tachycardia (SVT), junctional tachycardia (paroxysmal junctional tachycardia [PJT] or junctional ectopic tachycardia [JET]), and VT.

A. In SVT, the QRS is narrow, and P waves, if discernible, will be related to the QRS (see Fig. 3.6). Treatment of SVT can be divided into (i) immediate treatment to terminate the episode of SVT and (ii) treatment to prevent its recurrence.

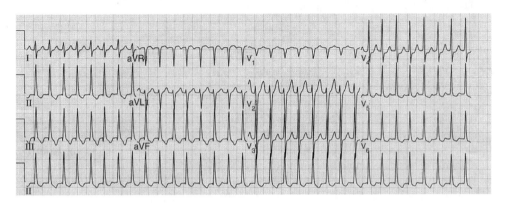

FIGURE 3.6 ● The electrocardiogram in SVT. The QRS is narrow, and P waves, if discernible, are related to the QRS.

There are several ways to terminate SVT. Because it is rarely life threatening, one can wait an hour or two for SVT to terminate on its own. The patient may be able to terminate SVT by doing a Valsalva maneuver, such as bearing down against a closed glottis and straining as if having a bowel movement. Carotid massage can be tried. Swallowing ice water will sometimes terminate SVT. If none of these works, immersing the patient's face in ice water may be effective but it is very uncomfortable. One of the most effective pharmacologic methods to terminate SVT is the intravenous use of adenosine. For the rare patient who is hemodynamically unstable while in SVT, electrical cardioversion is perhaps the best choice of treatment.

There are a variety of options to prevent recurrence of SVT. These include β-blockers, calcium channel blockers, amiodarone, and ablation of the atrial focus or the reentry circuit that is responsible for the arrhythmia. β-Blockers are certainly a safe choice. The use of other treatment methods should be guided by a cardiologist.

SVT may occur because a pacemaker other than the sinus node assumes the rhythm of the heart and has a faster intrinsic rate than the sinus node. This would be an *ectopic* atrial form of SVT. Another mechanism of SVT is *reentry*, in which there are two routes for conduction from the atria to the ventricles. One route usually is the normal atrioventricular (AV) node-His-Purkinje system and the second is an *accessory pathway* as seen in Wolff-Parkinson-White syndrome (see Fig. 3.7).

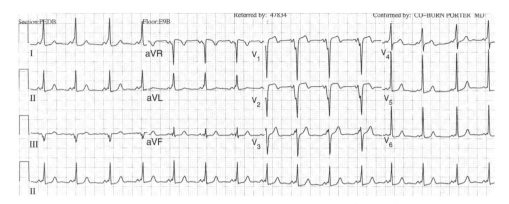

FIGURE 3.7 ● Wolff-Parkinson-White syndrome. Note delta waves in leads I, II, aVR, aVL, V₁ to V₆.

B. *JET* also is characterized by a narrow QRS complex but, in contrast to SVT, the P waves and QRS complexes are dissociated from one another (see Fig. 3.8). JET usually occurs in infants immediately following intracardiac surgery.

One usually is faced with treatment of JET in infants following cardiac operation. In this setting, one tries to minimize the use and dose of catecholamines. Cooling the patient may help. Currently, the drug of choice to control JET in the postoperative period is intravenous amiodarone.

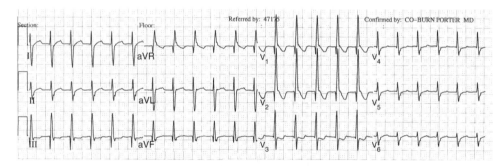

FIGURE 3.8 ● Junctional ectopic tachycardia characterized by a narrow QRS complex and by P waves and QRS complexes that are dissociated from one another.

C. *VT* is characterized by a wide QRS complex (usually >120 msecond) and AV dissociation (see Fig. 3.9). There is one *caveat* about the width of the QRS complex. If there is bundle branch block or other reasons for delayed ventricular depolarization, the QRS could be wide even though it originates from the atria or AV node region.

For treatment, see preceding text for discussion under "ventricular arrhythmias." In addition to these considerations, a new episode of VT can be treated with intravenous lidocaine, intravenous amiodarone, or electric cardioversion. The selection of the treatment will depend upon the cause of the VT and the urgency of the situation.

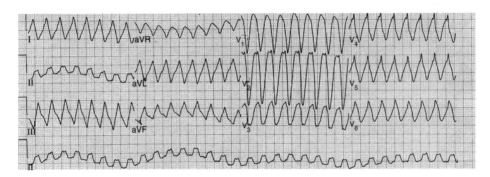

FIGURE 3.9 ● Ventricular tachycardia, characterized by a wide QRS complex (usually >120 msecond) and AV dissociation.

7. *Bradyarrhythmias* exist if the heart rate is slower than it should be on the basis of the patient's age and state of activity.

A. *Sinus bradycardia* exists if there is a P wave originating from the sinus node (upright P wave in leads I and aVF) (see Fig. 3.10). Sinus bradycardia can occur because of a high level of physical fitness, a variety of drugs, abnormalities of the sinus node, hypothyroidism, and anorexia, among others.

If there is an identifiable underlying cause of the bradycardia, it should be treated. It is unusual to have to treat the bradycardia itself, but in rare cases, it may be necessary to insert a pacemaker.

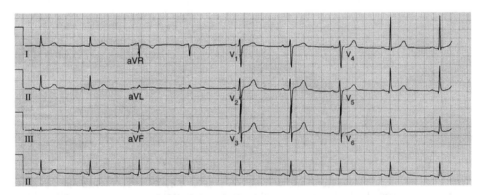

FIGURE 3.10 ● Sinus bradycardia, indicated by a P wave originating from the sinus node, upright P wave in leads I and aVF.

B. AV conduction abnormalities are frequently the cause of bradycardia.
    i. *First-degree AV block* exists if the PR interval is prolonged (the exact degree of prolongation that is considered to be abnormal depends upon the age of the patient) (see Fig. 3.11). First-degree AV block usually does not cause bradycardia and does not require treatment.
    ii. *Second-degree AV block* exists if P waves fail to conduct to the ventricle. There are two types of second-degree AV block: Mobitz I, or Wenckebach, (see Fig. 3.12) and Mobitz II (see Fig. 3.13). Mobitz I exists if the PR interval becomes progressively longer until a nonconducted P wave occurs and then the cycle recurs. Generally, as the PR interval lengthens, the R-R interval shortens (Fig. 3.12).

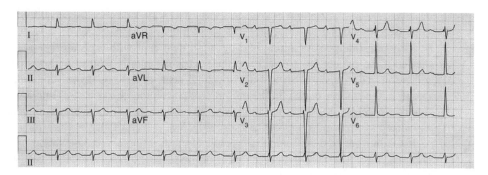

FIGURE 3.11 ● First-degree AV block, indicated when the PR interval is prolonged.

Mobitz II second-degree AV block exists if each QRS is preceded by more than one P wave.

Treatment is not usually indicated for Mobitz I, whereas Mobitz II block may require placement of a pacemaker if there are symptoms of lightheadedness, syncope, or congestive heart failure.

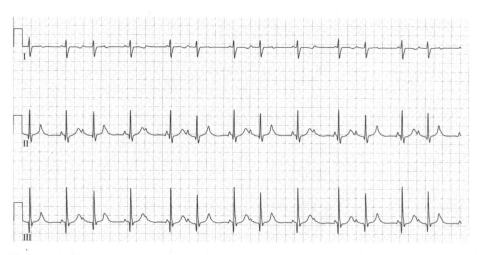

FIGURE 3.12 ● Mobitz I or Wenckebach type of second-degree AV block. This type exists when P waves fail to conduct to the ventricle and when the PR interval becomes progressively longer until a nonconducted P wave occurs and then the cycle recurs.

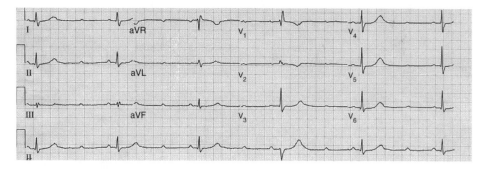

FIGURE 3.13 ● Mobitz II type of second-degree AV block. This type exists when P waves fail to conduct to the ventricle and each QRS is preceded by more than one P wave.

iii. *Third-degree or "complete" AV block* exists if P waves are not associated with QRS (see Fig. 3.14).

If the third-degree AV block is congenital, treatment with a pacemaker is indicated if the patient is an infant and the ventricular rate is <50 to 55 beats per minute in the absence of structural congenital heart disease or if the ventricular rate is <70 beats per minute in the presence of congenital heart disease. Implantation of a pacemaker is indicated in patients beyond infancy if there are significant associated symptoms, a wide QRS escape rhythm, or ventricular dysfunction.

If the third-degree AV block is a result of cardiac surgery, implantation of a pacemaker is indicted if the AV block is not expected to resolve or if it persists for at least 7 days postoperatively.

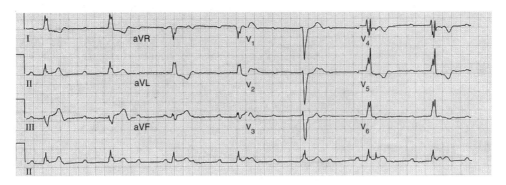

FIGURE 3.14 ● Third-degree or "complete" AV block. It exists if no P waves are associated with any QRS.

8. Prolonged QT-interval syndrome (see Fig. 3.15).

It is important to recognize prolonged QT-interval syndrome because it is a potentially lethal condition. The QT interval must be corrected for heart rate, and the formula is QTc = QT/square root of the R-R interval.

The treatment of prolonged QT-interval syndrome is evolving as additional ion channel defects are identified. The specific treatment will depend upon the specific ion channel defect and the family history. These patients are best referred to a specialist with experience in treating these patients.

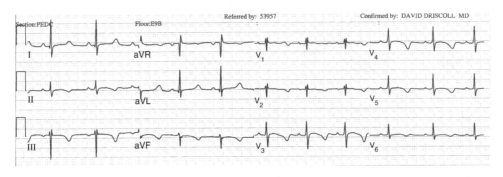

FIGURE 3.15 ● Prolonged QT-interval syndrome.

CARDIAC ENLARGEMENT AND HYPERTROPHY

1. Atrial Hypertrophy

   Classic teaching is that if the P wave exceeds 3 mm in height in limb lead II, then the right atrium is enlarged (right atrial enlargement [RAE]), and if the P wave is prolonged in limb lead II and has a negative deflection in lead V_1, then the left atrium is enlarged (left atrial enlargement [LAE]). However, echocardiographic correlation studies suggest that it is difficult to differentiate RAE from LAE using the ECG. Therefore, it may be more accurate to simply refer to "atrial enlargement," with no reference to "right" or "left."

2. Ventricular Hypertrophy

   Right ventricular hypertrophy (RVH) is determined by the combined voltages of the R wave in V_1 and the S wave in V_6 and by the R/S ratio in V_1. From birth to 4 days of age, the T wave is normally upright in V_1. After 4 days of age, it should become inverted and remain so until early adolescence. RVH exists if the T wave remains upright in V_1 between 4 days of age and early adolescence.

   The combined voltages of the S wave in V_1 and the R wave in V_6 indicate left ventricular hypertrophy (LVH).

   Because the normal values for voltage in V_1 and V_6 change with age, one must refer to a table of normal values to determine whether ventricular hypertrophy exists.

CHEST RADIOGRAPHY

Chest radiography is used to determine the size of the heart, the position of the heart in the chest, the shape of the heart, the presence of a right or left aortic arch, the status of the lungs (including over- or underperfusion of the lungs), abdominal situs, and spine and rib anomalies that may be associated with congenital heart defects. The important chest radiographic findings associated with various cardiac defects are discussed in the respective chapters on congenital heart defects. The following points, however, are instructive

The following points should be considered in a cyanotic newborn:

- The so-called classic "egg-on-a-string" appearance of transposition of the great arteries is rarely seen and is an unhelpful sign.
- If the heart is moderately enlarged and the pulmonary vascular markings are increased, consider transposition of the great arteries.
- If the heart is not enlarged and the pulmonary vascular markings are decreased and there is a systolic ejection murmur, consider tetralogy of Fallot (see Fig. 3.16). If there is not a systolic ejection murmur and there is a right aortic arch, consider pulmonary atresia with VSD.
- If the heart is massively enlarged, consider Ebstein anomaly (see Fig. 3.17), pulmonary atresia with intact ventricular septum, or pericardial effusion.
- If the stomach bubble is on the right and the heart is on the left, consider complex congenital heart disease (see Fig. 3.18).
- If there is a right-sided aortic arch, consider tetralogy of Fallot, pulmonary atresia with VSD, or truncus arteriosus.

The following points should be considered in acyanotic patients:

- Left-to-right shunts such as ventricular septal defect (VSD), atrial septal defect (ASD), and patent ductus arteriosus (PDA) cause a large heart and increased pulmonary vascular markings.

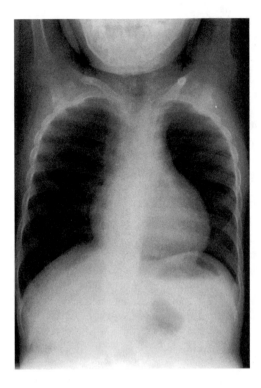

FIGURE 3.16 ● Typical chest x-ray of a patient with Tetralogy of Fallot. Note the normal heart size and dark lung fields indicative of reduced pulmonary blood flow.

- The degree of aortic insufficiency tends to correlate directly with heart size.
- The heart size is not helpful in assessing the degree of aortic or pulmonary valve stenosis.
- A very small heart can be a sign of Addison disease.
- If there is rib notching, consider coarctation of the aorta.
- The presence of a right aortic arch in the absence of intracardiac anomalies implies the presence of a vascular ring.

ECHOCARDIOGRAPHY

Echocardiography is one of the greatest advances to occur in the diagnosis of heart disease over the last 50 years. It allows accurate anatomic definition of essentially all forms of congenital and acquired heart diseases. With the addition of Doppler techniques, one can estimate pressure differences across valves and through septal defects. However, echocardiography is not a substitute for a thorough history and physical examination, chest radiography, ECG, and consultation with a pediatric cardiologist. Indeed, many health care dollars are wasted on unnecessary echocardiograms and on echocardiograms that are done improperly or interpreted incorrectly.

Although most echocardiogram reports suggest that intracardiac pressures can be obtained using Doppler, in fact, pressures are not measured. The velocity of blood flow is approximated and pressures are estimated using a number of mathematic assumptions. Also, cardiac structures are not actually "seen," but rather images of reflected sound waves are seen that bear some relationship to the structures from which these sound waves are reflected. Because of these issues, results of echocardiographic studies must be treated like those of any other test and interpreted in the light of all other findings.

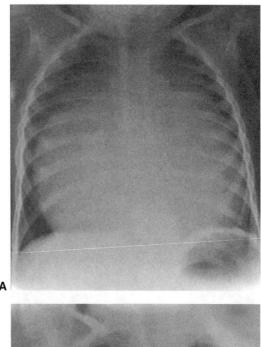

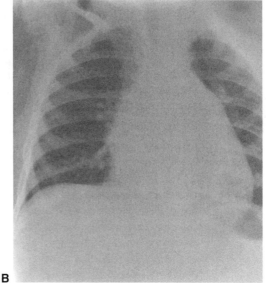

FIGURE 3.17 ● Chest x-ray from a child with Ebstein anomaly— Preoperative **(A)** and after repair **(B)**. **B**

CARDIAC CATHETERIZATION

Before the advent of echocardiography, cardiac catheterization was the primary tool for establishing a definitive diagnosis of congenital heart disease. Diagnostic information during cardiac catheterization is collected in three ways: (i) measurement of pressure, (ii) measurement of blood oxygen saturation, and (iii) angiograms. Using this information, the anatomy and pathophysiology of congenital cardiac defects can be determined with great accuracy.

Over the last several decades, interventional cardiac catheterization techniques have been described and have evolved. One of the earliest interventional techniques was the balloon septostomy described by Rashkind and Miller in 1966. In the early 1980s, dilation of blood

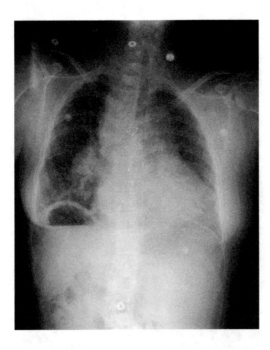

FIGURE 3.18 ● Chest x-ray of a patient with isolated levocardia and abdominal situs inversus. Note that the stomach bubble is on the right. This patient has a functional single ventricle. Also, note the aneurysmal enlargement of the right pulmonary artery.

vessels, pulmonary valves, and aortic valves and aortic coarctation were introduced and refined. Over the last 10 to 15 years, devices to close PDA, ASD, and VSD have been introduced and refined. Indeed, with the evolution of interventional cardiac catheterization techniques and echocardiography, cardiac catheterization is used more to treat cardiac defects than for their diagnosis.

SELECTED REFERENCES

Nihill M, Mullins C, Grifka R, et al. *An angiographic atlas of congenital cardiac abnormalities*, Boston, MA: Futura Publishing; 2003.

Zeigler V, Gillette P. *Practical management of pediatric arrhythmias*, Boston, MA: Blackwell Futura Publishing; 2001.

CHAPTER 4

Pediatric Exercise Testing

*"Those who think they have not time
for bodily exercise
will, sooner or later,
have to find time for illness"*

Accurate and reproducible measurement of work performance or exercise capacity provides a means to quantify a dimension of disease severity, to assess the effects of treatment and training, and, in some instances, to identify previously unrecognized disease.

DETERMINANTS OF EXERCISE PERFORMANCE

In humans, skeletal muscle sarcomere shortening is essential for work to be performed. Normal sarcomere shortening requires the presence of reasonably normal intracellular contractile proteins and, in addition, depends on the occurrence of a multitude of intracellular events. Because sarcomere shortening is an energy-requiring process, the presence of high-energy phosphate compounds and the reasonably normal functioning of mitochondria and intracellular energy transport systems are necessary. Although skeletal muscles can function anaerobically, the major energy requirements of working muscles involve aerobic processes.

For repetitive sarcomere shortening to occur, the working muscle must be supplied with oxygen (O_2) and energy sources including glucose and free fatty acids. Also, the by-products of cellular metabolism such as lactate and carbon dioxide (CO_2) must be removed from the cellular environment. The transport of supply and waste products is accomplished by the cardiovascular system. The rate at which the cardiovascular system can accomplish this task is dependent on cardiac output.

O_2 supply, CO_2 elimination, and, to some extent, thermal regulation are dependent upon appropriate pulmonary function. In addition, pH is modulated by changes in the rate of CO_2 elimination by the lungs. The rate of O_2 supply and CO_2 elimination depends on changes in respiratory rate, tidal volume, effective pulmonary blood flow, ventilation–perfusion matching or mismatching, diffusion capacity of O_2 at the blood–alveolar interface, appropriate functioning of breathing mechanisms, and large and small airway patency and size.

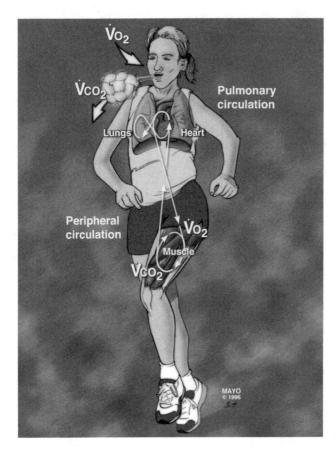

FIGURE 4.1 ● Illustration of the interaction of the lungs, heart, and musculoskeletal system during exercise.

The pulmonary, cardiovascular, and skeletal muscle systems are the three serially connected systems that are most important in facilitating work performance and instant-to-instant regulation of work performance (see Fig. 4.1). However, sustained and repetitive work cannot occur without appropriate renal function for eliminating additional waste products of oxidation and anaerobic metabolism, maintaining physiologic hydrogen ion concentration, and adjusting intracellular and extracellular plasma volume. In addition, because muscle contraction is a heat-producing process, the skin is critically important for thermal regulation.

Work performance requires a complex and intricate interaction of multiple organ systems. Abnormalities in any of these organ systems will affect and potentially limit work performance. When any one of these organ systems reaches maximal functional capacity, the performance of additional work will be limited.

WORK, POWER, AND MAXIMAL AEROBIC POWER

Exercise involves the performance of work and the application of power. *Work* is the application of force to move a mass for a given distance (work = force × distance). The unit of *force* is the Newton (force = mass × acceleration). One Newton is the force that gives a mass of 1 kg an acceleration of 1 m per second^2. A term that has been used to describe this force is the *kilopond* (kp). One kp is the force acting on a mass of 1 kg at the normal (i.e., earth) acceleration of gravity (1 kp is equal to approximately 10 N). Because work equals force multiplied by distance, the unit for work is Newton-meter, or joule (J). Because most exercise testing is done on earth, kilopond-meter (kpm) is frequently used as a unit of work for clinical exercise testing. *Energy* is necessary to perform work, and the relationship between energy and work is constant, described as 1 kilocalorie = 4.1868 J. *Power* is work performed per unit time. This can be expressed as kpm per second or J per second. A common conventional expression of power is watt (1 W = 1 J per second = 6.12 kpm per minute).

An important central issue to be addressed in exercise testing is the ability of an individual to perform work. The amount of work an individual can do could be used to define "exercise capacity," "fitness," or "aerobic power." However, it is difficult to measure work accurately. Although many different indices can be used to describe fitness or maximal exercise capacity, the maximum O_2 uptake ($\dot{V}O_2$ max) that can be achieved during exercise is, perhaps, the best index. The term *maximal aerobic power* has been used to indicate the highest achievable level of $\dot{V}O_2$ during exercise and is used throughout this chapter. Because energy is necessary to perform work, energy production requires combustion of fuel (food), and combustion of fuel requires O_2, there is a predictable relationship between work and $\dot{V}O_2$ (see Fig. 4.2).

Technically, $\dot{V}O_2$max is defined by the plateau of $\dot{V}O_2$ that occurs despite continued work (Fig. 4.2), which illustrates the fact that work can be performed using anaerobic mechanisms of energy production. But the amount of work that can be performed using anaerobic means is quite limited.

In assessing the cardiorespiratory responses to exercise, it is important to know the subjects' degree of effort. A maximal effort is necessary to accurately quantify $\dot{V}O_2$max, which is defined as the highest $\dot{V}O_2$ achieved despite continued work. Unfortunately, it is difficult to motivate many untrained subjects and most children to exercise to that point. Obviously, a subject is quite anaerobic at true $\dot{V}O_2$max, and continued exercise is uncomfortable. Because of this, the term *peak $\dot{V}O_2$*, *peak exercise study*, or *peak effort* has been coined to

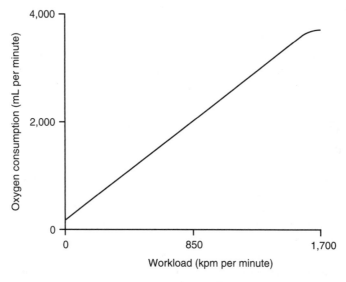

FIGURE 4.2 ● Illustration of the linear relationship of $\dot{V}O_2$ and work. Note the plateau of $\dot{V}O_2$ at the highest workload.

refer to a symptom- or discomfort-limited clinical exercise test. In such tests, a true $\dot{V}O_2$max may not have been attained.

At all ages, boys have a higher $\dot{V}O_2$max than girls. $\dot{V}O_2$max increases with increasing body mass. However, if $\dot{V}O_2$max is indexed to lean body mass, there is no difference between boys and girls in its achievable values. If $\dot{V}O_2$max is indexed to weight (kilograms), it remains relatively the same for boys aged between 6 and 18 years but declines over this age range for girls. This decline in girls probably represents the effect of increased body fat (or decreased lean body mass).

Investigators have searched for the best method of indexing $\dot{V}O_2$. Considerable controversy still exists about the best method, if, indeed, one exists. On the basis of the "dimensionality theory," some have proposed the use of an exponent of body length. Various investigators have proposed the use of an exponent from 1.5 to 3.2. However, the most commonly accepted method of indexing $\dot{V}O_2$ in clinical exercise testing is to use body weight (kilograms).

The maximum $\dot{V}O_2$ achieved during work will depend on the type of work performed. For example, one can repetitively flex one's index finger until the finger is exhausted and can no longer be flexed. However, maximum O_2 uptake during this maximum activity will not be very high because only a small muscle group is working. In contrast, $\dot{V}O_2$max will be considerably higher if one repetitively flexed a knee because larger muscle masses are working and more work is being performed. Similarly, one can achieve higher $\dot{V}O_2$max during treadmill than during cycle exercise because more muscle groups are working.

Over the last several years, considerable attention has been focused on the so-called anaerobic threshold as a measure of aerobic power. Theoretically, it might allow the assessment of exercise capacity using a submaximal exercise study, a potential advantage in children who have difficulty in achieving a true $\dot{V}O_2$max. The anaerobic threshold is defined as the $\dot{V}O_2$ at which there is a disproportionate increase in minute ventilation ($\dot{V}E$) relative to O_2 uptake (see Fig. 4.3(A)). In adults, there is frequently a disproportionate increase in lactate production at this point as well, hence the term *anaerobic threshold*. However, a disproportionate change in lactate level is not necessary for a disproportionate change in $\dot{V}E$ to occur. Therefore, the term *anaerobic threshold* may be a misnomer. Some investigators prefer to use the term *ventilatory anaerobic threshold* or *ventilatory threshold*. The anaerobic threshold is identified by an abrupt change in the slope of $\dot{V}E$ and the ventilatory equivalent for O_2 ($\dot{V}E/\dot{V}O_2$) without a concomitant change in the ventilatory equivalent for CO_2 ($\dot{V}E/\dot{V}CO_2$). In addition, there will be an increase in end-tidal PO_2 without an increase in PCO_2.

CARDIAC RESPONSES TO EXERCISE

HEART RATE

For healthy individuals, increased heart rate during exercise is the major determinant of increased cardiac output. There is a linear relationship between heart rate and $\dot{V}O_2$max (Fig. 4.3(B)). Each individual has a maximum heart rate (HR_{max}) that can be achieved but not exceeded during exercise. This HR_{max} is an important determinant of $\dot{V}O_2$max. For subjects aged between 5 and 20 years, HR_{max} is approximately 195 to 215 beats per minute. The HR_{max} for children younger than 5 years probably is similar, but it is difficult to motivate these young children to perform a truly maximal test. For subjects older than 20 years, $HR_{max} = 210 - 0.65 \times$ age. The reasons for the decline of HR_{max} with age are unclear but may be related to fibrosis and scarring of the sinoatrial node.

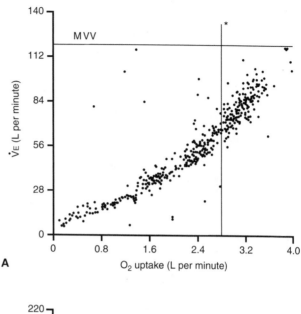

A

O_2 uptake (L per minute)

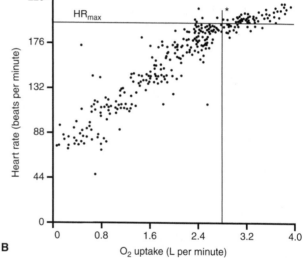

FIGURE 4.3 ● Graphic representation of the change of ventilation relative to $\dot{V}_{O_2}$ **(A)** and that of heart rate relative to $\dot{V}_{O_2}$ **(B)**. The horizontal and vertical lines represent the predicted normal for this subject. Note that the subject is very fit. The subject has exceeded the predicted $\dot{V}_{O_2}$max. MVV, maximum voluntary ventilation.

B

O_2 uptake (L per minute)

Maximum heart rate will vary slightly, depending on the exercise protocol used and the type of exercise performed. For example, a slightly higher HR_{max} is obtained for treadmill than for cycle exercise.

Four typical heart rate responses to exercise are illustrated in Figure 4.4. The "normal" graph represents the heart rate response of a healthy subject with an HR_{max} of 200 beats per minute and a $\dot{V}_{O_2}$max of 2.5 L per minute during exercise. When a heart rate of 200 beats per minute is attained, the subject stops exercising. Achieving HR_{max} could be considered indicative of achieving a maximum cardiorespiratory effort. However, technically it is not. Some very fit individuals can continue exercising while the heart rate remains at its maximum value for 1 to 2 minutes. Obviously, this can occur only at the expense of extreme anaerobiosis. The curve labeled *conditioned* illustrates the heart rate response if

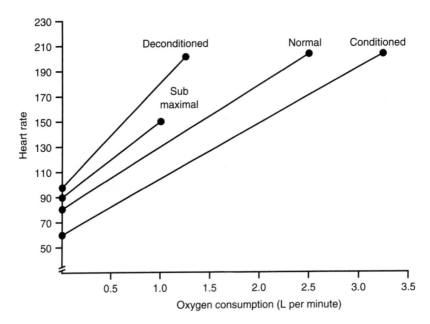

FIGURE 4.4 ● Illustration of the change of heat rate with increasing work or $\dot{V}O_2$. Four states are shown: (i) normal, (ii) deconditioned, (iii) conditioned, and (iv) submaximal effort.

the subject improves his or her physical fitness. With improved fitness, resting heart rate declines. Maximum heart rate does not increase but occurs at a higher $\dot{V}O_2$max. The curve labeled *deconditioned* illustrates the effect of deconditioning on heart rate. Resting heart rate is higher than that of the control, and HR_{max} occurs at a lower $\dot{V}O_2$. The curve labeled *submaximal* could represent simply a limited cardiorespiratory effort. This curve also is typical of patients with chronotropic insufficiency, that is, the HR_{max} is low. This occurs in many patients with heart disease with or without prior cardiac operation.

BLOOD PRESSURE

During isotonic exercise, systolic blood pressure increases (see Fig. 4.5). Diastolic blood pressure may vary within 10 mm Hg from its level at rest, but, on average, it remains the same during exercise. Larger-sized children have a higher blood pressure on submaximal and maximal exercise than smaller-sized children. Among similar-sized children, boys have higher peak systolic blood pressure than girls.

Blood pressure response to isometric exercise is quite different from that during isotonic exercise. With isometric exercise, both systolic and diastolic pressures increase. Indeed, with power weight lifting, systolic blood pressure may reach 320 to 480 mm Hg.

CARDIAC OUTPUT AND STROKE VOLUME

The essential function of the cardiovascular system is to propel blood to tissues. The basic measurement of this function is cardiac output. Cardiac output increases in a linear manner with increasing work or $\dot{V}O_2$. The relationship can be described as Cardiac Output = 4 + 0.006 × $\dot{V}O_2$.

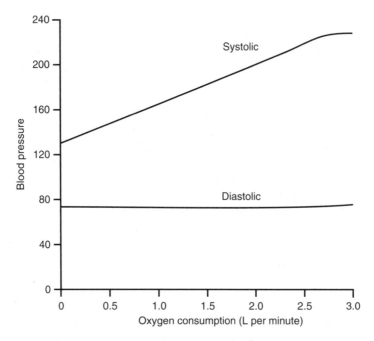

FIGURE 4.5 ● Illustration of the change of blood pressure with increasing work or $\dot{V}_{O_2}$. Systolic blood pressure increases but diastolic blood pressure does not.

Because cardiac output is the product of heart rate and stroke volume, cardiac output can change only if stroke volume and heart rate change. Stroke volume, in turn, is dependent upon left ventricular end-diastolic volume and ejection fraction. Therefore, the basic determinants of cardiac output are heart rate, end-diastolic volume, and ejection fraction.

Changes in stroke volume during exercise depend, to some extent, on the position in which exercise is performed. Stroke volume increases in humans when the supine position is assumed. Therefore, when supine exercise is performed, the increase in stroke volume is limited. Stroke volume increases primarily early in exercise and increases little thereafter. Therefore, the change in cardiac output resulting from change in stroke volume occurs early in exercise, and additional changes in cardiac output are heart rate dependent.

VENTILATORY RESPONSES TO EXERCISE

$\dot{V}_E$ increases with work. Ventilation increases because of increases in both tidal volume and breathing frequency. The relationship between $\dot{V}_E$ and work is relatively linear, but as described in the preceding text, the slope of the relationship between $\dot{V}_E$ and work changes when the ventilatory anaerobic threshold is attained.

$\dot{V}_E/\dot{V}_{O_2}$ describes the volume of air breathed relative to the volume of O_2 consumed. $\dot{V}_E/\dot{V}_{O_2}$ declines early in exercise as a result of better ventilation and blood flow matching in the lungs as pulmonary blood flow increases and flow redistributes to the apices of the lungs. The point during exercise when $\dot{V}_E/\dot{V}_{O_2}$ begins to increase describes the ventilatory anaerobic threshold. Simply speaking, after this point, ventilation increases disproportionately to $\dot{V}_{O_2}$ to eliminate relatively more carbon dioxide in an attempt to maintain arterial pH.

During intense work, CO_2 production increases disproportionately to $\dot{V}_{O_2}$ after the anaerobic threshold. $\dot{V}_E$ increases proportionately to CO_2 production but disproportionately to

$\dot{V}O_2$. Therefore, at the anaerobic threshold, the slope of $\dot{V}E/\dot{V}O_2$ increases but the slope of $\dot{V}E/\dot{V}CO_2$ does not. Later, during exercise, as acidosis continues to increase, $\dot{V}E$ increases disproportionately even to CO_2 production, resulting in a change in the slope of $\dot{V}E/\dot{V}CO_2$ and a reduction of $PaCO_2$ and end-tidal CO_2. This point has been termed the *threshold for decompensated metabolic acidosis*, and the period after this point has been termed as *respiratory compensation*.

Healthy subjects terminate exercise when cardiac output can increase no more. At this point, there is still some ventilatory reserve. This can be appreciated by examining the relationship between maximum voluntary ventilation (MVV) at rest and $\dot{V}E$ during exercise. When exercise is terminated, $\dot{V}E$ is 60% to 70% of rest MVV. Individuals with pulmonary disease who encroach upon this "ventilatory reserve" may reach a $\dot{V}E$ of >70% of MVV. One must be cautious, however, in assessing the relationship between $\dot{V}E$ during exercise and MVV at rest because obtaining a true measure of MVV at rest is dependent on the subject's effort. If the subject does not make a good effort, a factitiously low MVV will be recorded and its relationship with $\dot{V}E$ during exercise will be misleading. A true MVV should be approximately equal to forced expiratory volume in 1 second (FEV_1) × 40.

FITNESS

Improved fitness occurs with repetitive exercise. From a strict physiologic standpoint, improved fitness implies an increase in aerobic power ($\dot{V}O_2$max). In adults, there have been

TABLE 4.1

Changes That Occur with Increased Fitness

Ventilatory System	
Minute ventilation	
Submaximal	↓
Maximal	↑
Respiratory rate—submaximal	↓
Tidal volume—maximal	↑
Respiratory muscle endurance	↑
Muscle Metabolism	
Mitochondria (number and volume)	↑
Glycogen stores	↑
Triglyceride stores	↑
Myoglobin content	↑
Oxidative enzyme activity	↑
ATP content and utilization	↑
Creatine phosphate content and utilization	↑
Lactate (maximum)	↑
Anaerobic enzyme activity	↑

ATP, adenosine 5'-triphosphate; ↑, increase; ↓, decrease.

many studies demonstrating increases in $\dot{V}O_2max$ as a result of a conditioning or fitness program. In children, it has been more difficult to demonstrate this effect. This probably is due to the fact that "healthy children" simply are more fit than "healthy adults" to begin with; hence, it is more difficult to demonstrate a change in fitness in healthy children. It must be recognized that children can improve their performance in sports events without changes in aerobic power simply by improving their skill in the particular event, including simple running skill. As demonstrated in Figure 4.4, resting heart rate decreases with improved fitness, and maximum heart rate is achieved at a greater $\dot{V}O_2max$. As is apparent from Figure 4.4, the submaximal heart rate is lower at any $\dot{V}O_2$ in the fit individual as compared to the unfit individual. These adjustments of heart rate occur because of the increase in stroke volume that occurs with conditioning. Also, changes in the parasympathetic and sympathetic regulation of heart rate probably play an important role, with a relatively greater parasympathetic (vagal) influence on heart rate in the fit individual.

Changes in fitness or conditioning are not limited to changes in the function of the cardiovascular system. Important changes also occur in ventilatory function and subcellular changes occur in muscle; these are listed in Table 4.1.

Fitness can be improved with regular, sustained exercise. Conversely, deconditioning occurs if regular exercise is not done. Because children with heart disease may be sedentary, some component of reduced aerobic capacity in these patients may be due to deconditioning.

METHODOLOGY OF EXERCISE TESTING

TYPES OF EXERCISE AND ERGOMETERS

There are two types of exercise: Isotonic (dynamic) and isometric (static). Isotonic exercise implies alternate rhythmic contraction (shortening) and relaxation (lengthening) of muscles against a nonfixed resistance. Isometric exercise involves muscular contraction against a fixed resistance, with little, if any, muscle shortening. Clinical exercise testing can be done using either isotonic or isometric exercise. Usually, however, clinical exercise testing is done using isotonic forms of exercise such as cycling, walking, and running.

Treadmill and stationary cycles are the two most frequently used ergometers for clinical exercise testing. Neither is inherently superior to the other, each has advantages and disadvantages. Most individuals can walk reasonably efficiently, but not everyone can cycle efficiently. Children younger than 4 or 5 years may have more difficulty using a cycle ergometer than a treadmill. On the other hand, a treadmill may be more dangerous than a cycle because the subject can fall from the treadmill. Also, it is more difficult to hear Korotkoff sounds when the subject is running or jogging on a treadmill than when he or she is cycling. If the subject is connected to numerous monitoring devices, cycling may be preferable because it involves less movement of the trunk and extremities.

MEASUREMENT TECHNIQUES

HEART RATE AND ELECTROCARDIOGRAM

Heart rate, one of the basic indices of cardiac response to exercise, is measured from the electrocardiogram (ECG). This can be done manually by averaging several R-R intervals. Alternatively, the electrocardiographic signal can be processed through a tachometer and a direct recording of heart rate can be obtained on the basis of one or more R-R intervals.

At least three leads of the standard surface ECG should be displayed or recorded continuously during and for 5 to 10 minutes after completion of an exercise test. The examiner should have the option of viewing various combinations of leads so that inferior (leads II, III, and aVF), anterior right (V_1 or V_2), and anterior left (V_5 or V_6) cardiac events can be assessed. A complete ECG should be recorded at rest, at least once during each workload, and for several intervals after exercise. Ideally, the electrocardiograph should have several recording speeds. Obtaining an ECG at a speed of 50 mm per second facilitates the assessment of ST-segment changes. Continuous recording of the ECG at 5 mm per second paper speed facilitates the measurement of arrhythmias.

BLOOD PRESSURE

Blood pressure can be measured directly with an indwelling arterial catheter or, more commonly, indirectly with a cuff, sphygmomanometer, and stethoscope. The bladder of the cuff should completely encircle the arm, and the width of the cuff should be at least two thirds the length of the upper arm. It should be remembered that accurate measurement of diastolic blood pressure during exercise is very difficult. It is particularly difficult during treadmill exercise because the noise generated by the treadmill and by the contact of the feet with the treadmill make it very difficult to hear the Korotkoff sounds.

CARDIAC OUTPUT AND STROKE VOLUME

The two techniques used most frequently to make a relatively noninvasive measurement of cardiac output without the need for radioactive material are the CO_2 and the acetylene–helium rebreathing techniques. The CO_2 rebreathing technique is based on the Fick equation. The acetylene–helium rebreathing technique to measure cardiac output is based on the principle that acetylene diffuses from the alveolus to the pulmonary capillary. The concentration of acetylene in the rebreathing technique declines relative to the volume of effective pulmonary blood flow. This technique actually measures effective pulmonary blood flow rather than systemic blood flow, but in the absence of significant right-to-left or left-to-right intracardiac or intrapulmonary shunting, it is a reliable approximation of cardiac output.

MEASUREMENTS OF VENTILATION

The following indices of ventilation can be measured during exercise: Respiratory rate, tidal volume, $\dot{V}E$, $\dot{V}O_2$, $\dot{V}CO_2$, end-tidal CO_2, O_2, expired CO_2, and expired O_2. From these measurements, one can calculate the ventilatory equivalent for O_2 ($\dot{V}E/\dot{V}O_2$) and CO_2 ($\dot{V}E/\dot{V}CO_2$) and the respiratory quotient (R).

Noninvasive (ear or finger oximetry) measurement of blood O_2 saturation is useful to document the presence or absence of hypoxemia and to quantify the degree of hypoxemia.

CLINICAL APPLICATIONS OF EXERCISE TESTING IN PEDIATRIC CARDIOLOGY

AORTIC STENOSIS

Before the availability of Doppler echocardiographic techniques for the noninvasive estimation of the severity of aortic valve stenosis, investigators attempted to correlate indices of cardiac function during exercise to the severity of aortic stenosis.

Although exercise testing has been supplanted by Doppler echo techniques for the estimation of the severity of aortic stenosis, exercise testing is still useful in the following situations:

1. There is a subset of patients with aortic stenosis who, by pressure-gradient criteria, have mild or only moderately severe aortic stenosis but significant ST-segment depression with exercise. This suggests that these patients have compromised myocardial O_2 supply and may benefit from relief of aortic stenosis despite a transaortic pressure-gradient measurement *at rest* that implies only mild or moderate disease. However, one must be cautious in interpreting the significance of ST-segment change in postoperative patients who, because of abnormal repolarization of the ventricular mass, may have false-positive ST-segment changes.
2. Exercise testing may be useful in assessing whether patients with mild aortic stenosis or mild postoperative residual aortic stenosis can participate in vigorous physical activity or athletic competition.

COARCTATION OF THE AORTA

Exercise testing is useful in assessing patients who have had a repair of coarctation of the aorta. It may be helpful in establishing whether blood pressure is normal or excessive during exercise. Numerous investigators have used blood pressure response to exercise to help define the presence of significant recoarctation of the aorta. This task is hindered by the fact that there is no clear definition of significant, persistent, or recurrent coarctation of the aorta. Some investigators have reported a correlation between peak-exercise systolic blood pressure and the arm-to-leg blood pressure difference measured within 1 minute of exercise cessation. Other investigators have reported that exercise-induced systolic blood pressure >200 mm Hg, arm-to-leg blood pressure gradient >15 mm Hg during rest, and exercise-induced arm-to-leg systolic blood pressure gradient >35 mm Hg are associated with a ratio of the aortic diameter at the coarctation site to that at the diaphragm of <0.6. The role of exercise testing in the evaluation of patients after repair of coarctation of the aorta will remain unclear until it is understood what constitutes important, persistent, or recurrent coarctation of the aorta and what the indications are for reoperation or balloon dilation. The following points, however, are probably correct:

1. The presence of a normal upper-extremity systolic blood pressure response to exercise in a patient with little or no arm-to-leg blood pressure gradient at rest is consistent with an adequately repaired coarctation of the aorta.
2. Exercise-induced systolic hypertension can occur in the absence of significant, persistent, or recurrent coarctation of the aorta.
3. Significant, persistent, or recurrent coarctation of the aorta can be present despite a normal upper-extremity blood pressure at rest.
4. The postexercise arm-to-leg blood pressure gradient must be interpreted with caution because of variations in the rate of decrease in blood pressure after exercise and technical difficulties in measuring leg blood pressure.

PULMONARY ATRESIA WITH VENTRICULAR SEPTAL DEFECT

Patients with pulmonary atresia and ventricular septal defect (VSD) who have not been operated on or have had only a systemic-to-pulmonary artery anastomosis have reduced aerobic power, rest hypoxemia that is greater with exercise, and increased $\dot{V}E/\dot{V}O_2$ at rest and during exercise. The presence of a large right-to-left shunt that becomes even greater with exercise is a major determinant of this abnormal exercise response. Patients who have had augmentation of pulmonary blood flow after insertion of a right ventricular-to-pulmonary artery conduit (so-called first-stage procedure) have significant improvement in exercise tolerance and hypoxemia although the VSD remains open. After complete repair, exercise tolerance does not show much change compared to that after first-stage repair, but hypoxemia is essentially eliminated when the ventilatory response to exercise normalizes.

SINGLE VENTRICLE

The cardiorespiratory response to exercise in patients with unrepaired forms of functional single ventricle is typical for cyanotic forms of congenital heart disease. Maximum aerobic power is reduced, the rest hypoxemia is more marked with exercise, and ventilation is excessive relative to $\dot{V}O_2$.

After the modified Fontan operation, the maximum aerobic power increases but remains subnormal. The ventilatory response to exercise approaches but does not become completely normal, and hypoxemia is virtually eliminated, but rest systemic arterial blood O_2 saturation remains slightly, although significantly, less than normal. The mild persistent hypoxemia after the Fontan operation is due, most likely, to persistent pulmonary ventilation–perfusion mismatch. An additional source of mild systemic hypoxemia exists if the os of the coronary sinus is allowed to drain into the pulmonary venous atrium. After the Fontan operation, the cardiac output response to exercise is subnormal. This results from both subnormal heart rate and stroke volume responses to exercise. Abnormal stroke volume results from reduced systemic ventricular function in the absence of a subpulmonary ventricle.

PECTUS EXCAVATUM

Much has been written about the effects of pectus excavatum on cardiac function and the cardiorespiratory responses to exercise. Unfortunately, most observations on which conclusions were based were uncontrolled. These potentially erroneous conclusions include abnormal stroke volume response to exercise and increased maximum aerobic capacity after repair of pectus excavatum. However, Wynn et al., in a well-controlled study, demonstrated that there was no significant increase in maximum aerobic power after repair of pectus excavatum and that stroke volume response to exercise was normal. Patients with pectus excavatum may have below-normal aerobic capacity and develop the sensation of shortness of breath earlier than their peers with intense exercise because the total lung capacity is reduced in these patients. There are no data suggesting that repair of pectus excavatum during the teen years increases total lung capacity.

SELECTED REFERENCES

Andersen K, Seliger B, Rutenfranz J, et al. Physical performance capacity of children in Norway. II: Heart rate and oxygen pulse in submaximal and maximal exercises: Population parameters in a rural community. *Eur J Appl Physiol*. 1974;33:197–206.

Asmussen E. Growth in muscular strength and power. In: Rarick L, ed. *Physical activity, human growth, and development*. New York: Academic Press; 1973.

Asmussen E, Heebll-Nielsen KA. Dimensional analysis of physical performance and growth in boys. *J Appl Physiol*. 1955;7:593–603.

Astrand PO, Rodahl K. *Textbook of work physiology: Physiological basis of exercise*. New York: McGraw-Hill; 1977:450.

Balke J, Ware R. An experimental study of "physical fitness" of air force personnel. *US Armed Forces Med J*. 1959;10:675–688.

Barber G, Danielson G, Puga F, et al. Pulmonary atresia with ventricular septal defect: Preoperative and postoperative responses to exercise. *J Am Coll Cardiol*. 1986;7:630–638.

Bar-Or O. *Pediatrics sports medicine for the practitioner: From physiologic principles to clinical applications*. New York: Springer-Verlag; 1983.

Bar-Or O, Shephard R, Allen C. Cardiac output of 10- to 13-year-old boys and girls during submaximal exercise. *J Appl Physiol*. 1971;30:219–223.

Bar-Or O, Zwiren L, Ruskin H. Anthropometric and developmental measurements of 11- to 12-year-old boys as predictors of performance two years later. *Acta Pediatr Belgium*. 1974;28(Suppl):214–220.

Bruce R. Exercise testing in patients with coronary artery disease. *Ann Clin Res*. 1971;3:323–332.

Burmeister W, Rutenfranz J, Stresny W, et al. Body cell mass and physical performance capacity (W_{170}) of school children. *Int Z Angew Physiol Einschl Arbeits- phsiol*. 1972;31:61–70.

Davies C, Barnes C, Godfrey S. Body composition in maximal exercise performance in children. *Hum Biol*. 1972;44:195–214.

Driscoll D. Exercise rehabilitation programs for children with congenital heart disease: A note of caution. *Pediatr Exerc Sci*. 1990;2:191–196.

Driscoll D. Diagnostic use of exercise testing in pediatric cardiology: The noninvasive approach. In: Bar-Or O, ed. *Advances in pediatric sport sciences*. Champaign, IL: Human Kinetics; 1989:223–251.

Driscoll D, Danielson G, Puga F, et al. Exercise tolerance and cardiorespiratory response to exercise after the Fontan operation for tricuspid atresia or functional single ventricle. *J Am Coll Cardiol*. 1986;7:1087–1094.

Driscoll D, Heise C, Staats B. Techniques and goals of pediatric exercise testing. *CVP J Cardiovasc Pulm Tech*. 1983;11:13–23.

Driscoll D, Staats B, Beck K. Measurement of cardiac output in children during exercise: A review. *Pediatr Exerc Sci*. 1989;1:102–115.

Driscoll D, Staats B, Heise C, et al. Functional single ventricle: Cardiorespiratory response to exercise. *J Am Coll Cardiol*. 1984;4:337–342.

Driscoll D, Wolfe R, Gersony W, et al. Cardiorespiratory responses to exercise of patients with valvar aortic stenosis, pulmonary stenosis, and ventricular septal defect: Report of the Second Natural History Study of Congenital Heart. *Defects Circ*. 1993;87:I-102–I-113.

Fixler D, Laird W, Browne R, et al. Response of hypertensive adolescents to dynamic and isometric exercise stress. *Pediatrics*. 1979;64:579–583.

Freed M, Rocchini A, Rosenthal A, et al. Exercise-induced hypertension after surgical repair of coarctation of the aorta. *Am J Cardiol*. 1979;43:253–258.

Godfrey S. *Exercise testing in children*. London: WB Saunders; 1974.

James F, Kaplan S, Glueck C, et al. Responses of normal children and young adults to controlled bicycle exercise. *Circulation*. 1980;61:902–912.

Jones N, Cambell E. *Clinical exercise testing*, 2nd ed. Philadelphia, PA: WB Saunders; 1982.

MacDougall J, Tuxon D, Sale D, et al. Arterial blood pressure response to heavy resistance exercise. *J Appl Physiol*. 1985;58:785–790.

Markel H, Rocchini A, Beekman R, et al. Exercise-induced hypertension after repair of coarctation of the aorta: Arm versus leg exercise. *J Am Coll Cardiol*. 1986;8:165–171.

Rasmussen P, Staats B, Driscoll D, et al. Comparison of direct and indirect blood pressure during exercise. *Chest*. 1985;87:743–748.

Reybrouck T. The use of the anaerobic threshold in pediatric exercise testing. In: Bar-Or O, ed. *Advances in pediatric sports sciences*, Vol. 3. Champaign, IL: Human Kinetics; 1989.

Reybrouck T, Weymans M, Stijns H, et al. Ventilatory anaerobic threshold in healthy children: Age and sex differences. *Eur J Appl Physiol*. 1985;54:278–284.

Riopel D, Taylor A, Hohn A. Blood pressure, heart rate, pressure rate product, and electrocardiographic changes in healthy children during treadmill exercise. *Am J Cardiol*. 1979;44:697–704.

Triebwasser J, Johnson R, Burpo R, et al. Noninvasive determination of cardiac output by a modified acetylene rebreathing procedure utilizing mass spectrometer measurements. *Aviat Space Environ Med*. 1977;48:203–209.

Strong W, Miller M, Striplin M, et al. Blood pressure response to isometric and dynamic exercise in healthy black children. *Am J Dis Child*. 1978;132:587–591.

Wilmore J, Sigerseth PO. Physical work capacity of young girls 7 to 13 years of age. *J Appl Physiol*. 1967;22:923–928.

Wynn S, Driscoll D, Ostrom N, et al. Exercise cardiorespiratory function in adolescents with pectus excavatum: Observations before and after operation. *J Thorac Cardiovasc Surg*. 1990;99:41–47.

Yoshizawa S, Ishizaki T, Honda H. Physical fitness of children aged 5 and 6 years. *J Hum Ergol (Tokyo)*. 1977;6:311–314.

Zellers T, Driscoll D, Mottram C, et al. Exercise tolerance and cardiorespiratory response to exercise before and after the Fontan operation. *Mayo Clin Proc*. 1989;64:1489–1497.

Portions of the text have been published previously and are reproduced with permission of the publisher:

Driscoll DJ. Exercise testing. In: Emmanoulides G, Riemenschneider T, Allen H, et al. eds. *Moss and Adams' heart disease in infants, children and adolescents*, 5th ed. Baltimore, MD: Lippincott Williams & Wilkins; 1995.

Driscoll DJ. Exercise testing. In: Allen H, Gutgesell H, Clark E, et al. eds. *Moss and Adams' heart disease in infants, children and adolescents*, 6th ed. Baltimore, MD: Lippincott Williams & Wilkins; 2000.

CHAPTER 5

Innocent Murmurs

*"One needs to know what is normal before
one can know what is abnormal"*

Most children, at some time, will have a heart murmur. However, very few of these children will have heart disease. The physician's task is to determine whether the murmur is the result of a cardiac abnormality or is a so-called innocent or functional murmur.

Although an innocent murmur is not an obstacle to participation in sports and exercise, a pathologic murmur may necessitate restrictions on the child's physical activity. In view of the safety considerations and the importance of exercise and fitness, it is crucial to resolve any doubt about the nature of a murmur.

Innocent murmurs occur in all age-groups in the absence of structural heart disease. Their quality and intensity depend upon environmental conditions and the subject's state. For example, conditions that increase cardiac output, such as fever, anxiety, and exercise, will make an innocent murmur louder. The examiner's ability to hear a murmur depends on the presence of distracting ambient noise, patient cooperation, the examiner's hearing acuity, the quality of the stethoscope, and the thickness of the patient's chest wall.

The diagnosis of an innocent murmur is not made by exclusion, but rather is based on physical findings that indicate that the specific murmur is innocent. There are five innocent murmurs of infancy and childhood: (i) pulmonary flow murmur, (ii) Still's murmur, (iii) venous hum, (iv) carotid bruit, and (v) physiologic pulmonary branch stenosis of the neonate (see Figs. 5.1 and 5.2). All these murmurs usually are between 1 and 2 out of 6 on the intensity scale, and all feature normal first and second heart sounds, peripheral pulses, and precordial impulses.

PULMONARY FLOW MURMUR

Pulmonary flow murmur results from turbulent blood flow through an anatomically normal pulmonary valve. It probably is the most common innocent murmur of childhood and is more often heard in children and adolescents than in adults because of the relatively faster blood flow and thinner chest wall of young patients. Pregnant women often will have a pulmonary flow murmur because of the relatively hyperkinetic circulation and increased plasma volume during pregnancy.

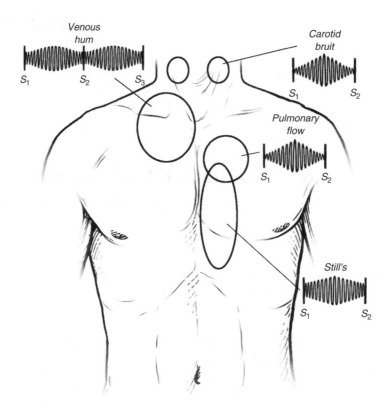

FIGURE 5.1 ● Location and characterization of four of the five innocent murmurs of childhood.

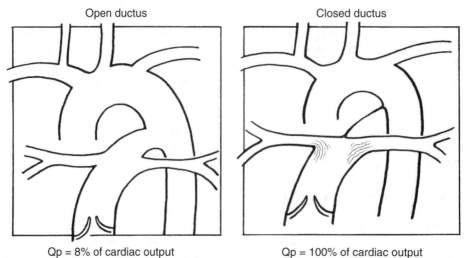

FIGURE 5.2 ● Illustration of the basis of physiologic pulmonary branch stenosis of the newborn. The murmur is similar to the innocent pulmonary flow murmur. It is heard best at the upper left sternal border and heard well in the axillae and over the back.

An innocent pulmonary flow murmur is best heard at the mid and left upper sternal border. It is a midfrequency, crescendo–decrescendo sound that occurs during systole. The murmur is louder with the patient in the supine rather than the upright position. The normal second heart sound distinguishes an innocent pulmonary flow murmur from that of an atrial septal defect, in which the second heart sound is widely split and relatively fixed during the respiratory cycle. The "right ventricular impulse" palpated at the lower left sternal border or subxiphoid area is normal.

STILL'S MURMUR

Still's murmur is very common in children and adolescents and can be heard in some infants. Described by George Still in the early 1900s, it was thought to originate from the vibration of the mitral valve chordae tendinea. Another theory was that it resulted from the vibration of a left ventricular false tendon, which is similar to a chordae tendinea but is connected to opposite walls of the left ventricle rather than the mitral valve. It is now known that the Still's murmur results from turbulence of blood being ejected from the left ventricle.

The pleasant quality of Still's murmur has been likened to the sound of a strummed bass fiddle, and it can occasionally be as loud as grade 3. It is low to midfrequency and crescendo–decrescendo. It is well localized to the lower and mid-left sternal border and is louder in the supine position. It occurs only in systole and is a very pleasant sound.

VENOUS HUM

This murmur results from turbulent flow of systemic venous return in the jugular veins and superior vena cava. It is best heard at the base of the neck or in the infra- or supraclavicular areas. It is more prominent on the right than the left side and is dependent on head and neck position. A change in the position of the patient's head can bring out or eradicate a venous hum. Digital compression of the jugular venous system also will obliterate the murmur. A venous hum disappears in the supine position because the influence of gravity on blood flow from the head to the heart is altered; presumably, the speed of flow, and hence turbulence, is reduced. With these maneuvers, an innocent venous hum can be distinguished from a murmur of a patent ductus arteriosus or an arteriovenous malformation.

A venous hum can occur in systole alone or in both systole and diastole. This high-frequency murmur is heard best with the diaphragm of the stethoscope. It sounds similar to the breeze blowing through the trees.

CAROTID BRUIT

Carotid bruits are very common in children and adolescents. One should routinely listen over the carotid arteries for this innocent murmur to become familiar with it and not attribute undue importance to it. A carotid bruit results from turbulence as blood leaves the relatively large-caliber aortic arch and enters the smaller-caliber brachiocephalic and carotid arteries. It is best heard over the carotid arteries and radiates to the head. An innocent carotid bruit occurs only during systole. It is a crescendo–decrescendo murmur. The carotid pulse volume, like other peripheral pulses, is normal.

One must distinguish this bruit from that associated with radiation of the murmur of aortic stenosis. As a rule, if aortic stenosis is present, the precordial murmur will be louder than the bruit that results from the radiation of the precordial murmur to the carotid arteries. In contrast, an innocent carotid bruit should be louder than any precordial murmurs that may be present. Other features of aortic stenosis, such as prominent apical impulse and an aortic ejection click, will not be heard with this bruit.

It is important not to confuse an innocent carotid bruit with the murmur that occurs with an intracranial arteriovenous malformation.

PHYSIOLOGIC PULMONARY BRANCH STENOSIS

Physiologic pulmonary branch stenosis is heard in infants <2 to 3 months old. It results from the turbulence of blood as it enters the right and left pulmonary arteries. *In utero*, approximately 92% of the blood entering the main pulmonary artery exits through the patent ductus arteriosus, and only 8% enters the branch pulmonary arteries. Therefore, at birth, the right and left pulmonary arteries are relatively small. With birth and lung expansion, and closure of the ductus arteriosus, all of the right ventricular output enters the branch pulmonary arteries. Turbulence occurs as blood travels from the relatively large main pulmonary artery to the smaller branch pulmonary arteries.

The murmur of physiologic branch stenosis is heard best at the upper left sternal border, the axillae, and over the back. It is a systolic crescendo–decrescendo murmur. Rarely, the murmur of physiologic pulmonary branch stenosis may be continuous. The murmur disappears by 2 to 3 months of age because of the growth of the branch pulmonary arteries. If it persists beyond 3 months of age, the murmur is not innocent but may be due to pathologic pulmonary branch stenosis.

ASSESSMENT OF INNOCENT MURMURS

Studies have shown that the innocent nature of a murmur can be determined through a careful history and physical examination done by an experienced pediatric cardiologist without the aid of an electrocardiogram (ECG), chest x-ray, or echocardiogram. The best way to determine the nature of a murmur by an inexperienced pediatric cardiologist or someone other than a cardiologist is less clear. From a cost effectiveness standpoint, referral to an experienced pediatric cardiologist is preferable to referral by the general physician or pediatrician for an echocardiogram.

Generally, if an asymptomatic patient's murmur is (i) grade 2 or less, (ii) occurs only in systole, (iii) is associated with a normal second heart sound, and (iv) the chest x-ray and ECG are normal, then the murmur probably is innocent or results from a condition that is not life threatening and can be reassessed at a later date (i.e., 6 to 12 months). Although some investigators have suggested that the ECG and chest x-ray add little value to making a specific cardiac diagnosis, they can be helpful and useful to the primary care physician when deciding which patients require further consultation.

Consultation with an experienced pediatric cardiologist should be sought if any of the following exist: The murmur is greater than grade 2 in intensity, there is a diastolic murmur (one exception to this is the venous hum), the patient is symptomatic, the second heart sound is abnormal, the chest radiogram or ECG is abnormal, or the examiner simply is unsure of the etiology and importance of the murmur.

A healthy level of skepticism is wise when assessing murmurs in infants because one would not want to misdiagnose a murmur that results from an important cardiac condition as an innocent murmur. It is prudent to have a low threshold for obtaining an echocardiogram in infants.

One should emphasize to the patient and the family that children with innocent murmurs do not have cardiovascular disease. These patients do not require endocarditis prophylaxis and should not be restricted from athletics or other exercise pursuits.

SELECTED REFERENCES

Danford DA. Cost-effectiveness of echocardiography for evaluation of children with murmurs. *Echocardiography*. 1995;12(2):153–162.

Danford DA. Effective use of the consultant, laboratory testing, and echocardiography for the pediatric patient with heart murmur. *Pediatr Ann*. 2000;29(8):482–488.

Danford DA, Martin AB, Fletcher SE, et al. Echocardiographic yield in children when innocent murmur seems likely but doubts linger. *Pediatr Cardiol*. 2002;23(4):410–414.

Newburger JW, et al. Noninvasive tests in the initial evaluation of heart murmurs in children. *N Engl J Med*. 1983;308(2):61–64.

Rosenthal A. How to distinguish between innocent and pathologic murmurs in childhood. *Pediatr Clin North Am*. 1984;31(6):1229–1240.

Yi M, Kimball T, Tsevat J, et al. Evaluation of heart murmurs in children: Cost-effectiveness and practical implications. *J Dev Behav Pediatr*. 2002;141(4):504–511.

Portions of the text have been published previously and are reproduced with permission of the publisher:
Driscoll DJ. Evaluation of cardiac murmurs in children. *Your patient and fitness*. 1991;3:13–18.

CHAPTER 6

Chest Pain

"The pathway to Hell
is not paved with good intention.
The pathway to Hell
is paved with uncontrolled clinical trials."

Abdominal pain, leg pain ("growing pains"), headache, and chest pain are common symptoms in children and adolescents. In a prospective study, 43 children with chest pain presenting to a children's hospital outpatient/emergency room over a 9-week period were evaluated. In this study, the occurrence rate per hospital visit was 0.288%, and in another study it was 0.249%. Chest pain accounts for 650,000 physician visits per year in patients aged 10 to 21 years.

Chest pain creates considerable angst among patients and their families because they assume that chest pain indicates heart pain. Indeed, most patients describe the pain as "my heart hurts" rather than "my chest hurts." Fortunately, chest pain in this age-group is rarely the result of a cardiac problem. Part of the treatment of the patient involves appropriate reassurance to him/her and the family about the benign nature of chest wall pain. Useful reassurance can be given only after a careful history and physical examination.

The mean age of children and adolescents who complain of chest pain is 9 to 14 years, but this complaint can occur in children as young as 4 years. Chest pain is slightly more common in men than in women.

The relative frequency and types of chest pain reported by several investigators are summarized in Table 6.1. The most common sources of chest pain in children and adolescents are the musculoskeletal structures of the chest cage and chest wall. Several specific types of chest cage and chest wall pain can be described.

COSTOCHONDRITIS

Costochondritis involves two to four contiguous costochondral or costosternal junctions. It is usually unilateral. More commonly, it involves the more cephalad joints. The pain usually is described as sharp, lasts several seconds to several minutes, and is exacerbated by deep

TABLE 6.1

Percentage Distribution of Causes of Chest Pain in Children and Adolescents

Study[a]	A	B	C	D	E	F	G
Idiopathic cause	—	13	46	55	28	—	21
Musculoskeletal disorder	—	16	13	—	15	45	15
Costochondritis	—	9	16	2	10	23	9
Asthma	64	12	—	3	4	—	7
Psychogenic cause	—	9	—	—	—	—	9
Trauma	—	7	3	—	4	—	5
Respiratory disorder	—	11	—	—	6	12.5	10
Pneumonia	—	6	—	—	2	—	4
Hyperventilation	—	—	23	—	—	—	—
Cardiac disease	—	4	—	6	—	—	4
Mitral prolapse	—	—	1	—	—	—	—
Arrhythmia	—	—	—	—	3	—	—
GI disease	—	3	3	2	7	—	4
Sickle cell disease	—	3	—	—	—	—	2
Breast-related disease	—	—	6	—	—	—	—
Functional cause	—	—	—	—	17	—	—
Miscellaneous	—	6	2	31	4	10	9

[a] Abstracted from Selected References.
GI, gastrointestinal.

breathing. The joints are not inflamed, and there is no swelling of the joints. Pushing on the joint can reproduce the pain.

TIETZE SYNDROME

Tietze syndrome is quite uncommon in children. It involves the inflammation of one costochondral junction. The area involved is warm, swollen, and tender.

NONSPECIFIC CHEST WALL PAIN (IDIOPATHIC CHEST PAIN)

Nonspecific chest wall pain may be the most common type of chest pain in children and adolescents. The pain usually is described as sharp. When asked to point to the site of pain, the patient usually will point to the center of the chest or the area below the left nipple. The pain lasts several seconds to several minutes and is exacerbated by deep breathing. Sometimes, squeezing the chest cage or gently pressing on the sternum can reproduce the pain. Frequently, the pain cannot be reproduced by palpating and pushing on various chest structures. The costochondral and costosternal joints are not tender.

PRECORDIAL CATCH SYNDROME

Precordial catch syndrome consists of a brief (several seconds) sharp pain inferior to the left nipple or at the lower left sternal border. It is frequently pleuritic and can be accentuated by bending forward. It frequently forces the patient to breathe shallowly. Its cause is unknown.

SLIPPING RIB SYNDROME

Slipping rib syndrome is quite rare and produces rather intense pain. It usually involves the eighth, ninth, and tenth ribs, which do not attach directly to the sternum but, rather, attach to each other. It has been postulated that trauma to the chest results in the disruption of the connection of these ribs to each other, and subsequent movement produces pain. A positive "hooking maneuver" is said to be characteristic of this problem. The "hooking maneuver" is performed by the examiner by placing his/her fingers under the inferior rib margin and pulling anteriorly. This will reproduce the pain and may produce a clicking sound.

HYPERSENSITIVE XIPHOID SYNDROME

Hypersensitive xiphoid syndrome is uncommon in children. It is easily diagnosed by applying digital pressure on the xiphoid process, which reproduces the pain.

TRAUMA AND MUSCLE STRAIN

Obviously, injury to the chest can produce chest wall pain. Usually, the pain can be reproduced on palpation of the chest.

One must be aware, of course, that significant trauma can produce a myocardial contusion and, possibly, a hemopericardium, both of which can cause chest pain.

SICKLE CELL DISEASE

Sickle cell crisis can produce chest wall bone pain. In addition, chest pain in patients with this disease can be of cardiac and pulmonary origin.

LESS COMMON CAUSES OF CHEST PAIN

Although chest wall pain is the most common cause of chest pain in children and adolescents, there is a long list of other, less common, causes of chest pain. These include the following:

ASTHMA

One group of investigators reported that laboratory evidence of asthma was detected in 73% of children evaluated for chest pain. Certainly, asthma or exercise-induced asthma can be associated with chest pain. In most clinicians' experience, this does not constitute the cause of chest pain in a large percentage of patients. However, reactive airway disease should be considered in patients with chest pain, particularly if there is a history of asthma, eczema, shortness of breath with exercise, exercise-associated chest pain, exertional cough, or wheezing, or a family history of asthma.

INFECTION

There are a number of infectious processes that can be associated with chest pain. Pneumonitis and bronchitis of all types can produce chest pain. Herpes zoster can produce chest pain, and frequently, pain can occur before the appearance of the typical skin eruption. Pleurodynia is a well-recognized cause of chest pain.

PERICARDITIS

Pericarditis causes chest pain. In general, the pain associated with pericarditis is more severe than the benign forms of chest wall pain and is usually intensified when the patient lies down and lessened when the patient leans forward. Pericarditis is associated with typical electrocardiographic findings of generalized ST-segment elevation.

GASTROINTESTINAL DISEASES

Gastroesophageal reflux and esophagitis can cause chest pain. In most studies, this constitutes a small percentage of chest pain in children and adolescents. It is possible that if gastrointestinal causes of chest pain were sought more vigorously, then the diagnosis would be made more frequently.

PNEUMOTHORAX

Among patients with chest pain, pneumothorax is uncommon. However, a pneumothorax always is associated with chest pain. A small pneumothorax may be difficult to detect by clinical examination. The abrupt onset of severe chest pain should alert the clinician to this diagnosis. Marfan syndrome is associated with spontaneous pneumothorax and should be considered in the differential diagnosis of pneumothorax.

CARDIAC CAUSES OF CHEST PAIN

In a population of children and adolescents with chest pain, the proportion of those with a cardiac origin for the chest pain will be very low. However, there are a number of cardiac conditions that can be associated with chest pain. These include hypertrophic cardiomyopathy, aortic stenosis, pericarditis, arrhythmias, coronary insufficiency, and mitral valve prolapse. Causes of coronary insufficiency in children include Kawasaki syndrome, William syndrome, anomalous origin of the coronary arteries, and coronary arteriovenous and coronary cameral fistulae.

Even in a population with these conditions, chest pain is an uncommon presenting symptom. It is important to identify patients who are at high risk for these conditions through historical information and identification of characteristics of pain so that appropriate diagnostic and therapeutic steps can be taken.

MEDICAL EVALUATION

The evaluation of chest pain requires a thorough history and careful physical examination. The family history should be explored for premature forms of heart or lung disease and instances of premature death. In addition, it may be helpful to know whether other family members have chest pain, such as a parent or grandparent who has angina. This might heighten the concerns of chest pain in the child. In most cases, the etiology of pain will be apparent after the history and physical examination. Most patients will not have a serious underlying medical problem, but the patients and their family may think that they do. A thorough and thoughtful history and physical examination is important for reassuring the patient and his/her family that there is no serious problem. As part of the examination, it is important to palpate the costochondral joints and other areas of the chest to elicit tenderness. As has been demonstrated by several investigators, in most cases, only a history and physical examination are necessary, and additional tests are not particularly helpful.

Very few patients truly have angina. If a history of angina is elicited, appropriate testing will be needed. A history of chest pain associated with lightheadedness or presyncope should make one more suspicious of a potentially serious underlying cause of chest pain such as aortic stenosis, hypertrophic cardiomyopathy, and anomalous origin of the right or left coronary artery from the wrong sinus of Valsalva. In these cases, appropriate investigations should be done.

TREATMENT

The specific treatment of chest pain, of course, will depend on the underlying cause of pain. For most patients with musculoskeletal causes of chest pain, such as costochondritis, nonspecific chest wall pain, and precordial catch syndrome, an explanation of the cause of pain and its benign nature is enough to reassure the patient and his/her family. By explaining the benign nature of the pain, the anxiety associated with it is relieved and the patient will tolerate the pain better with less fear. Mild analgesics can be prescribed, but in general, chest wall pain is relatively transient, and medication is usually unnecessary.

Exertional asthma can be treated with inhaled bronchodilators. Any specific cardiac cause of the chest pain, if present, should be treated.

OUTCOME

There have been two studies on the outcome of chest pain in children. One reported the follow-up of 149 patients and noted that the initial diagnosis was changed in 34%. Usually, a change in diagnosis indicated a nonorganic cause of the chest pain. A new organic cause was found in only 12 of the 149 patients. Only one child had a cardiac problem—mitral valve prolapse. Three children had asthma. The pain resolved in 57% of the patients. When the patients were questioned 4 weeks to 2 years after initial evaluation of the chest pain, one investigator found that the pain resolved in approximately 58% of patients.

SELECTED REFERENCES

Brown R. Costochondritis in adolescents. *J Adolesc Health Care*. 1981;1:198–201.
Coleman W. Recurrent chest pain in children. *Pediatr Clin North Am*. 1984;31:1007–1026.
Driscoll D, Glicklich L, Gallen W. Chest pain in children: A prospective study. *Pediatrics*. 1976;57:648–651.
Epstein S. Chest Wall Syndrome: A common cause of unexplained cardiac pain. *JAMA*. 1979;241:2793.
Fyfe D, Moodie D. Chest pain in pediatric patients presenting to a cardiac clinic. *Clin Pediatr*. 1984;23:321–324.
Lipkin M, Fulton L, Wolfson E. The syndrome of the hypersensitive xiphoid. *New Eng J Med*. 1955;253:591–597.
Miller A, Texidor T. "Precordial catch," a neglected syndrome of precordial pain. *JAMA*. 1955;159:1364–1365.
Pantell R, Goodman B. Adolescent chest pain: A prospective study. *Pediatrics*. 1983;71:881–887.
Porter G. Slipping Rib Syndrome: An infrequently recognized entity in children: A report of three cases and review of the literature. *Pediatrics*. 1985;76:810–815.
Selbst S. Chest pain in children. *Pediatrics*. 1985;75:1068–1070.
Selbst S, Ruddy R, Clark B. Chest pain in children: Follow-up of patients previously reported. *Clin Pediatr*. 1990;29:374–377.

Selbst S, Ruddy R, Clark B, et al. Pediatric chest pain: A prospective study. *Pediatrics*. 1988;82:319–323.

Wiens L, Sabath R, Ewing L, et al. Chest pain in otherwise healthy children and adolescents is frequently caused by exercise-induced asthma. *Pediatrics*. 1992;90:350–353.

Portions of the text have been published previously and are reproduced with permission of the publisher:

Driscoll DJ. Chest pain in children. In: Allen H, Gutgesell H, Clark E, et al. eds. *Moss and Adams' heart disease infants, children and adolescents*, 6th ed. Baltimore, MD: Lippincott Williams & Wilkins; 2000.

CHAPTER 7

Syncope and Sudden Death

"The coroner's jury sat upon the corpse, and, like sensible men, returned an unassailable verdict of 'sudden death.'"

Nathaniel Hawthorne, *The House of the Seven Gables*

SYNCOPE IN CHILDREN AND ADOLESCENTS

Does syncope identify a subset of patients at increased risk for sudden death? Certainly, some of the conditions such as hypertrophic cardiomyopathy, prolonged QT-interval syndrome, Brugada syndrome, Wolff-Parkinson-White (WPW) syndrome, and pulmonary hypertension are known to be associated with both syncope and sudden death. However, this does not mean that syncope, in a general population, is a precursor or predictor of sudden death.

Approximately 15% of adolescents faint at least once. We reported that syncope occurred in 90 to 166 of 100,000 females and in 48 to 93 of 100,000 males aged between 1 and 22 years, depending on the period when the patients were studied (see Fig. 7.1). Also, in this study, the long-term survival of children and adolescents was not different from that of an age-matched population. However, one patient had prolonged QT-interval syndrome and another died suddenly and unexpectedly. Both these patients had had syncope during exercise. Syncope during exercise may be a clue to identify patients who may have a serious underlying cause for syncope.

McHarg et al. studied 108 children ages 2 to 19 years who were referred to a pediatric neurologist or cardiologist for evaluation of syncope. They found that 75% of the patients had vasovagal syncope, 11% had migraine, 8% had seizures, and 6% had cardiac arrhythmias. Of the six patients with cardiac arrhythmias, two had long QT-interval syndrome, one had atrial flutter, two had ventricular tachycardia (one with associated endocardial fibroelastosis), and one had WPW syndrome. Only one patient, who had ventricular tachycardia, died. This was not a population-based study and had inherent ascertainment bias.

Although syncope is very common in children and adolescents, it does not appear that syncope in otherwise healthy children is a predictor of sudden death, except if the syncope occurs during exercise. What then is the appropriate evaluation for an otherwise healthy child or adolescent who faints? What is the role of echocardiography, electrocardiography, or tilt table testing?

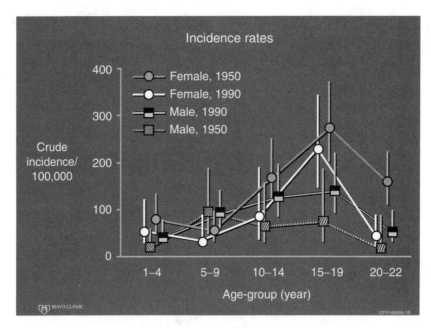

FIGURE 7.1 ● Occurrence rates of syncope in males and females. Syncope is more common in girls than in boys.

Most episodes of syncope in adolescents likely result from a "normal" autonomic imbalance that occurs in this age-group ("autonomic imbalance of adolescence") and is more common in girls than in boys. This results in a less well-tuned adjustment of heart rate and blood pressure to a number of situations such as postural changes, emotional stresses, relative hypovolemia, and certain tactile stimuli (e.g., having one's hair brushed or pulled). These episodes are what McHarg labeled *vasovagal* but now frequently are termed *vasodepressor* or *cardio inhibitory syncope*. Although one probably can classify these episodes further on the basis of the response to tilt table testing, the clinical usefulness of this testing remains to be proved.

When obtaining a history of syncope, it is important to be sure that the patient really had syncope and did not just have posture-related dizziness. Patients and their families frequently use the term *passed out* or *blacked out* although the patient did not lose consciousness.

It is important to determine whether the syncope occurred during or immediately after exercise. It is also important to know whether there is a family history of premature sudden death, cardiomyopathy, arrhythmia, drowning, and/or automobile accident–related deaths. It may be helpful to know whether the patient was injured as a result of the syncopal episode. In general, patients are not injured during a vasovagal episode but are more likely to be injured if the episode occurred because of an important underlying cardiac or neurologic problem. Patients are more likely to recall that they felt unwell and were about to faint before a vasovagal faint, whereas they are less likely to recall this if there was an important underlying cause of the event.

If the syncopal event had all the hallmarks of a vasovagal episode, the physical examination is completely normal (including a thorough cardiac and neurologic examination), and there is no family history of sudden death, then there is little data to suggest that additional testing is necessary. Some, however, would consider it prudent to do an electrocardiogram (ECG).

If the syncopal event was not typical of a vasovagal episode or occurred during or immediately after exercise, or there was a positive family history (see preceding text), then further testing is indicated. The specific tests would depend on the specific situation and might include (but not limited to) an ECG, echocardiogram, 24-hour ECG monitoring, exercise testing, blood glucose measurement, and appropriate neurologic testing.

Treatment, of course, depends on the underlying cause. However, one should not overtreat patients who have classical vasovagal presyncope. These patients are best treated with an explanation of the cause of the syncopal episode and with increased fluid intake and liberalized dietary salt. It is unclear if β-blockers, mineralocorticoids, or α-agonists are more effective than fluid and salt liberalization in preventing additional syncopal events in children.

SUDDEN DEATH IN CHILDREN AND ADOLESCENTS

One can categorize sudden death in children and adolescents as sudden infant death syndrome, sudden death in patients with known heart disease, or sudden death in presumably healthy children and adolescents exclusive of sudden infant death syndrome. This discussion is limited to sudden death in presumably healthy children older than 1 year and adolescents (i.e., exclusive of sudden infant death syndrome).

Sudden unexpected death in presumably healthy children and adolescents, as compared to that in adults, is relatively uncommon. We studied subjects in Olmsted County, Minnesota, ranging from 1 to 22 years of age. Sudden unexpected death occurred in 12 subjects (2.3%). This represented an incidence of 1.3 per 100,000 patient years. Kennedy et al. studied subjects in St. Louis County, Missouri, and reported the incidence of sudden unexpected death in children aged 1 to 9 years to be 2.5 and 8.5 per 100,000 patient years during 1981 and 1982 respectively. For subjects aged 10 to 19 years, the incidences were 2.4 and 5.3 for 1981 and 1982 respectively. Investigators (Neuspiel and Kuller) studying sudden deaths in Allegheny County, Pennsylvania, reported 207 cases of sudden unexpected death among a total of 948 nontraumatic deaths in individuals aged between 1 and 21 years, with an incidence of 4.6 per 100,000 patient years. The difference in the incidence rates between these studies may be accounted for by the different demographics of the populations studied and by differences in the interpretation of the definition of sudden unexpected death. In the first study, deaths from infectious disease identified before death, which can be associated with death (e.g., meningitis, epiglottitis), were not included, whereas these were included in the last study. Hence, the "real" incidence of sudden unexpected death in this age-group is somewhere between 1.3 and 4.6 per 100,000 patient years.

In addition to these three studies on the incidence of sudden unexpected death, there have been numerous non–population-based studies in which causes of sudden unexpected death have been cataloged. A number of these studies involved sudden deaths that occurred on the athletic field. The usual causes of nontraumatic athletic field deaths are listed in Table 7.1. In addition, in a significant number of cases, no apparent cause of death was found. One must suspect that in these cases, an arrhythmia may have caused the death; for example, the patient may have had prolonged QT-interval syndrome, WPW syndrome, or other underlying potentially fatal arrhythmias. One may not be able to extrapolate these findings to a general population. Because the subjects were athletes, one might presume that, in general, they were healthy and also had undergone prior preparticipation evaluations.

TABLE 7.1

Common Causes of Nontraumatic Death in Athletes

- Hypertrophic cardiomyopathy
- Anomalous origin of a coronary artery or its branches from the wrong sinus of Valsalva
- Idiopathic dilated cardiomyopathy
- Myocarditis
- Pulmonary vascular obstructive disease
- Fibrotic coronary artery occlusion

- Aortic stenosis
- Marfan syndrome
- Mitral valve prolapse
- Arrhythmogenic right ventricular dysplasia
- Tunneled left anterior coronary artery
- Atherosclerosis
- Subarachnoid hemorrhage

PREVENTION OF SUDDEN DEATH: SCREENING OF ATHLETES

There have been several reports of the utility of screening athletes, with particular emphasis on identifying disorders that could be associated with sudden death. Four studies included echocardiography screening (Feinstein [1993], Murray [1995], Weidenbener [1995], and Maron [1987]). A total of 6,684 high school, college, and Olympic athletes were screened. The following conditions were identified: Mitral valve prolapse (113 cases), bicuspid aortic valve (14 cases), small ventricular septal defect or aneurysm (five cases), increased left ventricular septal or wall thickness (but insufficient criteria for diagnosis of hypertrophic cardiomyopathy; four cases), aortic root dilation (but insufficient criteria for diagnosis of Marfan syndrome; four cases), and others (six cases). In none of the cases was it thought that the abnormality found put the subject at increased risk for sudden death.

Recently, a task force of the American Heart Association issued a statement about preparticipation screening of athletes. This expert panel concluded that "a complete and careful personal and family history and physical examination designed to identify those cardiovascular lesions known to cause sudden death or disease progression in young athletes is the best available and most practical approach to screening populations of competitive sports participants, regardless of age.... The cardiovascular history should include key questions designed to determine (1) prior occurrence of exertional chest pain/discomfort or syncope/near-syncope as well as excessive, unexpected, and unexplained shortness of breath or fatigue associated with exercise; (2) past detection of a heart murmur or increased systemic blood pressure; and (3) family history of premature death (sudden or otherwise), or significant disability from cardiovascular disease in close relatives younger than 50 years old or specific knowledge of the occurrence of certain conditions (e.g., hypertrophic cardiomyopathy, dilated cardiomyopathy, long QT syndrome, Marfan syndrome, or clinically important arrhythmias)." This task force did not recommend incorporating echocardiography or stress testing into a screening program.

ELECTROCARDIOGRAPHIC SCREENING OF CHILDREN

Studies on the utility of routine electrocardiographic screening of school children have been performed in Japan. Aihoshi et al. screened 14,227 school children and found nine cases of prolonged QT interval. In another study, 17,361 school children were screened, and 8 cases of left ventricular hypertrophy and 24 cases of WPW syndrome were found.

SCREENING ISSUES AND RECOMMENDATIONS

When considering screening for any problem, several issues must be considered, including: (i) The size of the population to be screened, (ii) the prevalence of the problem, (iii) false-positive results, (iv) false-negative results, (v) cost, and (vi) legal issues.

There are approximately 77,071,000 children in the United States aged between 1 and 19 years. The incidence of sudden unexpected death in this population is between one and four per 100,000 patient years. Therefore, one could expect 770 to 3,082 sudden unexpected deaths to occur in presumably healthy children each year.

The potential screening modalities include history, physical examination, chest x-ray, ECG, stress ECG, echocardiogram, and in the future perhaps, genetic screening using a blood specimen or other easily obtainable tissue.

The most common conditions causing sudden death in this population are cardiomyopathies and coronary artery anomalies. In athletes dying suddenly, these conditions account for approximately 73% of the deaths. Primary arrhythmias potentially account for 11% of sudden deaths. Therefore, to detect cardiomyopathy and coronary anomalies screening would require some sort of cardiac imaging such as echocardiography. In addition, electrocardiography would be needed to identify subjects with long QT-interval syndrome. Assuming that echocardiography costs $200 per study (a conservative estimate) and electrocardiography costs $25 per study, it would cost $17,340,975,000 to screen all children in the United States on one occasion. Knowing that the phenotype of hypertrophic cardiomyopathy may not be expressed at a young age, screening may have to be repeated. However, assuming only one screening encounter, it would cost from $5,626,533 to $22,520,746 per case of potential sudden death. There are likely to be very many false-positive and false-negative tests. This cost does not include the additional monetary, legal, and emotional cost of dealing with false-positive and false-negative tests.

One could consider routine ECG screening of children to detect potentially lethal cases of long QT syndrome and WPW. In athletes, this may account for 11% of the cases of sudden death on the athletic field. On the basis of Aihoshi's data, 0.06% of patients screened had long QT interval. Fukushige's data suggests that 0.04% of children screened had WPW (Fukushige JJ, personal communication, 1995).

Considering all these issues, the most prudent approach to screening a presumably healthy population of children and adolescents would be to incorporate the recommendations of the American Heart Association Task Force on Cardiovascular Preparticipation Screening of Competitive Athletes into the usual health maintenance evaluation of children and adolescents (see page 58). Currently, in the United States, echocardiographic screening of large populations does not appear to be cost effective or medically sound. Routine ECG screening could be performed, but there is insufficient data available to justify it at this time.

SELECTED REFERENCES

Aihoshi S, Yoshinaga M, Nakamura M, et al. Screening for QT prolongation using a new exponential formula. *Jpn Circ J*. 1995;59:185–189.

Driscoll JD, Edwards W. Sudden unexpected death in children and adolescents. *J Am Coll Cardiol*. 1985;5: 118B–121B.

Driscoll JD, Jacobsen S, Porter C, et al. Syncope in children and adolescents. *J Am Coll Cardiol*. 1997;29: 1039–1045.

Feinstein R, Colvin E, Kim O. Echocardiographic screening as part of a preparticipation examination. *Clin J Sports Med*. 1993;3:149–152.

Grubb B. Neurocardiogenic syncope. *N Engl J Med*. 2005;352:1004–1010.

Kennedy H, Whitlock J. Sudden death in young persons-an urban study (Abstract). *J Am Coll Cardiol*. 1984;3:485.

Kennedy H, Whitlock J, Buckingham T. Cardiovascular sudden death in young persons (Abstract). *J Am Coll Cardiol*. 1984;3:485.

Maron B, Bodison S, Wesley Y, et al. Results of screening a large group of intercollegiate competitive athletes for cardiovascular disease. *The Amer J Cardiol*. 1987;10:1214–1221.

Maron B, Thompson P, Puffer J, et al. Cardiovascular preparticipation screening of competitive athletes. *Circulation*. 1996;94:850–865.

Maron B, Zipes D, Driscoll D, et al. 36th Bethesda conference: Eligibility recommendations for competitive athletes with cardiovascular abnormalities. *J Amer Coll Card*. 2005;45:1313–1377.

McHarg M, Shinnar S, Rascoff H, et al. Syncope in childhood. *Pediatr Cardiol*. 1997;18:367–371.

Murray P, Cantwell J, Heath D, et al. The role of limited echocardiography in screening athletes. *Am J Cardiol*. 1995;76:849–850.

Neuspiel D, Kuller L. Sudden and unexpected natural death in childhood and adolescence. *JAMA*. 1985;254: 1321–1325.

Pelliccia A, Fagard R, Bjornstad H, et al. Recommendations for competitive sports participation in athletes with cardiovascular disease: A consensus document from the Study Group of Sports Cardiology of the Working Group at Cardiac Rehabilitation and Exercise Physiology and the Working Group of Myocardial and Pericardial Diseases of the European Society of Cardiology. *Eur Heart J*. 2005;26(14):1422–1445.

Weidenbener E, Krauss M, Waller B, et al. Incorporation of screening in echocardiography in the preparticipation exam. *Clin J Sports Med*. 1995;5:86–89.

Portions of the text have been published previously and are reproduced with permission of the publisher:

Driscoll DJ. Syncope sudden death, and sensible screening. In: Quan L, Franklin W, eds. *Ventricular fibrillation: A pediatric problem*. Armonk, NY: Futura Publishing Co; 2000:269–274.

CHAPTER 8

Principles of Inheritance and Genetics of Congenital Heart Disease

*"Pick a rare disease
and study it"*

PRINCIPLES OF INHERITANCE OF CONGENITAL HEART DISEASE

MULTIFACTORIAL INHERITANCE

Most forms of congenital heart disease (CHD) have a multifactorial etiology. This means that the development of a congenital heart malformation is determined by the interaction of several environmental and genetic factors. Although this may seem like a rather vague and imprecise mechanism, there are several principles of the multifactorial model that are borne out by empiric observations. These principles are useful for purposes of genetic counseling.

In the multifactorial model, the risk of occurrence, in general, is related to the frequency with which the defect occurs in the general population. For example, if one considers all CHDs, the frequency of their occurrence in the general population is approximately 0.7 of 100 live births. Therefore, if no members of a family have CHDs, the risk that a couple will have a child with CHD is approximately 0.7%.

The risk of an individual being born with CHD is increased if a first-degree relative (a parent or a sibling) has CHD. The risk is about 2% to 5%, assuming a multifactorial inheritance pattern. If it is a relatively common CHD such as ventricular septal defect (VSD), the recurrence risk will be at the higher end of this range, whereas if it is a relatively uncommon defect such as tricuspid atresia, it will be at the lower end of this range. The recurrence risk of CHD, if a first-degree relative has CHD, will depend on the specific defect and whether there is a gender predilection for the specific cardiac defect.

Much of the data on recurrence risk is based on empiric observational studies, and significant differences exist among different studies because of the manner in which the studies were performed (see Fig. 8.1). For example, an early study of the recurrence risk of aortic stenosis in children born to mothers with aortic stenosis suggested a recurrence risk as high as 26%. However, this study likely included significant ascertainment bias. In addition, the diagnosis of aortic stenosis in the children was based on physical examination only. The preponderance of the studies, however, suggests that the recurrence risk for aortic stenosis, pulmonary stenosis, and VSD in children of a mother or father with one of these defects is approximately 5% (see Table 8.1). In the second natural history study (NHS-2), there was minimal, if any, ascertainment bias, but the presence of CHD in the children was established

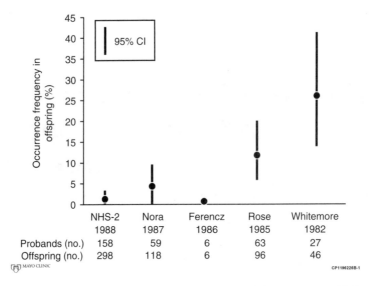

FIGURE 8.1 ● Comparison of the results of several studies of the recurrence risk for aortic valve stenosis. CI, confidence interval. See Driscoll D, Michels V, Gersony W, et al. Occurrence risk for congenital heart defects in children of patients with aortic stenosis, pulmonary stenosis, or ventricular septal defect: Report of the second natural history study of congenital heart defects. *Circulation.* 1993;87:1114–1120.

on the basis of history alone, and the recurrence rate was <5%. There have been several studies of atrioventricular septal defect (AVSD) suggesting that the recurrence risk is greater than the 5% that has been observed for aortic stenosis, pulmonary stenosis, and VSD.

Theoretically, if a CHD is more common in one gender than in the other, the risk of recurrence in the child will be higher if the defect is in the parent for whom the risk of incidence is lower. For example, aortic stenosis is more common in men than in women. Presumably, in a multifactorial model, if a woman has aortic stenosis, a greater load of

TABLE 8.1

Recurrence Rates for Aortic Stenosis, Pulmonary Stenosis, and Ventricular Septal Defect from the Second Natural History Study of Congenital Heart Disease

	Number of Parents	Number of Children	Percentage of Children with Congenital Heart Disease	Confidence Limits
Aortic stenosis	174	325	1.2	0.34–3.12
Pulmonary stenosis	204	387	2.8	1.43–5.03
VSD	353	722	2.9	1.81–4.41

VSD, ventricular septal defect.

environmental–genetic factors exists to cause the defect in the woman than in the man. This greater "environmental–genetic load" should increase the chances of the defect recurring in the child of that mother. However, empiric studies do not bear this out in all cases. It is not perfectly clear why the multifactorial model breaks down in this situation. It could probably be because not all cases of aortic stenosis, or for that matter any form of CHD, are explained by the multifactorial model. An important number of cases may be single gene defects, examples of the Knudson double hit hypothesis, a mixed model of multifactorial and single gene defects, or somatic gene mutations. Furthermore, empiric risk data have not been studied for all categories of recurrence risks relative to gender.

SINGLE GENE DEFECTS

Over the last 15 years, an increasing number of single gene defects have been discovered to be associated with isolated CHDs. Examples include supravalvar aortic stenosis (elastin gene), atrial septal defect (ASD) (genes that encode transcription factors TBX5, NKX 2.5, and GATA4, and the structural protein MYH6), hypertrophic cardiomyopathy (mutations in multiple genes that encode proteins of the cardiac sarcomere), and tetralogy of Fallot, as well as related defects (JAG, which is allelic to Alagille syndrome). If the CHD results from a single gene defect, recurrence risks would reflect a Mendelian pattern such as autosomal dominant or recessive. It is important to recognize these situations because the recurrence risks will be much greater than those if the inheritance pattern is multifactorial. Variable expression and incomplete penetrance need to be considered.

In addition to hereditary germ line mutations, somatic mutations in genes that relate to cardiac development have been demonstrated only in the heart tissue in some cases of sporadic CHD.

Marfan Syndrome

Marfan syndrome is an autosomal dominant condition with variable expression that results from a mutation in the gene that encodes for fibrillin-1. Less commonly, it is due to a mutation in transforming growth factor β (TGF β). It is characterized by tall stature, pectus excavatum or carinatum, reduced upper to lower body segment ratio (approximately <0.88, but it is age dependent), an arm span to height ratio >1.05, long thin fingers (arachnodactyly), pes planus, lax joints, long thin face, highly arched palate, myopia, dislocated lenses, skin stria, spontaneous pneumothorax, dural ectasia, mitral valve prolapse, aortic aneurysm, and aortic dissection. A strict clinical criteria (Ghent Criteria, see Table 8.2) must be used to make the diagnosis. Although assays for fibrillin-1 and TGF β are available, the results of these tests must be interpreted carefully because patients without identifiable gene defects can still have the features, risks, and complications of Marfan syndrome. Furthermore, gene variations of uncertain clinical significance may be detected. Therefore, it still is important to make a clinical diagnosis. The criteria listed in Table 8.3 are a useful guide in determining who likely has and who does not have Marfan syndrome.

The major cardiac issues in Marfan syndrome are aortic aneurysm and aortic dissection, aortic valve insufficiency, and mitral valve prolapse and insufficiency. The leading causes of death in Marfan syndrome are aortic rupture and aortic dissection. Hence, identification of patients with Marfan syndrome is important so that these problems can be diagnosed early and treated appropriately. There is clear evidence that treatment of patients with Marfan syndrome with β-blocking drugs slows the progression of aortic root dilation and reduces the risk of aortic rupture and dissection. There is general agreement that all patients with

TABLE 8.2

Diagnostic Criteria for Marfan Syndrome

Index Case
Major criteria in two different organ systems *and* involvement of a third system
Mutation present *and* one major criterion *and* involvement of a second organ system

Relative of Index Case
One major criterion in family history *and* one major criterion in an organ system *and* involvement
of a second organ system

Skeletal (presence of at least four of the following)
Major
    Pectus carinatum
    Pectus excavatum requiring surgery
    Upper to lower segment ratio
      (approximately <0.88) or arm span
      to height ratio >1.05
    Wrist and thumb signs Scoliosis of >20
      degrees or spondylolisthesis
    Reduced extension at the elbows
      (<170 degrees)
    Medial displacement of the medial
      malleolus, causing pes planus
    Protrusio acetabuli of any degree
      (ascertained on radiographs)

Skeletal
Minor
    Pectus excavatum
    Joint hypermobility
    Highly arched palate with crowding
      of teeth
    Facial
      Dolichocephaly
      Malar hypoplasia
      Enophthalmos
      Retrognathia
      Down-slanting palpebral
    Fissures

Ocular
Major
    Ectopia lentis

Ocular
Minor
    Flat cornea
    Increased axial length of globe (<23.5 mm)
    Hypoplastic iris *or* hypoplastic ciliary
      muscle causing decreased miosis

Cardiovascular
Major
    Dilatation of the ascending aorta with or
      without aortic regurgitation and
      involving at least the sinuses of
      Valsalva
    Dissection of the ascending aorta

Cardiovascular
Minor
    Mitral valve prolapse with or without mitral
      valve regurgitation
    Dilatation of the main pulmonary artery in
      the absence of valvular or peripheral
      pulmonic stenosis in patients younger
      than 40 y
    Calcification of the mitral annulus in
      patients younger than 40 y
    Dilatation or dissection of the descending
      thoracic or abdominal aorta in patients
      younger than 50 y

(continued)

TABLE 8.2 (Continued)

Dura	*Skin and Integument*
Major	Minor (only)
Lumbosacral dural ectasis by CT	Striae atrophicae
or MRI scans	Recurrent or incisional herniae
Pulmonary	*Pulmonary*
Major	Minor
None	Spontaneous pneumothorax
	Apical blebs (by chest x-ray)

Family/Genetic History

Having a parent, child, or sibling who meets these diagnostic criteria independently

Presence of a mutation in FBN1 that is known to cause the Marfan syndrome

Presence of a haplotype around FBN1, inherited by descent, known to be associated with
   unequivocally diagnosed Marfan syndrome in the family

CT, computed tomography; MRI, magnetic resonance imaging.
From De Paepe A, Devereux RB, Dietz HC, et al. Revised diagnostic criteria for the Marfan syndrome. *Am J of Med Genet.* 1996;62:417–426.

Marfan syndrome and aortic root or sinus of Valsalva dilatation should be treated with β-blockers unless there are comorbid contraindications. For patients who cannot be treated with β-blockers, it seems reasonable (but there are only limited studies) to use other agents to reduce blood pressure. Whether patients with Marfan syndrome without aortic dilation should be treated with β-blockers is controversial. Because aortic dilation is a progressive process, imaging of the aorta, at least annually, is necessary. More frequent imaging will be necessary in some patients. Because Marfan syndrome does not involve just the ascending aorta, it is important to periodically image the entire aorta.

In fully grown patients, aortic root replacement is indicated if the diameter of the aortic sinuses or the aortic root exceeds 4.5 to 5.5 cm. The exact size of the sinuses or root that

TABLE 8.3

Differential Diagnosis of Marfan Syndrome

- Homocystinuria
- Congenital contractural arachnodactyly
- Familial thoracic aortic aneurysm
- Familial aortic dissection
- Familial ectopia lentis
- Familial Marfan-like habitus
- MASS—**m**yopia, **m**itral valve prolapse, mild **a**ortic dilatation, **s**kin and **s**keletal (at least two, preferably three, criteria)

- Familial mitral valve prolapse syndrome
- Stickler syndrome
- Shprintzen-Goldberg syndrome
- Soto syndrome

would prompt surgery depends on the rate of enlargement of the aorta, the family history, the presence or absence of associated aortic valve insufficiency, and local medical/surgical beliefs and expertise. The size of the aorta that should prompt surgical intervention in children is unclear. Some believe that one should use the size of the aorta relative to normal age-matched data. Others, citing Laplace's law, contend that absolute measurements should be used because the risk of rupture should be related to wall tension, which is related to the radius of the aorta and aortic wall thickness. Surgery also may be indicated for significant aortic and/or mitral regurgitation.

Patients with Marfan syndrome who develop chest pain need careful evaluation to exclude aortic dissection or spontaneous pneumothorax as a cause of the chest pain.

Patients with Marfan syndrome should avoid competitive athletics, excessive weight lifting, and high-impact exercise activities that could result in joint injury and premature arthritis, increased risk of aortic rupture or dissection, and eye injury. Even in the absence of aortic root dilation, these activities should be avoided because aortic dissection can occur in the absence of aortic dilatation.

Pregnancy is a high-risk situation for women with Marfan syndrome and requires specific assessment and counseling.

Noonan Syndrome

Recently, PTPN11 has been described as the cause of Noonan syndrome. PTPN11 encodes for the nonreceptor protein tyrosine phosphatase SHP-2. Noonan syndrome is characterized by short stature, epicanthal folds, low-set ears, low posterior hairline, pectus excavatum, shield chest, broadly spaced nipples, cubitus valgus, webbing of the neck, cryptorchidism, and lymphedema. Lymphangiectasia can occur.

The classic cardiac manifestation is pulmonary valve stenosis, and usually, the valve is more dysplastic than when not associated with Noonan syndrome. Other structural heart diseases such as ASD can occur. Hypertrophic cardiomyopathy also occurs with Noonan syndrome.

Holt-Oram Syndrome

Holt-Oram syndrome results from a mutation of TBX5. As a single gene defect, it is inherited in an autosomal dominant manner with variable expression. It is characterized by triphalangeal thumbs or hypoplasia and proximal placement of the thumb, radial hypoplasia, and hypoplasia of the clavicles.

Occasionally, there may be phocomelia, small scapulae, and a skin tag over the lower sternum.

The classic cardiac manifestation is secundum ASD. However, a variety of CHDs have been reported to occur with this syndrome.

CHROMOSOMAL ABNORMALITIES

Aneuploidy

Down syndrome (Trisomy 21). Down syndrome was the earliest recognized chromosomal abnormality and results from nondisjunction or translocation of chromosome 21. It is important to determine whether the patient has trisomy 21 or 21 translocation. If the child has trisomy 21, the recurrence risk for the future siblings is approximately 1%. If it resulted from 21 translocation, the karyotype of the parents should be determined so that appropriate genetic counseling can be provided to them about the higher risk of their future children having Down syndrome.

Down syndrome occurs in 1 of 800 to 1,000 live births. It is manifested by poor muscle tone ("floppy baby"), flattened occiput, single transverse palmar creases, clinobrachydactyly of the fifth digit, wide spacing between the great and second toe, umbilical hernia, upslanting palpebral fissures, small oral cavity, and flat facies. Hypothyroidism is relatively common in Down syndrome and is difficult to recognize clinically. Hence, these patients should be screened for thyroid dysfunction on a regular basis.

Forty percent of patients with Down syndrome have congenital heart disease and 40% of these patients have a form of atrioventricular septal defect (AVSD). Of those with an AVSD, most will have a type C form of complete AVSD, which consists of an inlet VSD, an ostium primum ASD, and a common AV valve with a free floating (not attached to the ventricle or ventricular septum) anterior leaflet. Although this is the most common form of AVSD in Down syndrome, all types of AVSDs do occur.

The next most common CHDs in Down syndrome, in decreasing order of frequency, are VSD, tetralogy of Fallot, and ostium secundum ASD. The combination of complete AVSD and tetralogy of Fallot occurs in Down syndrome.

Some have suggested that pulmonary hypertension secondary to a left-to-right shunt is more common, more severe, and occurs at an earlier age in patients with Down syndrome compared to those without Down syndrome. However, this issue is confounded by the fact that it is relatively common to have chronic upper airway obstruction in patients with Down syndrome, and, hence, it is unclear whether these patients are more likely to have pulmonary hypertension because of the congenial heart disease or as a result of chronic upper airway obstruction or a combination of the two.

Because of the relatively high incidence of heart disease in patients with Down syndrome, the American Academy of Pediatrics recommends that all newborns with Down syndrome be screened using echocardiography for congenital heart disease. However, most babies in the first 3 days of life will have a patent ductus arteriosus and a patent foramen ovale. Obviously, an echocardiogram done during this period will reveal these conditions. This can lead to unnecessary referral for cardiac evaluation and repeated echocardiograms.

Turner syndrome. Turner syndrome results from a 45,X chromosome constitution. Some deletions and structural abnormalities of the X or Y chromosome also can cause Turner syndrome. It is manifested by short stature and a variable combination of neck webbing, low posterior hairline, broad chest, widely spaced nipples, hypoplastic or inverted nipples, absent secondary sexual characteristics, streak ovarian dysgenesis, lymphedema, short fourth metacarpal, pigmented nevi, renal anomalies, cardiac defects, and cubitus valgus. Intelligence is usually normal.

The usual cardiac manifestations are coarctation of the aorta and/or bicuspid aortic valve with or without aortic stenosis. Aortic aneurysm also occurs, and patients with Turner syndrome should have ongoing screening for aortic aneurysm. The American Academy of Pediatrics recommends that pediatric cardiology consultation be obtained as part of the initial evaluation of patients with Turner syndrome. The timing of screening echocardiograms is not well delineated and this should be decided by the pediatric cardiologist in concert with the primary care physician.

Microdeletion Syndromes

22q11.2 Microdeletion (Shprintzen/DiGeorge/Velocardiofacial syndromes). Before the recognition of microdeletions of 22q11.2, the clinical syndromes described by Shprintzen and DiGeorge, as well as velocardiofacial syndrome, were well recognized. Patients with Shprintzen and DiGeorge, as well as velocardiofacial syndromes shared the common features of CHDs; mental subnormality; mucosal cleft palate; hypernasal speech; feeding difficulties in infancy; medially displaced carotid arteries; long facies; digitalization of the thumb; and a nose that may appear bulbous, rectangular, or pear-shaped, or down-turned. Patients with DiGeorge syndrome, in addition, have thymic hypoplasia that is associated with significant immunodeficiency. Agenesis or hypoplasia of the thymus or frequent infections should suggest DiGeorge syndrome and prompt the assessment of immunologic function and adoption of appropriate precautions to avoid serious infections. Patients with this microdeletion may develop hypocalcemia, thrombocytopenia, and, less frequently, leukopenia and anemia.

With the identification of the 22q11.2 microdeletion, it became apparent that Shprintzen, DiGeorge, and velocardiofacial syndromes share this microdeletion. It still is unclear why some patients with this microdeletion have immunodeficiency, whereas others do not. However, there have been more than 30 genes mapped to this deleted region.

22q11.2 microdeletion is common, occurring in 1 of 4,000 to 5,000 live births. It is referred to as a *microdeletion* because the missing portion of the chromosome is too small to be detected by routine chromosome analysis. Therefore, a specific *FISH* (fluorescent *in situ* hybridization) probe must be used to detect this. The acronym "CATCH-22" had been attached to these syndromes but is a term that should not be used because of its negative connotations associated with the book *CATCH-22* by Joseph Heller. The acronym was intended to recall the association of *c*ardiac defects, *a*bnormal facial features, *t*hymic hypoplasia, *c*left palate, and *h*ypocalcemia with the 22 microdeletion. It is important to determine whether the parents of a child with 22q11.2 microdeletion also have the condition so that appropriate genetic counseling can be provided to the parents.

The most common CHDs associated with 22q11.2 microdeletion involve conotruncal abnormalities such as truncus arteriosus, pulmonary atresia/VSD, tetralogy of Fallot, absent pulmonary valve syndrome, interrupted aortic arch, and VSD. However, it can be associated with any type of CHD. The presence of subtle, clinically insignificant cardiac anomalies such as aberrant origin of a subclavian artery should suggest the possibility of 22q11.2 microdeletion. Patients with 22q11.2 microdeletion and pulmonary atresia with VSD tend to have very complex pulmonary artery anatomy with multiple systemic-to-pulmonary artery collateral vessels and nonconfluent pulmonary arteries.

Williams syndrome. Williams syndrome was previously known as *idiopathic hypercalcemia of the newborn*. At one time it was thought to be related to the vitamin D supplementation administered to pregnant women. However, it is now clear that Williams syndrome results from a microdeletion of chromosome 7q11.2 that encompasses the elastin gene. Interestingly, the initial description of elastin gene defects (intragenic deletion or mutations) was in families with supravalvar aortic stenosis but without other manifestations of Williams syndrome.

Because it is unusual for patients with Williams syndrome to reproduce, the pattern of inheritance was unrecognized until after the genetic defect was described. In practice, therefore, it is unusual for the parents of a patient with Williams syndrome to be affected. In most cases, Williams syndrome occurs because of a new mutation, and if a patient with Williams syndrome has children, the risk that they will be affected is 50%.

Williams syndrome is characterized by mental subnormality, prominent forehead, periorbital fullness, stellate iris, long philtrum, depressed nasal bridge, prominent lower lip, full sagging cheeks, enamel hypoplasia, a very engaging personality (sometimes referred to as a *cocktail party personality*), and CHDs.

Supravalvar aortic stenosis and peripheral pulmonary artery stenosis are the most characteristic cardiac features of Williams syndrome. In addition, these patients can have stenosis of any elastic artery. If there is stenosis of the renal arteries, the patient may have significant hypertension. Stenosis of the subclavian or carotid arteries can produce bruits over these vessels. The Coanda effect has been implicated as the cause for higher blood pressure in the right arm than in the left arm in patients with Williams syndrome. However, this blood pressure discrepancy could result from stenosis of the origin of the contralateral subclavian artery.

Important, but underappreciated, problems in Williams syndrome are cerebral vascular accidents and stenosis of the coronary arteries. Cerebral vascular accidents and myocardial infarction are very rare in infants and children, but when they occur, one must consider the diagnosis of Williams syndrome. Coronary artery stenosis is likely the explanation for the relatively high incidence of death associated with general anesthesia in patients with Williams syndrome.

For patients with significant supravalvar aortic stenosis, surgery is indicated to eliminate the area of obstruction. The recommendations for surgery are similar to those for aortic valve stenosis and are based on the pressure gradient across the obstruction and the degree of left ventricular hypertrophy.

Supravalvar pulmonary stenosis in Williams syndrome is frequently diffuse. At times, the entire pulmonary tree is hypoplastic. This makes it difficult to treat peripheral pulmonary valve stenosis in these patients. Certainly, if the stenoses are discreet, attempts to balloon dilate and stent the areas of stenoses are reasonable.

SELECTED REFERENCES

Allanson JE. Noonan syndrome. *J Med Genet*. 1987;24(1):9–13.

Ayeni TI, Roper HP. Pulmonary hypertension resulting from upper airways obstruction in Down's syndrome. *J R Soc Med*. 1998;91(6):321–322.

Baldini A. DiGeorge syndrome: An update. *Curr Opin Cardiol*. 2004;19(3):201–204.

Benson DW. The genetics of heart disease: A point in the revolution. *Cardiol Clin*. 2002;20(3):385–394.

Benson DW, Basson CT, MacRae CA. New understandings in the genetics of congenital heart disease. *Curr Opin Pediatr*. 1996;8(5):505–511.

Bossert T, Walther T, Gummert J, et al. Cardiac malformations associated with the Holt-Oram syndrome–report on a family and review of the literature. *Thorac Cardiovasc Surg*. 2002;50(5):312–314.

Bramswig JH. Expectation bias with respect to growth hormone therapy in Turner syndrome. *Eur J Endocrinol*. 1997;137(5):446–447.

Burn J. Closing time for CATCH22. *J Med Genet*. 1999;36(10):737–738.

Castiglia PT. Growth & development. Turner syndrome. *J Pediatr Health Care*. 1997;11(1):34–36.

Collod-Beroud G, Boileau C. Marfan syndrome in the third millennium. *Eur J Hum Genet*. 2002;10(11):673–681.

Committee on Genetics. American Academy of Pediatrics: Health care supervision for children with Williams syndrome. [erratum appears in *Pediatrics*. 2002;109(2):329]. *Pediatrics*. 2001;107(5):1192–1204.

Cooney TP, Thurlbeck WM. Pulmonary hypoplasia in Down's syndrome. *N Engl J Med*. 1982;307(19):1170–1173.

Cuneo BF. DiGeorge, velocardiofacial, and conotruncal anomaly face syndromes 22q11.2 Deletion syndrome: [erratum appears in *Curr Opin Pediatr*. 2002;14(2):286]. *Curr Opin Pediatr*. 2001;13(5):465–472.

Dean JC. Management of Marfan syndrome. *Heart (British Cardiac Society*. 2002;88(1):97–103.

Driscoll D, Michels V, Gersony W, et al. Occurrence risk for congenital heart defects in children of patients with aortic stenosis, pulmonary stenosis, or ventricular septal defect: Report of the second natural history study of congenital heart defects. *Circulation*. 1993;87:I114–I120.

Epstein JA, Buck CA. Transcriptional regulation of cardiac development: Implications for congenital heart disease and DiGeorge syndrome. *Pediatr Res*. 2000;48(6):717–724.

Feit LR. Genetics of congenital heart disease: Strategies. *Adv Pediatr*. 1998;45:267–292.

Francke U. Williams-Beuren syndrome: Genes and mechanisms. *Hum Mol Genet*. 1999;8(10):1947–1954.

Gelb BD. Molecular genetics of congenital heart disease. *Curr Opin Cardiol*. 1997;12(3):321–328.

Glorioso J Jr, Reeves M. Marfan syndrome: Screening for sudden death in athletes. *Curr Sports Med Rep*. 2002;1(2):67–74.

Goldmuntz E. The epidemiology and genetics of congenital heart disease. *Clin Perinatol.* 2001;28(1):1–10.

Goldmuntz E, Emanuel BS. Genetic disorders of cardiac morphogenesis. The DiGeorge and velocardiofacial syndromes [see comment]. *Circ Res.* 1997;80(4):437–443.

Grossfeld PD. The genetics of congenital heart disease. *J Nucl Cardiol.* 2003;10(1):71–76.

Halac I, Zimmerman D. Coordinating care for children with Turner syndrome. *Pediatr Ann.* 2004;33(3):189–196.

Horowitz PE, et al. Coronary artery disease and anesthesia-related death in children with Williams syndrome. *J Cardiothorac Vasc Anesth.* 2002;16(6):739–741.

Huang T. Current advances in Holt-Oram syndrome. *Curr Opin Pediatr.* 2002;14(6):691–695.

Kiess W, Dotsch J, Siebler T. Decreased sensitivity to insulin-like growth factor I as a cause of growth failure in Turner's syndrome? [comment]. *Eur J Clin Invest.* 1997;27(7):548–549.

Korenberg JR, et al. VI Genome structure and cognitive map of Williams syndrome. *J Cogn Neurosci.* 2000; 12(Suppl 1):89–107.

Lehner R, et al. Pedigree analysis and descriptive investigation of three classic phenotypes associated with Holt-Oram syndrome. *J Reprod Med.* 2003;48(3):153–159.

Loughlin GM, Wynne JW, Victorica BE. Sleep apnea as a possible cause of pulmonary hypertension in Down syndrome. *J Pediatr.* 1981;98(3):435–437.

Malec E, et al. Results of surgical treatment of congenital heart defects in children with Down's syndrome. *Pediatr Cardiol.* 1999;20(5):351–354.

Maron BJ, et al. Task Force 4: HCM and other cardiomyopathies, mitral valve prolapse, myocarditis, and Marfan syndrome. *J Am Coll Cardiol.* 2005;45(8):1340–1345.

Maslen CL. Molecular genetics of atrioventricular septal defects. *Curr Opin Cardiol.* 2004;19(3):205–210.

Meyers CM, et al. Gonadal (ovarian) dysgenesis in 46,XX individuals: Frequency of the autosomal recessive form. *Am J Med Genet.* 1996;63(4):518–524.

Mori AD, Bruneau BG. TBX5 mutations and congenital heart disease: Holt-Oram syndrome revealed. *Curr Opin Cardiol.* 2004;19(3):211–215.

Morris CA, Mervis CB. Williams syndrome and related disorders. *Annu Rev Genomics Hum Genet.* 2000;1: 461–484.

Nollen GJ, et al. Current insights in diagnosis and management of the cardiovascular complications of Marfan's syndrome. *Cardiol Young.* 2002;12(4):320–327.

Noonan JA. Noonan syndrome. An update and review for the primary pediatrician. *Clin Pediatr.* 1994;33(9): 548–555.

Noonan J, Connor WO. Noonan syndrome: A clinical description emphasizing the cardiac findings. *Acta Paediatr Jpn.* 1996;38(1):76–83.

Perez E, Sullivan KE. Chromosome 22q11.2 Deletion syndrome (DiGeorge and velocardiofacial syndromes). *Curr Opin Pediatr.* 2002;14(6):678–683.

Pyeritz RE. The Marfan syndrome. *Annu Rev Med.* 2000;51:481–510.

Reller MD, Morris CD. Is Down syndrome a risk factor for poor outcome after repair of congenital heart defects? *J Pediatr.* 1998;132(4):738–741.

Remulla JF, Tolentino FI. Retinal detachment in Marfan's syndrome. *Int Ophthalmol Clin.* 2001;41(4):235–240.

Robinson PN, Godfrey M. The molecular genetics of Marfan syndrome and related microfibrillinopathies. *J Med Genet.* 2000;37(1):9–25.

Robinson PN, et al. Mutations of FBN1 and genotype-phenotype correlations in Marfan syndrome and related fibrillinopathies. *Hum Mutat.* 2002;20(3):153–161.

Rose C, et al. Anomalies of the abdominal aorta in Williams-Beuren syndrome–another cause of arterial hypertension. *Eur J Pediatr.* 2001;160(11):655–658.

Saenger P. Turner's syndrome [see comment]. *N Engl J Med.* 1996;335(23):1749–1754.

Saenger P. Turner's syndrome. *Curr Ther Endocrinol Metab.* 1997;6:239–243.

Schiaffino S, Dallapiccola B, Di Lisi R. Molecular genetics of congenital heart disease. A problem of faulty septation. *Circ Res.* 1999;84(2):247–249.

Schultz RT, Grelotti DJ, Pober B. Genetics of childhood disorders: XXVI. Williams syndrome and brain-behavior relationships. *J Am Acad Child Adolesc Psychiatry.* 2001;40(5):606–609.

Sletten LJ, Pierpont ME. Variation in severity of cardiac disease in Holt-Oram syndrome. *Am J Med Genet.* 1996; 65(2):128–132.

Smith J. Brachyury and the T-box genes. *Curr Opin Genet Dev.* 1997;7(4):474–480.

Srivastava D. Developmental and genetic aspects of congenital heart disease. *Curr Opin Cardiol.* 1999;14(3): 263–268.

Suzuki K, et al. Pulmonary vascular disease in Down's syndrome with complete atrioventricular septal defect. *Am J Cardiol.* 2000;86(4):434–437.

Wilson SK, Hutchins GM, Neill CA. Hypertensive pulmonary vascular disease in Down syndrome. *J Pediatr.* 1979;95(5 Pt 1):722–726.

Winlaw DS, Sholler GF, Harvey RP. Progress and challenges in the genetics of congenital heart disease. *Med J Aust.* 2005;182(3):100–101.

Witt DR, et al. Lymphedema in Noonan syndrome: Clues to pathogenesis and prenatal diagnosis and review of the literature. *Am J Med Genet.* 1987;27(4):841–856.

Wouters CH, et al. Deletions at chromosome regions 7q11.23 and 7q36 in a patient with Williams syndrome. *Am J Med Genet*. 2001;102(3):261–265.

Zehr KJ, et al. Surgery for aneurysms of the aortic root: A 30-year experience. *Circulation*. 2004;110(11): 1364–1371.

CHAPTER 9

Left-to-Right Shunts

"A surgeon knows how to operate,
a good surgeon knows when to operate, and
an excellent surgeon know when not to operate"

A left-to-right shunt exists when blood from the left atrium, left ventricle, or aorta transits to the right atrium or its tributaries, the right ventricle, or the pulmonary artery. Because blood in the left atrium, left ventricle, and the aorta is normally fully oxygenated, left-to-right shunt lesions result in fully oxygenated blood recirculating through the lungs, a rather inefficient situation for gas exchange. Hence, the lungs receive all the deoxygenated blood from the systemic venous return (this is equal to cardiac output or systemic blood flow [Qs]) *plus* the volume of fully oxygenated blood that "short circuits" to the right side of the heart through the defect that allows the left-to-right shunt.

The magnitude of a left-to-right shunt can be expressed in terms of the ratio (Qp/Qs) of the volume of pulmonary flow (Qp) and systemic flow (Qs). Normally, this ratio is 1 because the volume of blood that is pumped to the lungs (Qp) is equal to the volume of blood that is pumped to the body (Qs). For patients with a left-to-right shunt, Qp/Qs will be >1. In general, Qp/Qs <1.5 is considered a small shunt, Qp/Qs = 1.5 to 2 is considered a moderate shunt, and Qp/Qs >2 is considered a large shunt. Qp/Qs can be calculated if the blood oxygen saturation is known for the mixed venous, pulmonary arterial, left atrial, and aortic blood (see Table 9.1).

The presence of a left-to-right shunt results in a volume overload of one or more cardiovascular chambers or structures. The chamber or structure that is volume overloaded depends upon the location of the anatomic defect causing the left-to-right shunt. With an atrial septal defect (ASD), blood passes from the left to right atrium. Hence, the left atrium, right atrium, right ventricle, and pulmonary artery are volume overloaded. After the blood transits the lungs and reaches the left atrium, some of the it again short circuits to the right atrium (by passing through the ASD), but a normal volume of blood goes through the mitral valve to reach the left ventricle. Therefore, the left ventricle is *not* volume overloaded.

In the presence of ventricular septal defect (VSD), blood passes from the left ventricle to the pulmonary artery. Technically, the blood transits the right ventricle, but because the right and left ventricle are contracting simultaneously, the right ventricle does not realize a

TABLE 9.1

Formula to Calculate the Ratio of Pulmonary and Systemic Blood Flow

$$Qp/Qs = (Sat_{AO} - Sat_{MV})/(Sat_{LA} - Sat_{PA})$$

Sat_{AO}, aortic blood oxygen saturation; Sat_{MV}, mixed venous blood oxygen saturation; Sat_{LA}, left atrial blood oxygen saturation; and Sat_{PA}, pulmonary artery blood oxygen saturation.

volume overload in this situation. The right atrium also does not realize a volume overload. However, the pulmonary artery is receiving an increased volume of blood as is the left atrium and left ventricle.

In the presence of patent ductus arteriosus (PDA), blood passes from the aorta to the pulmonary artery. Therefore, the pulmonary artery, left atrium, and left ventricle are volume overloaded but the right atrium and right ventricle are not.

The presence of a left-to-right shunt can result in pressure and volume overload of one or more cardiovascular chambers or structures. The presence of pressure overload will depend on the location and size of the left-to-right shunt and the pulmonary vascular resistance. ASDs that are not associated with increased pulmonary vascular resistance result in only a mild elevation of right ventricular (RV) and pulmonary artery pressure. A large VSD (i.e., one that is larger than the aorta) will result in elevated RV and pulmonary artery pressures that are equal to the pressure in the left ventricle. A small PDA will not cause significant elevation of the RV pressure, but a large PDA can cause elevated RV and pulmonary artery pressures equal to the pressure in the aorta.

ATRIAL SEPTAL DEFECTS

INCIDENCE, TYPES, AND EMBRYOLOGY

ASDs occur in 1 of 1,500 live births and constitute 6% to 10% of congenital cardiac defects. There is a female-to-male predominance of 2:1. There are four types of ASDs: (i) Ostium secundum, (ii) ostium primum, (iii) sinus venosus, and (iv) unroofed coronary sinus (see Figs. 9.1 and 9.2). There have been rare cases of familial ASD that have been associated with the genes encoding the transcription factors TBX5, NKX2.5, and GATA4, as well as the structural protein MYH6.

The most common form of ASD is the *ostium secundum*. This occurs in the region of the fossa ovalis. It results from excessive absorption of the septum primum or insufficient development of the septum secundum or both.

Ostium primum ASD is a type of atrioventricular sepal defect. It is located in the inferior aspect of the atrial septum contiguous with the tricuspid and mitral valves. It results from lack of closure of the ostium primum by the endocardial cushions. Because the endocardial cushions also form major portions of the mitral and tricuspid valves, it is not surprising that abnormalities of the atrioventricular (AV) valves are associated with ostium primum ASDs. A cleft in the septal leaflet of the mitral valve invariably is associated with ostium primum ASDs.

Sinus venosus ASDs occur in the posterosuperior aspect of the atrial septum. Frequently, there is associated partial anomalous drainage of the right upper pulmonary vein. This

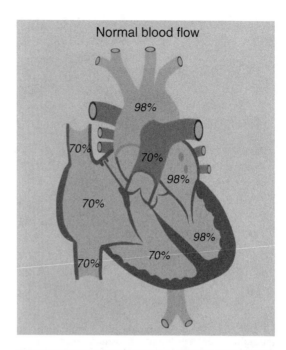

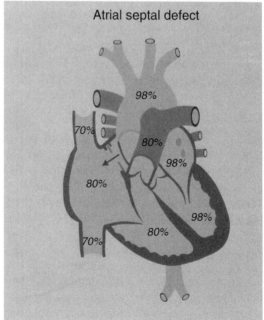

FIGURE 9.1 ● Diagrammatic representation of atrial septal defect (ASD). Note that because of the shunting of blood from the left to the right atrium, the saturation of the blood in the right atrium is higher than normal and higher than that in the superior vena cava (SVC).

vein can drain into the superior vena cava (SVC) or the right atrium. It is speculated that resorption of the wall between the vena cava and pulmonary veins results in the ASD. This also explains the anomalous drainage of the right upper pulmonary vein into the right atrium or SVC, commonly associated with sinus venous ASDs.

The most uncommon form of ASD is *the unroofed coronary sinus*. The coronary sinus is in apposition to the posterior aspect of the left atrium, but the orifice is in the right atrium. If

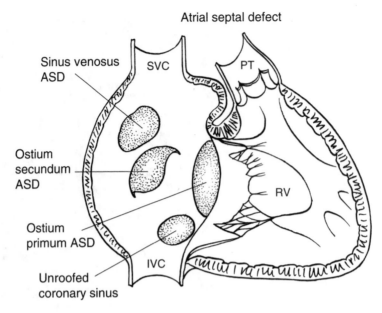

FIGURE 9.2 ● Diagrammatic representation of atrial septal defects (ASDs) as viewed from the right atrium. Note that the ostium secundum ASD is in the same location as the fossa ovalis or patent foramen ovale. Note the proximity of the ostium primum ASD to the atrioventricular valves. The sinus venosus ASD is located relatively posterior in the atrial septum. SVC, superior vena cava; PT, pulmonary trunk; RV, right ventricle; IVC, inferior vena cava.

a hole exists in the roof of the coronary sinus, the coronary sinus and the left atrium will be in continuity, and, therefore, the right and left atria will be in communication with each other.

CLINICAL PRESENTATION

Most patients with ASD are asymptomatic and seek medical attention when a heart murmur is detected. Frequently, the murmur is not appreciated to be a pathologic murmur until the child is as old as 3 to 5 years. In less than 10% of patients with ASD, symptoms of congestive heart failure (CHF) and growth failure can occur in infancy. If the ASD is associated with another defect such as PDA, CHF is much more common and the defect becomes apparent early in life.

PHYSICAL EXAMINATION

In patients with ASD, the RV impulse felt along the lower left sternal border or the subxiphoid area may be more forceful than normal. The first heart sound will be normal. The second heart sound will be more widely split than normal and does not become single with expiration, the so-called fixed splitting of S_2. There are several murmurs that can be heard in patients with ASD. All patients with ASD have a systolic ejection murmur, which is best heard along the left sternal border and is loudest at the upper left sternal border. This murmur is caused by excessive blood flow through the pulmonary valve, is similar to an "innocent pulmonary flow murmur," and probably explains why many patients with ASD are not diagnosed until several years of age. With moderate and large defects, a middiastolic murmur can be heard along the lower right or left sternal border. In some patients, this murmur is best heard over the xiphoid and is caused by excessive blood flow through the tricuspid valve. This murmur is not heard in patients with a small ASD. Generally, the Qp/Qs must be >1.5 for this murmur to be heard. In a patient with ASD, this murmur does not result from blood flowing through the ASD itself.

Patients with ostium primum ASD, in addition to the murmurs described in the preceding text, may have a murmur of mitral insufficiency because of the cleft in the septal leaflet of the mitral valve associated with this defect.

ELECTROCARDIOGRAPHIC FEATURES

The electrocardiographic (ECG) features of ASD depend on the size of the defect and the type of ASD. For secundum, sinus venosus ASDs, and the unroofed coronary sinus, the ECG can be normal if the defect results in only a small left-to-right shunt. The ECG may have an rSR' pattern in the right precordial leads that also is frequently found in healthy individuals. For patients with moderate to large defects resulting in moderate to large left-to-right shunts, the ECG will show evidence of right atrial and RV hypertrophy and right axis deviation. There is a rare form of autosomal dominant inherited secundum ASD that is associated with first-degree AV block.

Ostium primum ASDs can be distinguished from other types of ASDs electrocardiographically because, like other forms of endocardial cushion defects, they are characterized by an initial counterclockwise frontal plane loop and left axis deviation.

CHEST X-RAY

The findings on chest x-ray are helpful in judging the size of the left-to-right shunt in patients with ASD. With a small shunt, the chest x-ray will be normal. As the shunt increases in size, the chest x-ray will show increased heart size and increased pulmonary vascular markings. The chest x-ray is not helpful in distinguishing the various types of ASD.

ECHOCARDIOGRAPHIC AND CARDIAC CATHETERIZATION ISSUES

The diagnosis of ASD and its type can be confirmed by echocardiography. In addition, the degree of right atrial and RV enlargement and hypertrophy can be assessed. Elevation of pulmonary artery pressure can be approximated using Doppler techniques. It can be difficult to diagnose sinus venosus defects with transthoracic echocardiography, and, for some patients, transesophageal echocardiography may be necessary to confirm this diagnosis. However, a clue to the presence of a sinus venosus ASD, using transthoracic echocardiography, is increased blood flow in the SVC that results from the anomalous connection of the right upper pulmonary vein that is frequently associated with sinus venosus ASD.

In the era of echocardiography, it is rarely necessary to perform cardiac catheterization for the *diagnosis* of ASD. However, cardiac catheterization is now used to deliver and implant devices to close secundum ASDs without the need for open heart surgery.

TREATMENT

The treatment of ASD involves surgical or device closure. For secundum ASD, surgical closure can be accomplished by direct suture or patch closure and device closure by cardiac catheterization techniques. There are several types of devices to close secundum ASDs. It is important that a rim of septal tissue be present around the entire circumference of the defect to stabilize the device. Currently, device closure is the preferred method for closing secundum ASD in appropriately selected patients. However, the long-term outcome of this treatment remains unknown.

For ostium primum ASD, patch closure is invariably used, and in most cases, the cleft in the mitral valve leaflet is repaired. For sinus venosus ASD, the anomalous drainage of the right upper pulmonary vein is corrected, and the ASD is closed.

The usual age for closure of an uncomplicated ASD is 2 to 4 years. In rare cases of infants with ASD and heart failure, surgery should be performed during infancy.

Endocarditis prophylaxis is recommended for all types of ASDs except ostium secundum.

NATURAL HISTORY OF ATRIAL SEPTAL DEFECT AND OUTCOME OF TREATMENT

With the exception of ostium secundum, ASDs do not spontaneously close. It has been estimated that in children, up to 15% of ostium secundum ASDs close by 4 years of age.

Untreated ASDs, over time, can produce RV enlargement, fibrosis, and failure. They are associated with atrial enlargement, which, with time, can result in atrial arrhythmias. The presence of ASD can allow paradoxical embolization. Lastly, in some patients, there can be an association between ASD and pulmonary vascular obstructive disease. However, whether the ASD produces pulmonary vascular disease or whether the pulmonary vascular disease results in stretching of a patent foramen ovale is not clear.

The risk of death following surgical closure of an uncomplicated ASD is <1%. Murphy et al. reported a 25- to 30-year follow-up of patients who had undergone surgery for ostium secundum or sinus venosus ASD at the Mayo Clinic from 1956 to 1960. There were four perioperative deaths, and all these patients were older than 46 years and had pulmonary hypertension. Long-term survival of patients who had undergone surgery at <24 years of age was similar to that of the general population. Patients who had undergone surgery at >24 years of age had poorer survival than an age-matched control.

El-Najdawi et al. assessed the outcome of 334 patients who had undergone surgery for ostium primum ASD at the Mayo Clinic between 1956 and 1995. The surgical mortality was 3%; ten-year survival was 96%. Reoperation, usually for mitral valve malfunction or subaortic stenosis, was necessary for 38 patients.

VENTRICULAR SEPTAL DEFECTS

INCIDENCE, TYPES, AND EMBRYOLOGY

VSD occurs in 1.5 to 3.5 of 1,000 live births and constitutes 20% of congenital cardiac defects. There is no gender predominance. There are four types of VSD: (i) Perimembranous, (ii) supracristal (or subpulmonary or subaortic), (iii) inlet (VSD of the AV canal type), and (iv) muscular (see Figs. 9.3 and 9.4).

A *perimembranous VSD* is in the area of the membranous septum. This places it in the outflow tract of the left ventricle and immediately under the aortic valve. A perimembranous VSD can close spontaneously by apposition of the septal leaflet of the tricuspid valve to the defect.

A *supracristal VSD*, as the name implies, is located superior to the crista supraventric-ularis, that is, in the RV outflow tract and immediately below the right cusp of the aortic valve. This defect frequently is associated with prolapse of the right aortic valve cusp and aortic valve insufficiency. The prolapsed aortic cusp can partially or completely seal the defect.

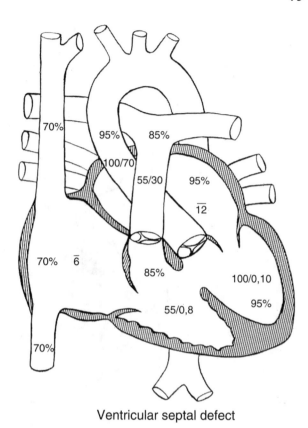

FIGURE 9.3 ● Diagrammatic representation of a large ventricular septal defect (VSD). Note that the saturation of blood in the right ventricle and pulmonary artery is greater than normal. Also, the pressure in the right ventricle is increased.

Ventricular septal defect

An *inlet VSD* is located posteriorly in the septum, just inferior to the tricuspid and mitral valves. This is a type of endocardial cushion defect, which never closes spontaneously.

A *muscular VSD* is located in the muscular ventricular septum. Patients can have more than one muscular VSD. This type of VSD has the highest rate of spontaneous closure.

The ventricular septum is formed from four sources. Muscular invagination forms the major portion of the muscular septum. The outlet portion of the ventricular septum is formed from the conotruncal septum. The inlet septum is formed from the endocardial cushions. The aorta, by connecting to the left ventricle, is the fourth component of the ventricular septum. Imperfections in these progenitors of the ventricular septum result in the various types of VSDs.

CLINICAL PRESENTATION

The clinical presentation of patients with VSD depends primarily on the size of the VSD and, to a much lesser extent, on the type of VSD. The size of the VSD can be expressed in terms of the actual size of the defect (in centimeters) or the volume of the resultant left-to-right shunt (Qp/Qs). If the VSD is as large as the aorta, it is considered to be a large VSD because, in this case, the resistance to flow through the VSD would be the same as that through the aortic valve. In terms of Qp/Qs, a small VSD will be associated with a Qp/Qs <1.5, a moderate VSD with a Qp/Qs of 1.5 to 2, and a large VSD with a Qp/Qs >2. However, the size of the left-to-right shunt is determined not just by the size of the VSD. If the VSD itself is unrestrictive to blood flow, then the downstream resistance of the RV outflow tract or the

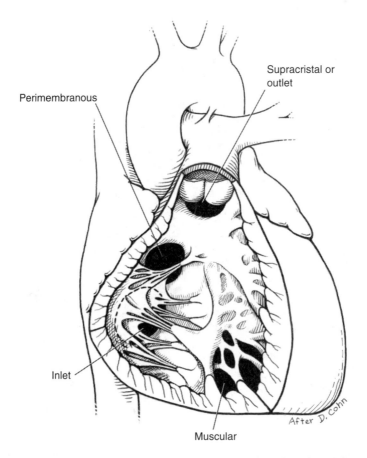

FIGURE 9.4 ● View of the different types of ventricular septal defects (VSDs) from the right side of the ventricular septum.

pulmonary microcirculation will determine the volume of pulmonary blood flow. In newborns, the pulmonary resistance is elevated, and this will reduce the left-to-right shunt in a patient with a large nonrestrictive VSD. As the pulmonary resistance declines, the left-to-right shunt will increase, and the symptoms of pulmonary edema and CHF will appear.

The type of VSD may influence the clinical presentation. For example, a patient with a supracristal VSD may present primarily with aortic valve insufficiency.

Patients with a small or moderate VSD present with a cardiac murmur. Infants with a large VSD also initially may present only with a murmur. However, as pulmonary resistance declines, they will develop signs and symptoms of pulmonary edema, pulmonary venous hypertension, and CHF. This is manifested by tachypnea, tachycardia, pallor, poor feeding, and poor weight gain.

PHYSICAL EXAMINATION

The physical findings for a patient with VSD depend on the size of the VSD, the magnitude of the left-to-right shunt, and the level of RV and pulmonary artery hypertension.

A small VSD with a Qp/Qs <1.5 and normal or only slightly elevated RV and pulmonary artery pressures is characterized by normal precordial impulses and normal first and second heart sounds. The murmur is holosystolic. In muscular VSDs, this murmur may be best heard over the lower sternal area. If the jet of blood through the VSD is directed toward the pulmonary artery, as is the case with many perimembranous and supracristal VSDs, the murmur radiates to the upper left sternal border. Frequently, a precordial thrill is palpable.

For moderate and large VSDs, the RV impulse, felt at the lower left sternal border or the subxiphoid region, is prominent. In addition, the left ventricular impulse will be displaced laterally and has increased activity. The first heart sound will be normal. As the degree of pulmonary hypertension increases, the intensity of the pulmonary component of S_2 will increase. There will be a holosystolic midfrequency murmur. In patients with Qp/Qs >2, there will be a middiastolic mitral flow murmur (this produces the so-called gallop rhythm), in addition to the systolic murmur, as a result of increased volume of blood flowing from the left atrium to the left ventricle. A precordial thrill and the closure of the pulmonary and aortic valves may be palpable. Infants with a large VSD will be tachypneic. In addition, infants with severe CHF may have pallor, poor feeding, and failure to gain weight.

ELECTROCARDIOGRAPHIC FEATURES

For small VSDs, the ECG will be normal. For moderate VSDs, left ventricular hypertrophy will occur because of left ventricular volume overload. For large VSDs, left ventricular and/or RV hypertrophy will occur. Because inlet VSDs are forms of endocardial cushion defects, the ECG will show left axis deviation.

CHEST X-RAY

In case of small VSDs, the chest x-ray will be normal. As the size of the VSD increases, the heart size will enlarge and the pulmonary vascular markings will become more prominent.

ECHOCARDIOGRAPHIC AND CARDIAC CATHETERIZATION ISSUES

The diagnosis of VSD can be confirmed using echocardiography. The location and size of the defect can be defined and associated anomalies can be identified. Using Doppler techniques, RV and pulmonary artery pressures can be estimated.

Cardiac catheterization is rarely necessary for patients with uncomplicated VSD and without evidence for pulmonary vascular obstructive disease. In patients suspected of having pulmonary vascular obstructive disease, cardiac catheterization is essential to accurately measure pulmonary vascular resistance to determine whether the patient is a candidate for closure of the VSD.

TREATMENT

The goals of treatment are to ensure adequate growth of the patient, prevent the development of pulmonary vascular obstructive disease, prevent chronic right and left ventricular dysfunction, and prevent bacterial endocarditis. Small VSDs do not require surgical closure unless they are supracristal. Infants with moderate to large VSDs associated with CHF are treated with digoxin and diuretics. High caloric formula can be used to optimize growth if growth failure results from the CHF. If, despite these measures, growth failure continues, the defect should be closed surgically. The decision to perform surgery in these circumstances will usually be made when the infant is 1 to 4 months of age.

For infants with pulmonary hypertension, the VSD should be closed before the infants are 6 to 9 months of age to prevent the development of irreversible pulmonary vascular obstructive disease.

Some young children will have a moderate VSD and normal growth and only mild elevation of pulmonary artery pressure, but a significant left-to-right shunt. If these defects are associated with cardiomegaly and there is evidence of ventricular hypertrophy, they should be surgically closed.

Patients who have a large VSD that was not closed early in life will develop pulmonary vascular obstructive disease (Eisenmenger syndrome). Once pulmonary vascular obstructive disease has developed, the VSD should not be closed.

All patients with VSD need endocarditis prophylaxis. If there are no residual cardiac defects after the defect is closed, endocarditis prophylaxis can be discontinued.

NATURAL HISTORY OF VENTRICULAR SEPTAL DEFECT AND OUTCOME OF TREATMENT

Approximately 50% to 80% of VSDs are small to begin with or become so small that surgical closure is unnecessary. For patients who do require surgery, the surgical mortality is <5%.

In a long-term follow-up study of 1,280 patients with VSD, 25-year survival was 87%. For patients with small defects, the survival was 95.9% at 25 years. For patients with moderate and large defects, the 25-year survivals were 86.3% and 61.2% respectively. For patients with Eisenmenger syndrome, the 25-year survival was 41.7%. For patients who had surgical closure of the defect, only 5.5% required a second surgery to close a residual or recurrent VSD.

PATENT DUCTUS ARTERIOSUS

INCIDENCE AND EMBRYOLOGY

The ductus arteriosus represents the distal portion of the sixth embryonic aortic arch. This structure is patent in the fetus but, normally, should close within several days of birth (see Fig. 9.5).

The ductus arteriosus remains patent (PDA) in 1 of 2,500 to 5,000 live births, but, in infants born prematurely, the incidence is 8 of 1,000 live births. PDA occurs in 45% of infants born weighing <1,750 g and in 80% of infants born weighing <1,200 g. It represents 9% to 12% of congenital heart defects. The incidence of PDA is 30 times greater for babies born at high altitude than for those born at sea level.

CLINICAL PRESENTATION

In term infants and children, the presence of PDA is suspected when a typical cardiac murmur is detected. In premature infants too, a murmur is usually the presenting feature, but the character of the murmur is different from that heard in term infants and children. Because of the greater incidence of PDA in preterm infants, the level of suspicion for the presence of PDA should be high in this group. For preterm infants with respiratory distress syndrome, the presence of PDA may be heralded by worsening of the baby's respiratory status.

Although it is unusual for PDA to present with CHF in a term baby, this can occur and usually means that the ductus arteriosus is quite large.

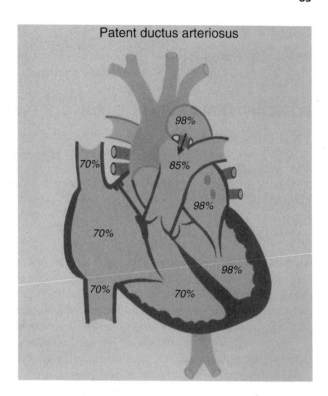

Patent ductus arteriosus

FIGURE 9.5 ● Diagrammatic representation of a patent ductus arteriosus (PDA). Note that the saturation of blood in the pulmonary artery is greater than normal and greater than that in the right ventricle (RV).

PHYSICAL EXAMINATION

For patients who have PDA but no CHF, the respiratory rate will be normal. Patients with a small PDA will have normal precordial impulses, but those with a moderate or large ductus may have a prominent left ventricular and, at times, an RV impulse. The peripheral pulses will be prominent ("bounding") because of widened pulse pressure. Typically, the murmur of PDA is continuous and heard best at the left infraclavicular area. However, in preterm and newborn infants, the murmur may be heard only in systole and can easily be confused with the murmur of VSD. Indeed, it has been said that "if one hears VSD murmur in a newborn, it probably is a PDA." In patients with a large PDA, a diastolic mitral flow murmur may be heard between the left lower sternal border and the apex, which results from a greater than normal volume of blood flowing from the left atrium to the left ventricle.

There are several conditions that can produce a murmur similar to that of PDA. Any arteriovenous connection within the chest can produce a continuous murmur. These include coronary arteriovenous fistulae, coronary cameral fistulae, pulmonary arteriovenous fistulae, chest wall arteriovenous fistulae, and so on. The radiation of a murmur produced by cerebral arteriovenous fistulae can sound like PDA. A venous hum could be confused with a murmur of a PDA. The former should disappear when the patient is supine and the latter should not.

ELECTROCARDIOGRAPHIC FEATURES

In most cases of PDA, the ECG will be normal. With a large PDA there may be left or biventricular hypertrophy. The QRS axis will be normal or rightward.

CHEST X-RAY

Patients with a small PDA will have a normal chest x-ray. Patients with moderate and large PDA may have cardiomegaly and increased pulmonary vascular markings.

ECHOCARDIOGRAPHIC AND CARDIAC CATHETERIZATION ISSUES

The presence and size of PDA can be confirmed using echocardiography before measures are undertaken to close the defect. Doppler techniques can be used to estimate the pulmonary artery pressure.

The use of cardiac catheterization is no longer necessary to diagnose the presence of PDA but can be used to close PDAs (see in the subsequent text).

TREATMENT

All PDAs that are apparent by physical examination should be closed. This applies even to very small PDAs with typical physical findings because the risk of closure is less than the risk of endocarditis. Whether to close very small PDAs that are detected serendipitously by echocardiography in the absence of typical physical findings is controversial.

There are several ways of closing a PDA. In preterm infants, the ductus can be closed, in most cases, using indomethacin. If indomethacin does not work or if there are contraindications to using indomethacin, the ductus can be closed surgically.

PDA can be closed with a variety of devices at the time of cardiac catheterization. For small ducti, the delivery of metal coils (Gianturco coils) through a catheter into the ductus works well. For larger ducti, devices other than coils can be used quite successfully. For patients with CHF, digitalis and diuretics can be used until the ductus can be closed.

All patients with PDA should observe endocarditis prophylaxis, but after the ductus is completely closed, this no longer is necessary.

NATURAL HISTORY OF PATENT DUCTUS ARTERIOSUS AND OUTCOME OF TREATMENT

The risks associated with persistent patency of the ductus arteriosus include endocarditis, calcification of the ductus, aneurysm of the ductus, and, for large PDAs, CHF and pulmonary vascular obstructive disease. If the PDA is closed before any of these complications occur, the outcome is excellent and life span should be normal. There are, however, potential complications associated with surgical closure and coil occlusion of the PDA. For surgical closure, the left pulmonary artery can inadvertently be ligated, the recurrent laryngeal nerve can be damaged and, if the PDA is ligated but not divided, recanalization can occur. For coil occlusion, the coil can embolize into the pulmonary artery or the aorta, the catheter can damage the femoral artery, and recanalization of the ductus can occur.

ATRIOVENTRICULAR SEPTAL DEFECTS

INCIDENCE, TYPES, AND EMBRYOLOGY

Atrioventricular septal defects (AVSDs) consist of a number of specific cardiac malformations that result from abnormal development of the endocardial cushions. AVSDs occur in 0.19 of 1,000 live births and constitute 4% to 5% of congenital heart defects. Forty percent of patients with Down syndrome and congenital heart disease will have AVSD.

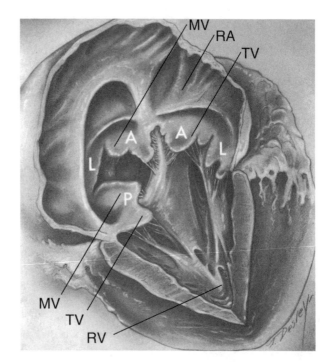

FIGURE 9.6 ● Illustration of a complete atrioventricular septal defect. Note that the atrial septal defect (ASD) and ventricular septal defect (VSD) are contiguous. There is a common atrioventricular valve rather than a mitral and tricuspid valve. Essentially, the center of the heart is missing. MV, mitral valve; RA, right atrium; TV, tricuspid valve; RV, right ventricle; A, anterior; P, posterior; L, lateral.

AVSDs can be categorized as (i) incomplete (or partial), (ii) complete (see Fig. 9.6), and (iii) intermediate (or transitional).

Incomplete AVSDs include ostium primum ASD, common atrium, cleft mitral valve, and defects of the AV septum producing a left ventricular to right atrial shunt (Gerbode defect).

Complete AVSD is a condition in which the inferior portion of the atrial septum and the posterior portion of the ventricular septum are absent. These two defects are contiguous. In addition, instead of two separate AV valves, there is one large common AV valve. Hence, the entire central portion of the heart is missing (Fig. 9.6).

Intermediate or transitional AVSDs consist of an ostium primum ASD, a restrictive posterior VSD, but two complete AV valve rings. Therefore, the ASD and VSD are not contiguous.

The structures deficient in AVSDs are structures formed by the endocardial cushions.

CLINICAL PRESENTATION AND PHYSICAL EXAMINATION

The presentation and clinical examination of patients with ostium primum ASD and common atrium are the same as those for ASD and are discussed in the preceding text. The presentation and clinical examination of patients with complete AVSDs are similar to those for patients with a large VSD and are discussed in the preceding text.

ELECTROCARDIOGRAPHIC FEATURES

In most cases, the ECG associated with AVSDs has an initial counterclockwise frontal plane loop and a left or superior QRS axis. The presence of a counterclockwise frontal plane loop is apparent on the surface ECG by Q waves in leads I and aVL.

The presence of ventricular hypertrophy will depend on the volume of the left-to-right shunt, whether there is an ASD or VSD, the degree of pulmonary hypertension, and the degree of AV valve insufficiency.

CHEST X-RAY

The findings on chest x-ray are helpful in judging the size of the left-to-right shunt in patients with an ostium primum ASD. With a small shunt, the chest x-ray will be normal. As the shunt increases in size, the chest x-ray will show increased heart size and increased pulmonary vascular markings.

The chest x-ray in most patients with complete AVSD reveals cardiomegaly and increased pulmonary vascular markings. If the patient has elevated pulmonary artery resistance, the heart may not be enlarged and the pulmonary vascular markings may be normal. However, in this situation, the main pulmonary artery segment and the proximal right and left pulmonary arteries may be enlarged.

ECHOCARDIOGRAPHIC AND CARDIAC CATHETERIZATION ISSUES

The diagnosis and type of AVSD, as well as associated anomalies, can be determined using echocardiography. Using Doppler techniques, RV and pulmonary artery pressures can be estimated.

Cardiac catheterization is rarely necessary for the management of patients with partial or incomplete forms of AVSD or for infants with uncomplicated complete AVSDs. For patients with complete AVSDs who may have pulmonary vascular obstructive disease, cardiac catheterization is essential to determine whether the patient is a candidate for complete repair.

TREATMENT

The same guidelines for treatment of ASD can be applied to patients with incomplete or partial AVSDs. The same treatment guidelines for VSD can be applied to patients with complete AVSDs.

All patients with AVSDs should receive endocarditis prophylaxis both before and after repair.

NATURAL HISTORY OF ATRIOVENTRICULAR SEPTAL DEFECTS AND OUTCOME OF TREATMENT

The natural history of patients with AVSDs is similar to the natural history of ASD for patients with incomplete or partial AVSDs. One point that differs is the effect of the malformed AV valve apparatus on the natural history of patients with AVSDs. Mitral insufficiency and/or stenosis can be a problem for patients with AVSDs, and this problem may require valve repair or replacement. Also, patients with AVSDs can develop subaortic stenosis after repair.

From a surgical standpoint, the mortality associated with repair of a complete AVSD is greater than that for a simple VSD because of the more complex repair of the AV valve apparatus and the need to repair at a young age.

AORTICOPULMONARY WINDOW

Aorticopulmonary (AP) window is a rare cause of left-to-right shunt. It consists of a connection of the ascending aorta and the main pulmonary artery immediately above the sinotubular junction (see Fig. 9.7). Because there is little length to this connection, it results in a large left-to-right shunt and symptoms and signs of severe CHF in infancy. Repair of this defect

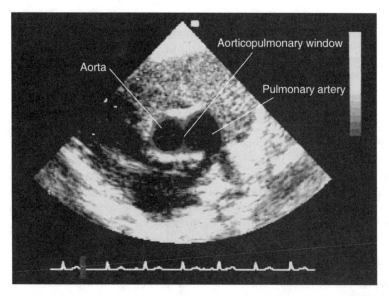

FIGURE 9.7 ● Echocardiogram of an aorticopulmonary window. Note the lack of a wall between the aorta and the pulmonary artery. Note how close the defect is to the aortic valve.

usually is necessary in the first few months of life. The long-term results of surgery usually are excellent.

ORIGIN OF ONE PULMONARY ARTERY FROM THE AORTA

The origin of one pulmonary artery from the aorta is also a relatively rare cause of left-to-right shunt. It results in a large left-to-right shunt, pulmonary hypertension in the ipsilateral lung, and, paradoxically, pulmonary hypertension in the contralateral lung. Without repair, this condition is lethal, and repair should be performed as soon as possible after the diagnosis is made. In general, long-term results of surgery are excellent. Some authors have referred to this condition as *hemitruncus*, which obviously is a misnomer because there is no VSD.

TRUNCUS ARTERIOSUS

In truncus arteriosus, there is only one semilunar valve (the truncal valve) and a VSD, and the pulmonary arteries arise from the ascending aorta (technically, from the truncus arteriosus). Frequently associated anomalies include interrupted aortic arch, truncal valve insufficiency or stenosis, and microdeletion of chromosome 22q11.2 (velocardiofacial, Shprintzen, and DiGeorge syndromes). Although truncus arteriosus usually is classified as a "cyanotic" form of congenital heart disease (see Chapter 10), it also can result in a large left-to-right shunt and significant pulmonary congestion and CHF. The need for surgery stems from the problems created by the left-to-right shunt rather than by the cyanosis. Because of the large left-to-right shunt and pulmonary hypertension, these patients develop pulmonary vascular obstructive disease at a very early age if the defect is not repaired. Therefore, truncus arteriosus needs to be repaired before 6 months of age. In the absence of truncal valve stenosis and/or insufficiency and the absence of interruption of the aortic arch, the results of the surgery are good. The surgery consists of closing the VSD, removing the pulmonary arteries from the aorta, and connecting the pulmonary arteries to the right ventricle using a conduit containing a valve. The conduit needed to connect the pulmonary arteries to the right ventricle will need to be replaced in the future. The outcome for patients with truncus arteriosus and associated anomalies is poorer than that in the absence of associated anomalies.

ARTERIOVENOUS FISTULA

Any large arteriovenous fistula can cause CHF. The large fistulae associated with CHF usually occur in the brain, liver, or heart. Cardiac AV fistulae usually involve a coronary artery to coronary vein connection or a coronary artery to right atrial or RV connection. Fistulae associated with CHF need to be closed either surgically or using interventional catheterization techniques. The outcome depends upon the complexity of the arteriovenous fistula and the amenability to disrupting the fistula.

SELECTED REFERENCES

El-Najdawi E, Driscoll D, Puga F, et al. Operation for partial atrioventricular septal defect: A 40-year review. *J Thorac Cardiovasc Surg*. 2000;119:880–889.

Feldt R, McGoon D, Ongley P, et al. eds. *Atrioventricular canal defect*. Philadelphia, PA: WB Saunders; 1976.

Fukazawa M, Fukushige J, Ueda K. Atrial septal defects in neonates with reference to spontaneous closure. *Am Heart J*. 1988;116:123–127.

Gabriel HM, Heger M, Innerhofer P, et al. Long-term outcome of patients with ventricular septal defect considered not to require surgical closure during childhood. *J Am Coll Cardiol*. 2002;39(6):1066–1071.

Gunther T, Mazzitelli D, Haehnel CJ, et al. Long-term results after repair of complete atrioventricular septal defects: Analysis of risk factors. *Ann Thorac Cardiovasc Surg*. 1998;65(3):754–759, discussion 759–760.

Kidd L, Driscoll D, Gersony W, et al. Second natural history study of congenital heart defects: Results of treatment of patients with ventricular septal defects. *Circulation*. 1993;87:I–38–I–51.

Murphy J, Gersh B, McGoon M, et al. Long-term outcome after surgical repair of isolated atrial septal defect. *N Engl J Med*. 1990;323:1645–1650.

Nakanishi T. Interventional catheterization. *Curr Opin Cardiol*. 2000;15(4):211–215.

Patel HT, Cao QL, Rhodes J, et al. Long-term outcome of transcatheter coil closure of small to large patent ductus arteriosus. *Catheter Cardiovasc Interv*. 1999;47(4):457–461.

Pearl JM, Laks H. Intermediate and complete forms of atrioventricular canal. *Semin Thorac Cardiovasc Surg*. 1997; 9(1):8–20.

Permut LC, Mehta V. Late results and reoperation after repair of complete and partial atrioventricular canal defect. *Semin Thorac Cardiovasc Surg*. 1997;9(1):44–54.

Prifti E, Bonacchi M, Leacche M, et al. A modified 'single patch' technique for complete atrioventricular septal defect correction. *Eur J Cardiothorac Surg*. 2002;22(1):151–153.

Radzik D, Davignon A, van Doesburg N, et al. Predictive factors for spontaneous closure of atrial septal defects diagnosed in the first 3 months of life. *J Am Coll Cardiol*. 1993;22:851–853.

Spangler J, Feldt R, Danielson G. Secundum atrial septal defect encountered in infancy. *J Thorac Cardiovasc Surg*. 1976;71:398–401.

Suzuki K, Yamaki S, Mimori S, et al. Pulmonary vascular disease in Down's syndrome with complete atrioventricular septal defect. *Am J Cardiol*. 2000;86(4):434–437.

Tanoue Y, Sese A, Ueno Y, et al. Surgical management of aortopulmonary window. *Jpn J Thorac Cardiovasc Surg*. 2000;48(9):557–561.

*

Portions of the text have been published previously and are reproduced with permission of the publisher:
Driscoll D, Left-to-right shunt lesions. *Pediatr Clin North Am*. 1999;46:355–368.

CHAPTER 10

Right-to-Left Shunts

"Loeb's Four Rules of Medicine

1. If the patient is getting better, keep doing what you are doing
2. If the patient is getting worse, change something
3. If you are not sure what you are doing, do nothing
4. Try to keep the patient out of the operating room"

Cyanosis is a physical sign characterized by a slate-blue color of the mucous membranes, nail beds, and skin. It results from the presence of deoxygenated hemoglobin in the blood at a concentration of at least 5 g per dL. At this or a slightly less concentration, deoxygenated hemoglobin may not be associated with cyanosis or may produce only a "ruddy" appearance. Cyanosis is less likely to occur in a patient with severe anemia because the hemoglobin levels may be too low to produce the color. In contrast, patients with erythrocythemia may exhibit a ruddy appearance or cyanosis despite a normal arterial partial pressure of oxygen (PaO_2). Because cyanosis is a physical sign, detecting it depends on the observer's acuity. It may be more difficult to appreciate the presence of cyanosis in patients who have heavily pigmented skin.

Hypoxemia is a state of abnormally decreased arterial blood oxygen concentration. It is recognized by measuring PaO_2 or arterial blood oxygen saturation (SaO_2). The degree of hypoxemia may or may not correlate with the physical signs of cyanosis, depending on the blood hemoglobin concentration and the ability of the examiner to detect cyanosis. A newborn, because of erythrocythemia, may appear plethoric or cyanotic despite a normal PaO_2 and the absence of cardiac or pulmonary disease.

The relationship between PaO_2 and SaO_2 is important in understanding the determinants of cyanosis, hypoxemia, and tissue oxygenation. An arterial SaO_2 of 88% (the level at which cyanosis is apparent to most observers) can be achieved with PaO_2 ranging from 30 to 85 mm Hg, depending on the fetal hemoglobin concentration, pH, temperature, and level of 2,3-diphosphoglycerate (2,3-DPG).

Normally, all the systemic venous return flows from the right atrium to the right ventricle (RV) and to the pulmonary artery. The volume of blood flowing into the pulmonary

TABLE 10.1

Tissue Oxygenation and Blood Oxygen Content

1. Tissue oxygenation = Systemic arterial blood oxygen content × Cardiac output
2. Systemic arterial blood oxygen content = (Hb in g/dL × 1.36 in mL O_2/g/Hb × HbO_2 saturation in percentage) + (PaO_2 in mm Hg × 0.003 mL O_2/dL per mm Hg) where the second term, PaO_2 × 0.003, represents oxygen dissolved in the blood, unattached to hemoglobin
3. Systemic (Qs), pulmonary (Qp), and effective pulmonary (Qep) blood flow

$$Qs = \frac{VO_2}{[(Hb \times 1.36 \times SaO_2) + (PaO_2 \times 0.003)] - [(Hb \times 1.36 \times SmvO_2) + (PmvO_2 \times 0.003)]}$$

$$Qp = \frac{VO_2}{[(Hb \times 1.36 \times SpvO_2) + (PpvO_2 \times 0.003)] - [(Hb \times 1.36 \times SpaO_2) + (PpaO_2 \times 0.003)]}$$

$$Qep = \frac{VO_2}{[(Hb \times 1.36 \times SpvO_2) + (PpvO_2 \times 0.003)] - [(Hb \times 1.36 \times SmvO_2) + (PmvO_2 \times 0.003)]}$$

Where		
	VO_2 = Oxygen uptake, L/min	mv = Mixed venous
	Hb = Hemoglobin, g/dL	pa = Pulmonary artery
	1.36 = mL O_2/g Hb	pv = Pulmonary vein
		PaO_2 = Partial pressure of arterial oxygen
	0.003 = mL O_2/dL/mm Hg	SaO_2 = O_2 saturation in aorta

artery is the same as the volume of blood that travels through the lungs to the left atrium and left ventricle and into the aorta. The volume of blood flowing into the aorta represents the systemic blood flow or Qs. The terms Qs and *cardiac output* are frequently used interchangeably. "Effective pulmonary blood flow," or "Qep," is the volume of systemic venous return that travels through the pulmonary vascular bed *and becomes oxygenated* (i.e., volume of pulmonary blood flow that is *effective* in participating in gas exchange in the lung). In the normal situation, the systemic, pulmonary, and effective pulmonary blood flows are equal—Qp = Qep = Qs. The formulae for calculating these volumes are listed in Table 10.1. The denominator of each of these equations merely describes oxygen extraction or addition to blood as it passes through either the systemic or the pulmonary vascular bed. For patients with cyanotic congenital heart disease, Qp, Qs, and Qep are usually *not* equal. The physiologic consequences of a specific defect can be understood and described by the values of Qp, Qs, and Qep and by the relationship among them.

In addition, the concepts of left-to-right and right-to-left shunts are useful in understanding and describing the physiologic consequences of cyanotic forms of congenital heart defects. A left-to-right shunt exists when oxygenated blood from the lungs returns to systemic veins, the right atrium, the RV, or the pulmonary artery rather than going to the left atrium, left ventricle, and aorta. A right-to-left shunt exists when a volume of deoxygenated blood (systemic venous return) travels directly to the left atrium, left ventricle, or aorta instead of traveling through the lungs to be oxygenated.

An important concept in understanding the physiologic consequences of cyanotic forms of congenital heart defects is the relationship between the volume of pulmonary blood flow and the degree of hypoxemia. Tetralogy of Fallot (TOF), pulmonary atresia with ventricular septal defect (VSD), truncus arteriosus, and tricuspid atresia are four defects in which the volume of pulmonary blood flow may be abnormally low and there is a communication between the two ventricles. In these instances, the lower the Qp, the more cyanotic the patient will be, and the higher the Qp, the less cyanotic the patient will be (see Fig. 10.1). Why is this? Consider TOF. SaO_2 in the ascending aorta will depend on the relative volume of deoxygenated blood reaching the aorta from the RV and the volume of oxygenated blood reaching the aorta from the left ventricle. The volume of deoxygenated blood in the RV is relatively fixed and depends on systemic venous return to the atrium. However, the volume

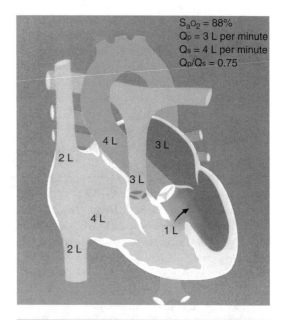

$S_aO_2 = 88\%$
$Qp = 3$ L per minute
$Qs = 4$ L per minute
$Qp/Qs = 0.75$

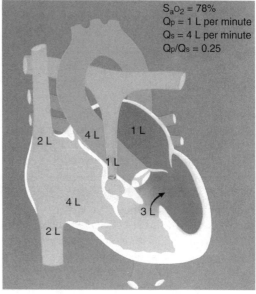

$S_aO_2 = 78\%$
$Qp = 1$ L per minute
$Qs = 4$ L per minute
$Qp/Qs = 0.25$

FIGURE 10.1 ● Illustration of the relationship of the volume of pulmonary blood flow and systemic arterial blood oxygen saturation for a patient with tetralogy of Fallot. Top, the pulmonary blood flow is 3 L per minute and the systemic arterial blood oxygen saturation is 88%. Bottom, the pulmonary blood flow is only 1 L per minute and the systemic blood oxygen saturation is 78%.

of oxygenated blood in the left ventricle represents the volume of blood it receives from the left atrium, which in turn depends on the volume of pulmonary blood flow. In TOF, the volume of pulmonary blood flow depends on the degree of restriction of blood flow into the pulmonary artery from the right ventricular outflow tract obstruction.

A second important concept is the anatomic relationship of the systemic veins (inferior and superior vena cavae and coronary sinus) and the pulmonary veins with the aorta and the pulmonary artery. Normally, the inferior and superior vena cavae are connected to the pulmonary artery through the right atrium and ventricle, and the pulmonary veins are connected to the aorta through the left atrium and ventricle. Deoxygenated blood is directed to the lungs, and oxygenated blood is directed to the body.

In d-transposition of the great arteries (d-TGA) (see Fig. 10.2), these relationships are unusual in that the inferior and superior vena cavae connect with the aorta through the right atrium and RV, and the pulmonary veins connect with the pulmonary artery through the left atrium and left ventricle. Therefore, deoxygenated blood is directed to the aorta, and oxygenated blood is directed to the pulmonary artery. Obviously, a communication must exist between these two circuits for survival. In this instance, the size of the communication and the degree of blood mixing through the communication determines the degree of cyanosis and hypoxemia, more than the volume of pulmonary blood flow. Indeed, in patients with TGA without a VSD, pulmonary blood flow, characteristically, is more than normal, but cyanosis is intense.

Total anomalous pulmonary venous return is another example of cyanotic congenital heart disease that results from an inappropriate relationship of the pulmonary venous drainage and the pulmonary artery (see Fig. 10.3). In this case, both the systemic and pulmonary venous return enters the pulmonary artery through the right atrium and RV.

With these concepts in mind, two questions must be answered to understand the anatomy and physiology of cyanotic forms of congenital heart disease: (i) What are the sources, reliability, and volume of pulmonary blood flow? and (ii) What is the relationship between the venous drainage to the heart and the arterial exit from the heart? The answers to these questions are critical in the clinical management of these patients.

Cardiac, pulmonary, metabolic, and hematologic diseases can produce cyanosis in the newborn. Any condition that causes cardiac shock can produce cyanosis, even in a patient with a structurally normal heart. When evaluating a cyanotic newborn, first consider the source of the cyanosis. Is it cardiac, pulmonary, metabolic, or hematologic (although methemoglobinemia rarely occurs in newborns) in origin?

The most common causes of cyanosis in newborns are cardiac and pulmonary diseases. Beginning with a thorough history, these two diseases must be distinguished. For a premature infant, respiratory distress syndrome is an important cause of cyanosis. If meconium aspiration occurred before or during delivery, pneumonia should be considered. In general, infants with cyanosis and pulmonary disease are more tachypneic and appear to have greater respiratory distress than those with cyanotic congenital heart disease, particularly in the first 24 to 48 hours of life. Newborns with cyanotic congenital heart disease are tachypneic but to a lesser extent than those with pulmonary disease. Significant pulmonary edema associated with a congenital cardiac defect can be misinterpreted as primary pulmonary disease. Many pulmonary causes of cyanosis are readily apparent from the chest radiograph, which should be obtained early in the evaluation of the cyanotic infant (see Table 10.2).

The use of echocardiography greatly simplifies the distinction of pulmonary from cardiac disease in infants. When echocardiography is not available, the "hyperoxia test" is useful and is performed by measuring and comparing PaO_2 while the baby breaths room air and while the baby breaths 100% O_2. It is important to measure the PaO_2 and not just blood

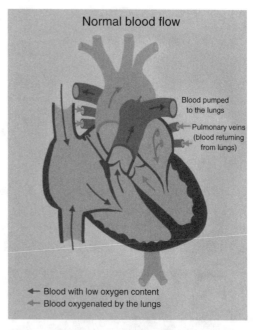

Normal blood flow

Blood pumped
to the lungs

Pulmonary veins
(blood returning
from lungs)

Blood with low oxygen content
Blood oxygenated by the lungs

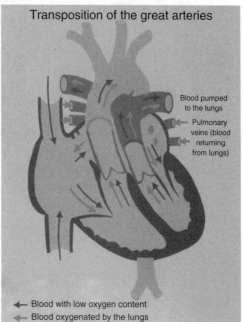

Transposition of the great arteries

Blood pumped
to the lungs

Pulmonary
veins (blood
returning
from lungs)

Blood with low oxygen content
Blood oxygenated by the lungs

FIGURE 10.2 ● Diagrammatic representation of d-transposition of the great arteries.

oxygen saturation. For an infant breathing room air, PaO_2 may be depressed to a similar level by pulmonary disease and by congenital heart disease. In cyanotic congenital heart disease, the PaO_2 is decreased because of right-to-left shunting of blood; that is, systemic venous return (blood that is low in oxygen content) travels to the left side of the heart and into the aorta without going through the lungs to participate in gas transfer. Regardless of the

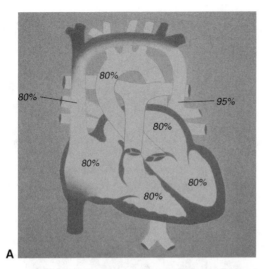

A

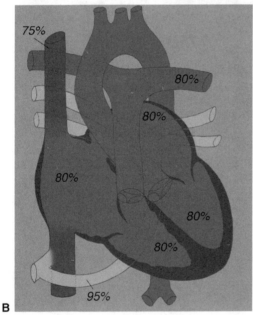

B

FIGURE 10.3 ● Diagrammatic representation of **(A)** supracardiac totally anomalous pulmonary venous return (TAPVR) and **(B)** infradiaphragmatic TAPVR.

effectiveness of ventilation and the amount of oxygen delivered to each alveolus, the blood that is shunting from right to left cannot participate in gas transfer and cyanosis will persist.

In pulmonary disease, all the systemic venous return passes through the lungs, but, because of the pulmonary disease, not all the alveoli are ventilated appropriately. Blood passing through the unventilated alveoli cannot participate in gas exchange. However, if the fraction of inspired oxygen (FIO_2) is increased and the patient is ventilated optimally, ventilation of these alveoli improves, gas exchange with the pulmonary blood flow improves, and PaO_2 increases. As a rule of thumb, if PaO_2 increases above 150 mm Hg when $FIO_2 = 1$ and the baby is adequately ventilated, cyanotic cardiac disease is unlikely. However, if PaO_2 fails to increase above 100 mm Hg, cyanotic congenital heart disease is probably the cause

TABLE 10.2

Pulmonary Causes of Cyanosis

Respiratory distress syndrome of the newborn	Anatomic airway obstruction
Pneumonia	Pulmonary telangiectasis
Meconium aspiration	Bronchogenic cyst
Pulmonary hypoplasia	Labor emphysema
Chylothorax	Pleural effusion
Diaphragmatic hernia	Hemothorax

of the cyanosis. If PaO_2 is between 100 and 150 mm Hg, cardiac disease is likely to be the cause, but the diagnosis is uncertain.

APPROACH TO DIAGNOSIS

The goal of the primary care physician is to recognize the presence of significant heart disease in the infant. Utilizing the history, physical findings, chest radiography, and electrocardiography, one can make a reasonable assessment of the physiologic manifestations of the underlying congenital heart defect (increased or decreased pulmonary blood flow or presence or absence of a shunt). However, it is difficult to determine the underlying anatomic defect without the aid of echocardiography, cardiac catheterization, angiography, or a combination of these.

HISTORY

The family history and pregnancy and delivery history may be helpful in some cases. If there is a strong family history of congenital heart disease, one may be more likely to suspect this in the infant. Maternal diabetes or parental congenital heart disease is associated with a higher than normal incidence of the disease in the children. Perinatal problems such as meconium staining or aspiration may make pulmonary disease a more likely explanation than cardiac disease for cyanosis in the newborn.

PHYSICAL EXAMINATION

The respiratory pattern and frequency are helpful in distinguishing pulmonary from cardiac disease in newborns with cyanosis. The baby with cyanotic congenital heart disease will usually be tachypneic but will not have significant respiratory distress or retraction. An exception to this is the baby with obstructed totally anomalous pulmonary venous return (TAPVR) who will have significant respiratory distress resulting from pulmonary edema.

Careful palpation of the carotid, brachial, and femoral pulses is important in excluding associated coarctation of the aorta or interruption of the aortic arch. The quality of the precordial activity should be noted. Most forms of cyanotic congenital heart disease are associated with pressure or volume overload of the RV, and a prominent impulse will be apparent at the lower left sternal border or subxiphoid region.

The first heart sound is usually normal. The second heart sound is usually single in newborns with cyanotic congenital heart disease but, if widely split, Ebstein anomaly should be considered. The absence of a cardiac murmur does *not* exclude the presence of significant cyanotic congenital heart disease. A systolic pulmonary ejection murmur may suggest TOF; a harsh to-and-fro murmur would suggest absent pulmonary valve syndrome. A systolic murmur of tricuspid insufficiency and a tricuspid diastolic murmur may suggest Ebstein anomaly. A systolic murmur of tricuspid insufficiency can be heard in the infant if the delivery was stressful. In the newborn, the murmur of tricuspid insufficiency is easy to confuse with that of a VSD. However, it is unusual for the murmur of a VSD to be audible in the first 2 days of life when transient tricuspid insufficiency of the stressed newborn is heard.

CHEST RADIOGRAPH

The chest radiograph is important in evaluating a newborn with cyanosis. It is most helpful in excluding noncardiac causes of cyanosis (Table 10.2). Except for certain classical appearances, the chest radiograph has limited use in defining the exact nature of a congenital cardiac defect. TGA often is associated with cardiomegaly and increased pulmonary vascular markings, but this is quite variable. The so-called egg on a string appearance of the cardiac silhouette is not very useful in the diagnosis of TGA (see Fig. 10.4). A chest radiograph showing a normal heart size and paucity of pulmonary vascular markings suggests TOF or pulmonary artery atresia with VSD, especially if there is also a right-sided aortic arch. Marked cardiomegaly and decreased pulmonary vascular markings suggests Ebstein anomaly or pulmonary atresia with intact ventricular septum.

ELECTROCARDIOGRAM

The electrocardiogram of a healthy newborn is characterized by right ventricular dominance. Left axis deviation and an initial counterclockwise frontal plane loop are abnormal and, in a cyanotic infant, are consistent with tricuspid atresia or complete atrioventricular septal defect with associated pulmonary stenosis (see Fig. 10.5).

d-TRANSPOSITION OF THE GREAT ARTERIES

d-TGA is the most common form of congenital heart disease that presents with cyanosis in the newborn. It constitutes 3.8% of all congenital cardiac defects. d-TGA results from abnormal conotruncal septation such that the aorta arises from the RV and the pulmonary artery arises from the left ventricle. Forty percent of patients with d-TGA have an associated VSD. Among patients with d-TGA, 6% of those with intact ventricular septum and 31% of those with VSD have associated pulmonary stenosis.

In d-TGA, systemic venous return (blood with low oxygen content) is returned to the RV and is then pumped to the body through the aorta without passing through the lungs for gas exchange. The pulmonary venous return (oxygenated blood) to the left ventricle is pumped back to the lungs. The effective pulmonary blood flow (the volume of deoxygenated blood that participates in gas exchange in the lungs) is very low, although total pulmonary blood flow is increased. d-TGA is incompatible with life unless a communication exists between the two circuits to allow the mixing of oxygenated and deoxygenated blood. This mixture occurs at the patent foramen ovale (or atrial septal defect [ASD]), the ductus arteriosus (if patent), and the VSD (if present). This is a tenuous situation for a patient with an intact

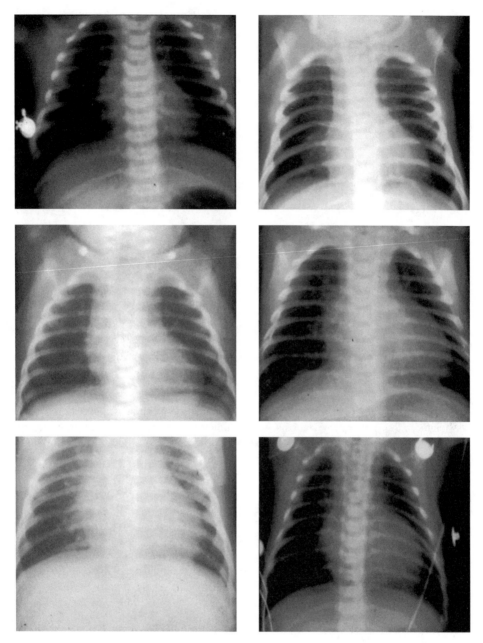

FIGURE 10.4 ● Chest radiograms from six different infants with d-transposition of the great arteries. Note the great variability of the radiographs. The bottom left x-ray would be considered most typical.

ventricular septum and no true ASD because mixing of the two circuits will decrease as the patent ductus arteriosus closes and the patent foramen ovale becomes sealed.

Cyanosis, a prominent precordial impulse at the lower left sternal border ("right ventricular impulse"), and a single and loud second heart sound are common findings in babies with d-TGA. There are no physical findings that are pathognomonic of d-TGA. There may

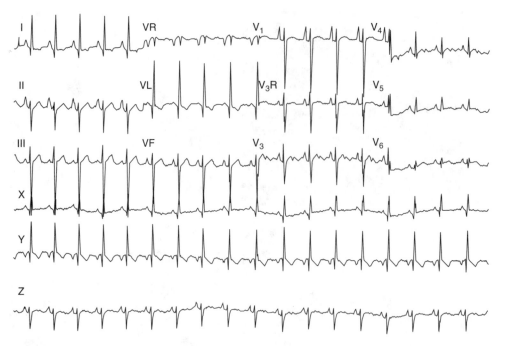

FIGURE 10.5 ● An electrocardiogram demonstrating left axis deviation and atrial enlargement. This would be most characteristic of tricuspid atresia.

be no cardiac murmur or there may be a systolic ejection murmur, which can result from an associated VSD, pulmonary stenosis, or dynamic left ventricular outflow tract obstruction. Physical examination is important for excluding the presence of associated anomalies such as coarctation of the aorta.

The chest radiograph shows cardiomegaly with increased pulmonary vascular markings in most patients with d-TGA and intact ventricular septum. Patients with d-TGA, VSD, and pulmonary stenosis may have decreased pulmonary vascular markings.

A newborn with d-TGA represents a medical emergency. It is critical to establish or exclude this diagnosis and to document and ensure adequate sites for mixing between the parallel systemic and pulmonary circuits of d-TGA. The diagnosis of d-TGA and most associated malformations can be established using two-dimensional echocardiography. The presence of a patent ductus arteriosus can be determined, but the ductus arteriosus cannot be relied upon as a stable source of mixing because it likely will close. The ductus arteriosus can be maintained patent by infusion of prostaglandin E_1, and this should be done if the baby is extremely hypoxemic (PaO_2 <25 mm Hg), acidotic, or to be transferred to another institution.

MANAGEMENT OF d-TRANSPOSITION OF THE GREAT ARTERIES WITH NO VENTRICULAR SEPTAL DEFECT

Arterial Switch (Jatene) Procedure

This procedure represents the best option for managing infants with d-TGA, intact ventricular septum or VSD, and a normal pulmonary valve. In this operation, the aorta and pulmonary artery are transected cephalad to their respective valves. The ostia of the coronary arteries are removed from the stump of the aorta and sewed to the stump of the pulmonary artery (the neoaorta). The distal portion of the aorta is anastomosed to the proximal stump of the pulmonary artery, and the distal portion of the pulmonary artery is anastomosed to the stump of the aorta (see Fig. 10.6). The mortality for this procedure is 10% or less, and the long-term results are quite good. This procedure must be done early (<3 weeks of age), before

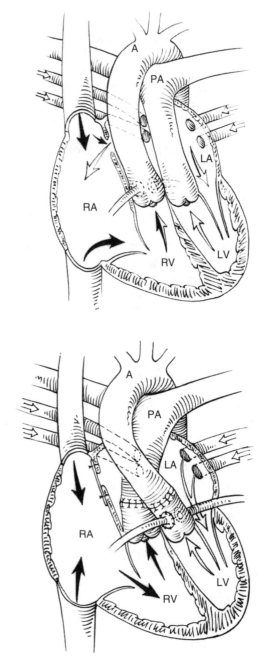

FIGURE 10.6 ● Diagrammatic representation of the arterial switch (Jatene) operation for d-transposition of the great arteries. Note the suture lines that connects the proximal stump of the pulmonary artery to the aorta and the second suture connecting the stump of the aorta to the pulmonary artery. A, aorta; PA, pulmonary artery; LA, left atrium; LV, left ventricle; RV, right ventricle; RA, right atrium.

the thickened left ventricular walls involute as pulmonary arterial resistance decreases. In many institutions, the operation is performed without preoperative cardiac catheterization. Prostaglandin E_1 is infused preoperatively to maintain patency of the ductus arteriosus and preserve the acid-base stability of the patient.

Atrial Switch (Senning or Mustard) Procedure

The Senning and Mustard operations were described in the 1960s and predate the arterial switch operation. These are alternatives to the arterial switch procedure. They are used if the pulmonary valve is abnormal such that it would not work as the neoaortic valve following a Jatene (arterial switch) procedure. With these procedures, systemic and pulmonary venous returns are rerouted in the atrium. The systemic venous return from the superior and inferior vena cavae is directed through the mitral valve and into the left ventricle (and subsequently to the pulmonary artery). The pulmonary venous return is directed through the tricuspid valve (and subsequently to the aorta). This is accomplished by sewing a baffle in the atrium (see Fig. 10.7). In essence, TGA is treated by creating "transposition" of the venous return to the heart.

The Senning and Mustard operations usually are performed in patients 6 months to 1 year of age, but some surgeons will perform the operation in the newborn period. If one of these methods of operation is to be utilized, an adequate interatrial communication must be established in the newborn period. This is accomplished by a Rashkind balloon atrial septostomy. A catheter with an inflatable balloon at its tip is advanced from the femoral or umbilical vein to the right atrium through the patent foramen ovale and into the left atrium. The balloon is inflated in the left atrium, and withdrawn rapidly into the right atrium, producing a rent in the atrial septum.

The Senning and Mustard operations have a low operative mortality but significant intermediate and long-term problems. These include obstruction of systemic and pulmonary venous return by the baffle, atrial arrhythmias, tricuspid insufficiency, and right ventricular failure.

MANAGEMENT OF d-TRANSPOSITION OF THE GREAT ARTERIES WITH VENTRICULAR SEPTAL DEFECT

When a significant VSD coexists with d-TGA, the systemic and pulmonary venous returns can mix through the VSD. In general, babies with associated VSD but without pulmonary stenosis are less hypoxemic than those with intact ventricular septum. d-TGA and VSD without pulmonary stenosis can be managed by an arterial switch procedure (Jatene) plus VSD closure. The presence of a large VSD prevents left ventricular pressure and wall thickness from declining as pulmonary resistance decreases. Therefore, in contrast to patients with d-TGA and no VSD, the arterial switch procedure can be delayed until 1 to 2 months of age.

MANAGEMENT OF d-TRANSPOSITION OF THE GREAT ARTERIES WITH VENTRICULAR SEPTAL DEFECT AND PULMONARY STENOSIS OR ATRESIA

The physiology of d-TGA with VSD and pulmonary stenosis is different from that of d-TGA without pulmonary stenosis because pulmonary blood flow is limited by the pulmonary stenosis. The degree of hypoxemia in these patients will be determined both by the extent of mixing of the systemic and pulmonary venous returns and by the volume of pulmonary blood flow. In these patients, the sources and adequacy of the pulmonary blood flow must

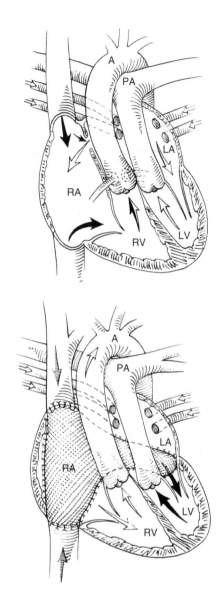

FIGURE 10.7 ● Diagrammatic representation of the Mustard operation for d-transposition of the great arteries. The atrial septum has been removed and a baffle has been sutured into the atrium such that systemic venous return (blue blood) is diverted to the left ventricle and pulmonary venous return (red blood) is diverted to the right ventricle. A, aorta; PA, pulmonary artery; LA, left atrium; LV, left ventricle; RV, right ventricle; RA, right atrium.

be determined. With severe pulmonary stenosis or pulmonary artery atresia, the ductus arteriosus may be contributing significantly to the pulmonary blood flow. When the ductus arteriosus closes, severe hypoxemia and acidosis may ensue. In the presence of an abnormal pulmonary valve, these patients are not candidates for an arterial switch (Jatene) procedure. Eventually, repair is best accomplished using the Rastelli procedure, which involves closing the VSD so that blood exits the left ventricle through the VSD and enters the aorta. The pulmonary artery is divided, the proximal stump is oversewn, and a conduit is placed from the RV to the distal portion of the main pulmonary artery. This operation has the disadvantage of using a prosthetic extracardiac conduit, which eventually will fail and need to be replaced. To allow the placement of a reasonably large conduit, this operation usually is delayed until age 4 to 6 years. Before 4 to 6 years of age, it may be necessary to establish a systemic-to-pulmonary artery shunt to augment pulmonary blood flow.

OUTCOME OF TREATMENT OF d-TRANSPOSITION OF THE GREAT ARTERIES

Treatment outcome is dependent on the type of operation used to repair the defect. The results of treatment for patients who had a Jatene (arterial switch) procedure are excellent. The operative mortality ranges from 5% to 17%. Mid- to long-term postoperative problems include supravalvar pulmonary and aortic stenosis, aortic insufficiency, and loss of branches of the coronary arteries. Fortunately, these problems are relatively uncommon.

Patients with VSD and pulmonary stenosis who have had a Rastelli procedure may experience failure of the right ventricular to pulmonary artery conduit, necessitating periodic replacement of the conduit. Failure of the conduit can occur because of stenosis of the conduit or stenosis or insufficiency of the valve within the conduit. In general, these conduits last 5 to 20 years and then need to be replaced.

The long-term results of the Senning or Mustard procedure are worse than that for the Jatene or Rastelli procedure. Because the RV remains the systemic ventricle after the Senning and Mustard procedures, failure of the RV is a late complication. This eventually may necessitate cardiac transplantation. Also, because of extensive suturing in the atria, atrial arrhythmias are a common long-term problem.

TETRALOGY OF FALLOT

TOF consists of (i) VSD, (ii) pulmonary stenosis (which may be valvular, subvalvar and/or supravalvar), (iii) an aorta that "overrides" the VSD, and (iv) right ventricular hypertrophy (see Figs. 10.8 and 10.9). TOF represents 4% to 8% of congenital cardiac defects. It results from unequal conotruncal septation. Babies with TOF are cyanotic because of the right-to-left shunt through the VSD and decreased pulmonary blood flow. The degree of hypoxemia is proportional to the volume of pulmonary blood flow, which is related to the severity of the obstruction of right ventricular outflow tract and any additional sources of pulmonary blood flow (including a patent ductus arteriosus and systemic-to-pulmonary artery collateral vessels). If the degree of right ventricular outflow obstruction is mild, cyanosis may not be apparent (so-called pink TOF). Also, if a significant portion of the pulmonary blood flow results from patency of the ductus arteriosus, cyanosis and hypoxemia will increase when the ductus arteriosus closes.

For most patients with TOF, cyanosis is apparent soon after birth. There is an increased right ventricular impulse at the lower left sternal border. There is a systolic ejection murmur along the left sternal border. In the classic case, the chest radiograph will reveal a normal heart size and decreased pulmonary vascular markings. In approximately 25% of patients, a right aortic arch will be apparent on the chest radiograph. There may be a small main pulmonary artery segment. Hypoplasia of the main pulmonary artery and right ventricular hypertrophy may produce the *coeur en sabot* (boot-shaped) configuration of the cardiac silhouette, but this is not a particularly helpful sign in an infant. Because of normal right ventricular dominance in newborns, the electrocardiogram is usually not distinctly abnormal. The diagnosis of TOF, the presence and size of the patent ductus arteriosus, and the size of the main and central right and left pulmonary arteries can be established using two-dimensional echocardiography. Angiography may be necessary to ascertain the size and distribution of the peripheral pulmonary arteries, the presence or absence of peripheral pulmonary stenosis, and the presence of additional VSDs.

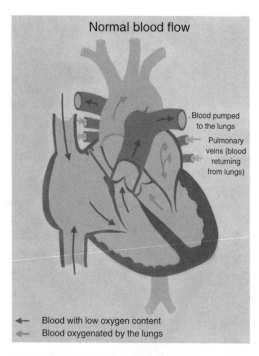

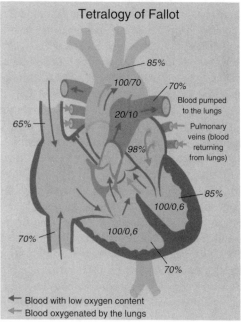

FIGURE 10.8 ● Diagrammatic representation of tetralogy of Fallot. Note the ventricular septal defect (VSD), subpulmonary stenosis, and overriding aorta.

MANAGEMENT OF TETRALOGY OF FALLOT

Initial management of patients with TOF involves establishing important details of the anatomic diagnosis and treating the hypoxemia and acidosis if they are significant. Severely hypoxemic infants should be treated with an infusion of prostaglandin E_1 to reopen the ductus arteriosus or

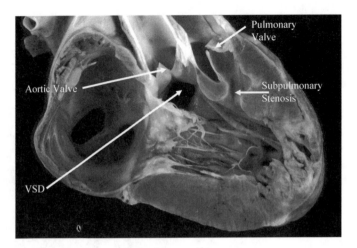

FIGURE 10.9 ● Pathologic specimen of tetralogy of Fallot. Note that the ventricular septal defect (VSD) is directly below the aortic valve. There is subvalve as well as pulmonary valve stenosis.

maintain its patency. If pulmonary blood flow is inadequate, a systemic-to-pulmonary artery anastomosis should be established surgically. A Blalock-Taussig (subclavian artery to pulmonary artery anastomosis) or modified Blalock-Taussig (interposition of a Gore-Tex tube from the subclavian artery to the pulmonary artery) is the procedure of choice. Intracardiac repair of TOF is usually performed between ages 3 and 12 months, depending on the size and distribution of the pulmonary arteries and the presence or absence of associated anomalies (such as anomalous origin of the left anterior descending coronary artery from the right coronary artery and/or multiple VSDs). Intracardiac repair involves closure of the VSD and relief of the pulmonary stenosis. The latter may necessitate patch enlargement of the right ventricular outflow tract, pulmonary annulus, or both.

Hypercyanotic or "tetralogy" spells can occur in all forms of congenital heart disease in which there is obstruction to pulmonary blood flow and a communication between the subpulmonary and subaortic ventricles. These spells initially were associated with TOF and hence the name tetralogy spells. Hypercyanotic spells consist of the abrupt onset of increased cyanosis, hypoxemia, dyspnea, and agitation. If left untreated, they can lead to profound hypoxemia, acidosis, seizures, and death. They rarely occur before the age of 2 months. Hypercyanotic spells tend to occur more frequently in the morning, within hours of the child awakening, but can occur at any time. The cause of hypercyanotic spells is multifactorial. Physiologically, there is an increased right-to-left shunt and decreased pulmonary blood flow. Restlessness and agitation may lead to crying, which increases pulmonary vascular resistance, further decreasing pulmonary blood flow and accentuating the hypoxemia. The hypoxemia may produce acidosis, which leads to a vicious cycle of further pulmonary vasoconstriction, decreased pulmonary blood flow, and increased hypoxemia. Hypercyanotic spells are treated in a stepwise manner, as outlined in Table 10.3. Once the spell resolves, the patient should undergo an operation to establish a systemic-to-pulmonary artery shunt or complete repair.

OUTCOME OF TREATMENT OF TETRALOGY OF FALLOT

The long-term outcome of treatment of TOF depends primarily on the size and anatomy of the pulmonary arteries and whether a competent native pulmonary valve remains after

TABLE 10.3

Stepwise Treatment of Hypercyanotic Spells

Comfort child and place in knee–chest position

Administer oxygen by face mask

Give morphine, 0.01–0.1 mg/kg, subcutaneously

Begin intravenous fluid replacement and volume expansion (if child is anemic, administer blood)

Treat acidosis with sodium bicarbonate

Repeat morphine, 0.01–0.1 mg/kg, intravenously

Increase systemic vascular resistance by intravenous administration of phenylephrine; titrate dose to increase systemic systolic blood pressure by 20%

Administer propranolol, 0.1 mg/kg, intravenously

Administer general anesthesia

Operate to repair defect or to establish systemic-to-pulmonary artery anastomosis

---

operation. Patients with normal-sized pulmonary arteries that are normally distributed and a competent pulmonary valve have an excellent long-term prognosis postoperatively.

For patients with hypoplastic pulmonary arteries and/or peripheral pulmonary artery stenoses, the long-term prognosis depends upon the postoperative level of the pulmonary artery pressure. After repair, the RV pressure will be inversely related to the size of the pulmonary arteries and directly related to the severity of pulmonary arterial stenoses. The higher the postoperative RV pressure, the greater the likelihood of eventual right ventricular failure and the occurrence of significant arrhythmias.

Patients with significant postoperative pulmonary regurgitation, particularly if associated with residual pulmonary artery stenosis, can develop right ventricular failure and arrhythmias. These patients may benefit from insertion of a valve in the pulmonary position if significant arrhythmias or right ventricular failure occurs.

PULMONARY ARTERY ATRESIA WITH VENTRICULAR SEPTAL DEFECT

Although pulmonary atresia with VSD has been described by some as "severe TOF" or "TOF with pulmonary atresia," the management of these patients and the morbid anatomy of the pulmonary artery tree can be considerably different from that of TOF (see Fig. 10.10). In contrast to TOF, with pulmonary atresia and VSD, there is usually no systolic ejection murmur. There may be a continuous murmur resulting from blood flow through the ductus arteriosus or the systemic-to-pulmonary artery collateral vessels. As in TOF, it is important to establish the sources and reliability of the pulmonary blood flow. If the sources are insufficient or considered to be unreliable, a systemic-to-pulmonary artery anastomosis should be created. It is important to determine, as accurately as possible (usually by angiography), the anatomic features of the pulmonary artery tree before surgery because the entire pulmonary artery tree may not be confluent. Patients with nonconfluent pulmonary arteries usually

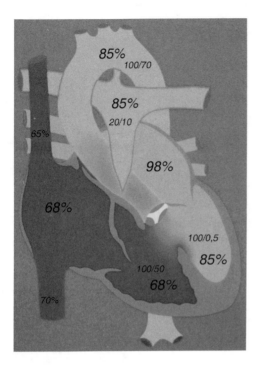

FIGURE 10.10 ● Diagrammatic representation of pulmonary atresia and ventricular septal defect (VSD).

will have multiple aortico-pulmonary collateral arteries (MAPCAs) that provide pulmonary blood flow. These patients are very likely to have a 22q11.2 microdeletion.

Eventual repair of pulmonary artery atresia/VSD involves closure of the VSD and establishing continuity between the RV and the pulmonary artery. The feasibility of accomplishing this depends on the size, distribution, and confluence or nonconfluence of the pulmonary artery tree. If the pulmonary arteries are too small, the VSD must not be closed because the patient will then have an unacceptably elevated RV pressure. This will lead to right ventricular failure, serious arrhythmias, and premature death.

OUTCOME OF TREATMENT OF PULMONARY ATRESIA AND VENTRICULAR SEPTAL DEFECT

The long-term outcome of treatment of pulmonary atresia and VSD depends primarily on the size and anatomy of the pulmonary arteries. Patients with normal-sized pulmonary arteries that are normally distributed have a good long-term prognosis.

For patients with hypoplastic pulmonary arteries and/or peripheral pulmonary artery stenoses, the long-term prognosis depends upon the level of the pulmonary artery and RV pressures that exists postoperatively. The higher the postoperative RV pressure, the greater the likelihood of eventual right ventricular failure and occurrence of significant arrhythmias.

The valve containing the conduit used to connect the RV to the pulmonary arteries will eventually fail and require replacement. Failure of the conduit can occur because of stenosis of the conduit or stenosis or insufficiency of the valve within the conduit. In general, these conduits last 5 to 20 years and then need to be replaced.

TRUNCUS ARTERIOSUS

Truncus arteriosus consists of a VSD and only one great artery ("the truncus") arising from the heart (see Figs. 10.11 and 10.12). This great artery is positioned above the VSD and gives rise to the coronary arteries, the pulmonary arteries, and the aortic arch. There are three types of truncus arteriosus: (i) Both pulmonary arteries arise as a single vessel from the truncus arteriosus, (ii) the right and left pulmonary arteries arise from separate orifices but from the same side of the truncus arteriosus, and (iii) the right and left pulmonary arteries arise from separate orifices on opposite sides of the truncus arteriosus. Significant associated anomalies include truncal valve insufficiency and interrupted aortic arch. Truncus arteriosus constitutes approximately 0.7% of all congenital heart defects. It results from abnormal conotruncal septation. There is a relatively common association between microdeletion of 22q11.2 and truncus arteriosus, especially if there is interruption of the truncal valve.

Babies with truncus arteriosus may present with cyanosis or severe congestive heart failure. Cyanosis occurs because of a right-to-left shunt at the level of the VSD and is dependent upon the volume of pulmonary blood flow. The volume of pulmonary blood flow is related to the pulmonary arteriolar vascular resistance, the absence or presence of proximal pulmonary artery stenosis, and the severity of the pulmonary artery stenoses. These patients have a prominent right ventricular impulse at the lower left sternal border. Usually, there is a systolic ejection murmur at the left sternal border. There may be an apical aortic ejection click and increased pulse pressure. If there is truncal valve insufficiency, there will be a decrescendo diastolic murmur. If there is associated interruption of the aortic arch, the femoral pulses may be decreased or absent.

The chest radiograph is not particularly distinctive, usually revealing cardiomegaly and increased pulmonary vascular markings. The electrocardiogram reveals the usual right ventricular dominance of infancy. The diagnosis is made by echocardiography.

In infancy, as pulmonary arteriolar resistance decreases, significant congestive heart failure develops. The initial management consists of medical treatment of the congestive heart failure (using digitalis, diuretics, and, perhaps, afterload-reducing agents). Surgery is necessary to correct truncus arteriosus and should be performed before 3 months of age. Surgical correction involves closure of the VSD, separation of the pulmonary arteries from the truncus, and establishing continuity between the RV and pulmonary arteries with a conduit. Early surgical correction is necessary to prevent the development of pulmonary vascular obstructive disease and to treat the congestive heart failure.

OUTCOME OF TREATMENT OF TRUNCUS ARTERIOSUS

The initial operative mortality for repair of truncus arteriosus depends upon the presence of associated problems such as interrupted aortic arch and truncal valve stenosis or insufficiency. As compared to patients with none of these associated anomalies, those with one or more of these anomalies have a significantly increased operative mortality and poorer long-term prognosis.

In the ideal cases of patients with truncus arteriosus and no associated anomalies repaired in the first 3 months of life, the mortality should be <10%.

Because correction of this defect is necessary in infancy and requires use of an extracardiac conduit, reoperation to replace the conduit will be necessary when the patient outgrows the relatively small conduit or if the conduit fails. Failure of the conduit can occur because

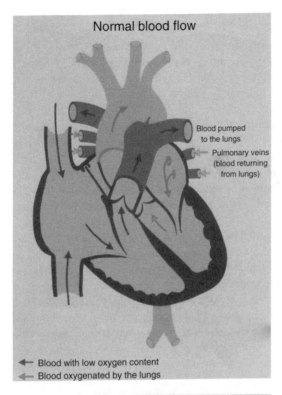

Normal blood flow

Blood pumped
to the lungs

Pulmonary veins
(blood returning
from lungs)

◄— Blood with low oxygen content
◄— Blood oxygenated by the lungs

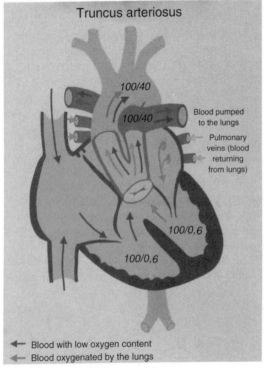

Truncus arteriosus

100/40

100/40

Blood pumped
to the lungs

Pulmonary
veins (blood
returning
from lungs)

100/0,6

100/0,6

◄— Blood with low oxygen content
◄— Blood oxygenated by the lungs

FIGURE 10.11 ● Diagrammatic representation of type 1 truncus arteriosus.

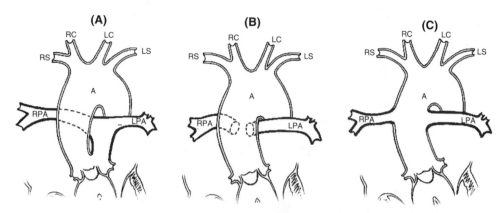

FIGURE 10.12 ● Diagrammatic representation of **(A)** type 1 truncus arteriosus, **(B)** type 2 truncus arteriosus, and **(C)** type 3 truncus arteriosus. A, aorta; RPA, right pulmonary artery; LPA, left pulmonary artery; RC, right carotid artery; LC, left carotid artery; RS, right subclavian artery; LS, left subclavian artery.

of stenosis of the conduit or stenosis or insufficiency of the valve within the conduit. In general, these conduits last 5 to 20 years and then need to be replaced.

TRICUSPID ATRESIA

In tricuspid atresia, there is no direct communication between the right atrium and the RV (see Fig. 10.13). Tricuspid atresia constitutes 2.7% of all forms of congenital heart disease. The initial survival of infants with tricuspid atresia depends upon the presence of an interatrial communication to allow egress of blood from the right atrium to the left atrium. Tricuspid atresia occurs in combination with normally related or transposed great arteries and with or without pulmonary stenosis or atresia. The clinical presentation, physiologic manifestations, and treatment depend, to a large extent, on the relationship of the great arteries (normal or transposed) and the presence or absence of pulmonary stenosis or atresia.

Infants with tricuspid atresia usually present with cyanosis and frequently have a murmur. The apical impulse may be overactive. The presence of a systolic ejection murmur can result from associated pulmonary stenosis or a restrictive VSD. The second heart sound may be single or split. A middiastolic apical cardiac murmur may be present, particularly if there is increased pulmonary blood flow and congestive heart failure.

The chest radiograph reveals cardiomegaly, and the pulmonary vascular markings may be normal, increased, or decreased, depending on the degree of pulmonary stenosis. The right atrium (right border of the heart) may be prominent on a chest radiograph.

The electrocardiogram is quite helpful in suggesting this diagnosis (Fig. 10.5). It is characterized by left axis deviation and an initial counterclockwise frontal plane loop. There may be left ventricular hypertrophy.

The diagnosis of tricuspid atresia and delineation of most of the associated anomalies are made by echocardiography. Because tricuspid atresia can be associated with pulmonary stenosis and pulmonary atresia, it is important to establish the sources and reliability of the pulmonary blood flow. If these are not readily apparent by echocardiography, cardiac catheterization and angiography may be necessary. Rarely, the interatrial communication is too small for adequate egress of blood from the right atrium, and balloon atrial septostomy is necessary to enlarge this communication.

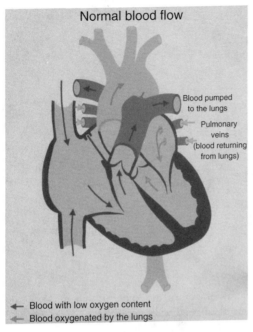

Normal blood flow

Blood pumped
to the lungs

Pulmonary
veins
(blood returning
from lungs)

← Blood with low oxygen content
← Blood oxygenated by the lungs

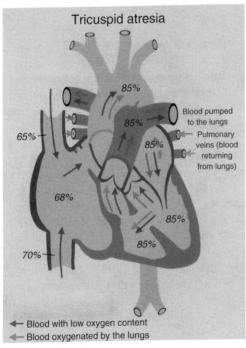

Tricuspid atresia

85%

85%

65%

85%

68%

85%

70%

85%

Blood pumped
to the lungs

Pulmonary
veins (blood
returning
from lungs)

← Blood with low oxygen content
← Blood oxygenated by the lungs

FIGURE 10.13 ● Diagrammatic representation of tricuspid atresia and normally related great arteries.

The initial management of babies with tricuspid atresia involves treatment of the congestive heart failure, if present, with digitalis and diuretics. In addition, it is essential to establish a reliable source of pulmonary blood flow if it is insufficient and if significant hypoxemia and acidosis are present. This can be accomplished with an infusion of prostaglandin E_1 while one prepares to surgically create a systemic-to-pulmonary artery shunt.

TRICUSPID ATRESIA WITH NORMALLY RELATED GREAT ARTERIES

Almost invariably, tricuspid atresia with normally related great arteries is associated with pulmonary stenosis or a restrictive VSD (that frequently becomes even more restrictive with time). Therefore, the course of these patients is characterized by progressive decrease of pulmonary blood flow and increase of cyanosis. Many of these patients eventually will require surgical placement of a systemic-to-pulmonary artery anastomosis to augment pulmonary blood flow. Rarely, a patient with tricuspid atresia and normally related great arteries will not have subpulmonary stenosis or a restrictive VSD. These patients will have increased pulmonary blood flow, pulmonary hypertension, and congestive heart failure. Eventually, pulmonary vascular obstructive disease will develop unless a pulmonary artery band is placed to decrease pulmonary blood flow and pulmonary hypertension.

TRICUSPID ATRESIA WITH TRANSPOSED GREAT ARTERIES

Usually, tricuspid atresia with transposed great arteries is associated with unrestricted pulmonary blood flow that is increased, pulmonary hypertension, and striking congestive heart failure. Surgical banding of the pulmonary artery is necessary to decrease the volume of pulmonary flow and pulmonary hypertension, and to control the symptoms of congestive heart failure. A disadvantage of pulmonary artery banding is the possible acceleration of VSD closure, which can result in subaortic stenosis.

TRICUSPID ATRESIA WITH PULMONARY ARTERY ATRESIA

As in all forms of congenital heart disease associated with pulmonary atresia, the sources and reliability of pulmonary blood flow must be established (usually by cardiac catheterization and angiography). Surgical creation of a systemic-to-pulmonary artery shunt is necessary to augment pulmonary blood flow in the patients, with insufficient pulmonary blood flow.

DEFINITIVE TREATMENT OF TRICUSPID ATRESIA

Definitive treatment of tricuspid atresia is accomplished using the modified Fontan procedure (see Fig. 10.14). Since its original description, the Fontan operation has undergone numerous modifications. The goal of the Fontan operation is to direct all the systemic venous return (blue blood) to the pulmonary artery without passing through a ventricle. Currently, the most popular modification of the Fontan operation is the bicaval connection. In this procedure, the superior vena cava is disconnected from the heart and anastomosed, in an end-to-side manner, to the right pulmonary artery. The inferior vena cava is connected to the underside of the right pulmonary artery using an interposition graft that is positioned either outside the heart or within the right atrium. This separates systemic and pulmonary venous returns and decreases ventricular volume overload.

In some patients, a small communication ("fenestration") is created between the inferior vena cava to pulmonary artery connection and the pulmonary venous atrium. Patients who have had a "fenestrated Fontan" operation continue to have a right-to-left shunt and are mildly cyanotic. The fenestration reduces some of the postoperative complications and may reduce the risk of late development of protein-losing enteropathy.

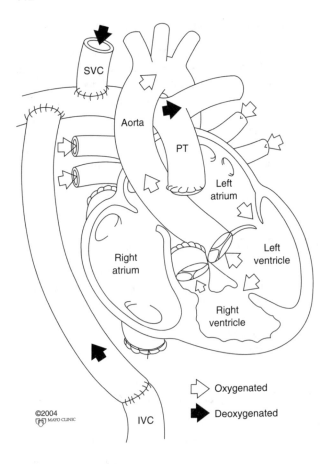

FIGURE 10.14 ● Diagrammatic representation of a bicaval modification of the Fontan operation for tricuspid atresia. All systemic venous return is directed to the pulmonary arteries without passing through the heart. SVC, superior vena cava; PT, pulmonary trunk; IVC, inferior vena cava.

SVC

Aorta

PT

Left atrium

Right atrium

Left ventricle

Right ventricle

▷ Oxygenated

◀ Deoxygenated

©2004 MAYO CLINIC

IVC

OUTCOME OF TREATMENT OF TRICUSPID ATRESIA

The outcome after the Fontan operation depends upon the number of risk factors for poor outcome that existed prior to the Fontan operation (see Table 10.4). Because patients with tricuspid atresia have only one functional ventricle, this ventricle is used to pump blood into the aorta. There is no ventricle to pump blood into the pulmonary artery. For blood to flow into the pulmonary artery, it has to be normal in size and there must be normal pulmonary arterial resistance. In addition, left ventricular filling pressure and ejection fraction must be normal, and there must be no significant mitral valve stenosis or insufficiency. It is preferable if there are no significant abnormalities of systemic and venous return. It is advantageous for these patients to have sinus rhythm.

The long-term survival for patients who are ideal candidates for the Fontan operation is excellent and may exceed 85% 10 years after the operation. However, as the number of risk factors for poor outcome increases, the long-term outcome worsens (see Fig. 10.15). Long-term complications after the Fontan operation include atrial arrhythmias, protein-losing enteropathy, and left ventricular dysfunction.

UNIVENTRICULAR HEART

All human hearts have two ventricles. However, since one of the ventricles can be hypoplastic, there are a number of congenital heart defects in which there is a physiologic

TABLE 10.4

Factors that May Adversely Affect Outcome after Fontan Operation

Operation at age <2 y	Common AV valve
Absence of sinus rhythm	Ventricular hypertrophy
Anomalous systemic venous return	Valved RA–PA connection
Anomalous pulmonary venous connection	Hypoplastic left ventricle
Mean pulmonary artery pressure >15 mm Hg	Nontricuspid atresia forms of single ventricle
Pulmonary arteriolar resistance >4 $\mu \cdot m^2$	Heterotaxia syndromes
Ratio of pulmonary artery diameter to aorta diameter <0.75	Incompetent atrioventricular valve
Left ventricular ejection fraction <60%	

AV, atrioventricular; RA, right atrium; PA, pulmonary atresia.

or functional single ventricle (or "univentricular heart"). Tricuspid atresia is one of these. Others include double-inlet left ventricle, unbalanced atrioventricular septal defect, mitral atresia with VSD, double-outlet RV with straddling atrioventricular valve, and hypoplastic left heart syndrome (HLHS) among others. The principles outlined in the preceding text for the management of tricuspid atresia can be applied to the management of other forms of univentricular heart. One must establish an anatomic diagnosis (usually with echocardiography), define the status of pulmonary perfusion (too much or too little), and determine the sources and reliability of pulmonary blood flow. If pulmonary blood flow is insufficient,

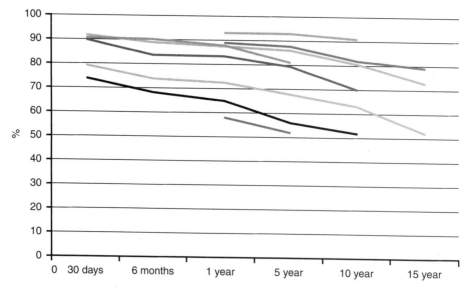

FIGURE 10.15 ● Survival curves from several studies of patients who have had the modified Fontan operation. In general, the curves depicting poorer survival had a relatively larger representation of patients with hypoplastic left heart syndrome (HLHS).

a systemic-to-pulmonary artery shunt is needed. If pulmonary blood flow is excessive, a pulmonary artery band is placed. Eventual definitive palliation is accomplished using the modified Fontan procedure.

OUTCOME OF TREATMENT OF UNIVENTRICULAR HEART

As alluded to in the preceding text, the outcome of patients who undergo the Fontan operation is related to the number of "risk factors" for poor outcome that the patient has before the operation. One of the "risk factors" is a single ventricle of right ventricular morphology. Except for tricuspid atresia and double-inlet left ventricle, most other forms of univentricular heart have a morphologically right single ventricle. Hence, the long-term outcome for these patients will not be as good as that for patients with a morphologically left single ventricle.

TOTALLY ANOMALOUS PULMONARY VENOUS RETURN

TAPVR can be divided into four anatomic groups: (i) Supracardiac (Fig. 10.3A), (ii) cardiac, (iii) infracardiac (Fig. 10.3B), and (iv) mixed. It also can be divided into two physiologic types: Nonobstructed and obstructed. Instead of connecting to the left atrium, the pulmonary veins connect to the systemic venous system. Consequently, pulmonary venous blood (fully oxygenated) returns to the right atrium instead of the left atrium. The locations of the connection of the pulmonary veins to the systemic veins (in order of frequency of occurrence) are the left vertical vein, innominate vein, coronary sinus, right atrium, umbilicovitelline system (i.e., portal vein, ductus venosus, inferior vena cava, and hepatic vein), and superior vena cava. In "mixed" TAPVR, a combination of the above occurs. For example, the left pulmonary veins may connect to the left vertical vein and the right pulmonary veins connect directly to the right atrium. Obviously, to allow survival, a communication must exist between the right atrium and left atrium to allow blood to reach the left atrium, left ventricle, and aorta. Relatively complete mixing of the systemic and pulmonary venous returns occurs in the right atrium such that SaO_2 values in the right atrium, left atrium, RV, pulmonary artery, left ventricle, and aorta are similar.

If there is an adequate interatrial communication and no significant obstruction to pulmonary venous return, the patient will have mild cyanosis and evidence of increased pulmonary blood flow. Examination reveals an increased right ventricular impulse at the lower left sternal border and a systolic ejection murmur. The chest radiogram may reveal mild to moderate cardiomegaly and increased pulmonary vascular markings. The electrocardiogram is not particularly helpful. The diagnosis can be established by echocardiography but may need to be confirmed by cardiac catheterization and angiography.

The clinical picture is completely different if there is obstruction to pulmonary venous return. Characteristically, this occurs with infradiaphragmatic forms of total anomalous pulmonary venous return. In this case, there is pulmonary edema and respiratory stress. This is a surgical emergency and immediate emergent repair is indicated. The clinical picture and chest radiographic findings can be confused with those of the respiratory distress syndrome of the newborn. In the infant with atypical respiratory distress syndrome, obstructed total anomalous pulmonary venous return should always be suspected, and the possibility of lack of connection of the pulmonary veins to the left atrium should be investigated.

The technique of surgical repair of TAPVR depends on the anatomic type of TAPVR. However, in one manner or another, the drainage of the pulmonary veins must be rerouted to the left atrium.

OUTCOME OF TREATMENT OF TOTALLY ANOMALOUS PULMONARY VENOUS RETURN

Patients with unobstructed supracardiac or cardiac types of TAPVR have excellent long-term survival and results. In general, operative mortality is <5%. Unfortunately, mortality for babies with obstructed infradiaphragmatic types of TAPVR is much higher. Without operation, mortality is essentially 100% and with operation it may be as high as 20% to 40%.

The major long-term problem for patients who survive operation is stenosis of the surgical connection that is made to establish the connection of the pulmonary veins to the left atrium.

THE HYPOPLASTIC LEFT HEART SYNDROME

The HLHS includes aortic valve atresia, mitral valve atresia with intact ventricular septum, and hypoplasia of the mitral and aortic valves and left ventricle. It is perhaps the most serious form of congenital heart disease. Neonates with HLHS may appear normal for several hours or up to 3 to 5 days after birth or may display mild cyanosis. Several hours after birth, a systolic murmur may become apparent, and the signs and symptoms of congestive heart failure occur. The right ventricular impulse at the lower left sternal border is increased. If the patent ductus arteriosus is closing, the peripheral pulses will be diminished or absent. The presence of normally palpable pulses does not exclude the diagnosis of HLHS because the pulses can be normal as long as the ductus arteriosus is patent. The diagnosis of HLHS is made using echocardiography. Most patients with HLHS will have associated coarctation of the aorta.

When left untreated, HLHS is a lethal malformation. After diagnosis, these patients require prostaglandin E_1 infusion to maintain patency of the ductus arteriosus. This is followed by the Norwood procedure, in which the hypoplastic ascending aorta and the pulmonary artery are opened and connected in a longitudinal manner and any coarctation of the aorta is repaired. The pulmonary artery confluence is disconnected from the main pulmonary artery and a systemic-to-pulmonary shunt is constructed as a source of pulmonary blood flow. With this arrangement, the source of systemic blood flow is the blood ejected from the RV into the pulmonary artery, which now is the neoaorta. At approximately 6 months of age, a second operation is done to establish a bidirectional Glenn anastomosis, remove the systemic-to-pulmonary shunt, and correct any distortion of the right and left pulmonary arteries. Babies who survive the Norwood procedure and the bidirectional Glenn anastomosis are candidates for a modified Fontan operation or cardiac transplantation. Neonatal cardiac transplantation has been successful as initial surgical treatment in a limited number of babies with HLHS.

OUTCOME OF TREATMENT OF HYPOPLASTIC LEFT HEART SYNDROME

The mortality for the Norwood procedure ranges from 10% to 40%. There will be an additional 5% to 10% mortality associated with the bidirectional Glenn anastomosis and another additional 5% to 15% mortality associated with the modified Fontan operation. Indeed, one study showed a better survival for infants with HLHS undergoing cardiac transplantation than those undergoing the Norwood operation. However, the greater survival after transplantation has to be tempered by the long-term problems associated with this procedure, such as rejection, infection, graft vasculopathy, and post-transplant lymphoproliferative disease.

EBSTEIN ANOMALY

Ebstein anomaly is a malformation of the tricuspid valve in which the anterior and septal leaflets are abnormally attached to the endocardial surface of the RV (see Figs. 10.16 and 10.17). The valve usually is incompetent or, rarely, stenotic or both. Thirty percent to 78% of patients with Ebstein anomaly have an associated ASD and are cyanotic because of a right-to-left shunt through the ASD.

The physical examination findings are characterized by an easily recognizable split first and second heart sounds. The chest radiograph reveals a large heart with a prominent right-sided border and decreased pulmonary blood flow. The electrocardiogram is characterized by tall P waves in limb lead II (indicating right atrial enlargement) and a right bundle branch block pattern. Approximately 30% of patients with Ebstein anomaly have Wolff-Parkinson-White syndrome. The diagnosis of Ebstein anomaly can be confirmed by echocardiography.

There is a broad spectrum of severity of Ebstein anomaly. In very mild cases, there may be minimal tricuspid regurgitation and minimal cardiomegaly. These patients can live a perfectly normal life and never require cardiac surgery. On the other hand, there is a subset of newborn infants with massive cardiomegaly who do poorly, and the best way to manage this group of infants is as yet unclear. Some investigators have recommended surgical repair although there may be a high mortality for these babies.

A second subset of newborn infants will be stable but intensely cyanotic for several days until the pulmonary vascular resistance declines. As pulmonary vascular resistance decreases, pulmonary blood flow increases and cyanosis lessens. Prostaglandin E$_1$ infusion

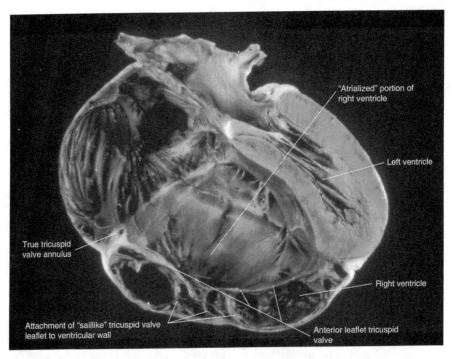

FIGURE 10.16 ● Pathologic specimen of Ebstein anomaly. The leaflets of the tricuspid valve are plastered to the walls of the right ventricle. Because of the large size of the right ventricle, the ventricular septum is deviated toward the left ventricle. A large atrial septal defect also is apparent.

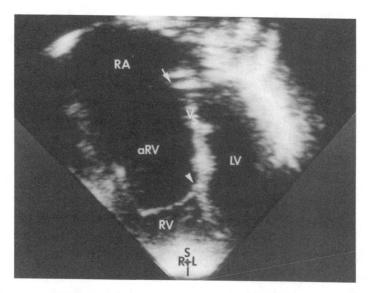

FIGURE 10.17 ● Echocardiogram from a patient with Ebstein anomaly. Note how the sepal leaflet of the tricuspid valve is plastered against the ventricular septum and the free edge of the leaflet is displaced deep into the right ventricle. RA, right atrium; aRV, atrialized portion of the RV; RV, right ventricle; LV, left ventricle.

can be used, if necessary, to augment pulmonary blood flow for these patients until pulmonary resistance decreases. Patients with Ebstein anomaly, normal pulmonary arteries, and no pulmonary stenosis usually do well during the newborn period without surgical treatment.

Infants with Ebstein anomaly and right ventricular outflow tract obstruction are difficult to manage, but establishment of a systemic-to-pulmonary artery shunt may be helpful in these patients. Certainly, if pulmonary atresia exists, a systemic-to-pulmonary artery shunt must be established surgically.

For patients with significant tricuspid insufficiency or stenosis and cardiomegaly, operation can be done to repair or replace the tricuspid valve and close the ASD. The indications for operation include: Cardiomegaly with a cardiothoracic (C/T) ratio >65%, progressive cardiomegaly, significant right-to-left shunt, increasing exercise intolerance, and decreasing left ventricular function.

OUTCOME OF TREATMENT OF EBSTEIN ANOMALY

There is a small subset of babies with very severe forms of Ebstein anomaly who have a very high mortality shortly after birth. Except for this very small group of patients, the outcome of most patients with Ebstein anomaly is good. The operative mortality for patients undergoing repair or replacement of the tricuspid valve is 5%. If valve replacement is necessary, future operations will be necessary to re-replace the tricuspid valve prosthesis. Most surgeons prefer to use a bioprosthesis for tricuspid valve replacement.

PULMONARY ATRESIA WITH INTACT VENTRICULAR SEPTUM

Pulmonary atresia with intact ventricular septum is less common and completely different from pulmonary atresia with VSD. There is nothing particularly characteristic about the physical findings, but the chest radiograph reveals marked cardiomegaly with a prominent right atrium, similar to the appearance of Ebstein anomaly. The electrocardiogram reveals tall P waves in limb lead II, indicative of right atrial enlargement. The diagnosis can be confirmed by echocardiography.

An unrestrictive ASD is necessary for survival. If the ASD appears to be restrictive, cardiac catheterization and balloon atrial septostomy will be necessary. The patent ductus arteriosus is the only source of pulmonary blood flow, and patency of the ductus arteriosus should be maintained with prostaglandin E_1 infusion until a more stable source of pulmonary blood flow can be established. The spectrum of severity of pulmonary atresia with intact ventricular septum is defined by the size of the RV and the tricuspid valve. Patients with an extremely hypoplastic RV may have coronary to right ventricular fistulae and coronary artery stenoses or atresia. The presence of coronary artery to right ventricular fistulae is important when planning the surgical management of patients with this lesion.

The surgical approach to this lesion depends on the size of the RV, whether the RV is tripartite, the size of the tricuspid valve, and the presence or absence of coronary artery stenoses. If the RV is tripartite and the tricuspid valve is of reasonable size, complete repair can be accomplished by reconstructing the right ventricular outflow tract and closing the ASD. If the RV and tricuspid valve are too small to allow complete repair, the right ventricular outflow tract is reconstructed and a systemic-to-pulmonary artery shunt is constructed but the ASD is left open. At a later date, if the tricuspid valve and RV grow, the ASD and the systemic-to-pulmonary shunt can be closed. If the RV and/or the tricuspid valve fail to grow, a Fontan operation provides definitive palliation.

If there are coronary to right ventricular fistulae and coronary artery stenoses or atresia, then the RV outflow tract should not be opened because decompression of the RV can lead to coronary insufficiency and myocardial infarction. Indeed, usually, if there are coronary artery to RV fistulae, the RV is too small for a two-ventricle repair to be performed, and the patient will eventually require a Fontan operation.

OUTCOME OF TREATMENT OF PULMONARY ATRESIA AND INTACT VENTRICULAR SEPTUM

The outcome of treatment depends upon the severity of the tricuspid and right ventricular hypoplasia and the presence or absence of coronary artery stenoses and coronary artery to right ventricular fistulae. These factors, in turn, dictate whether repair results in a two-ventricle arrangement, a single-ventricular arrangement (Fontan procedure), or a one-and-a-half ventricular arrangement (bidirectional Glenn anastomosis, ASD closure, and right ventricular outflow tract reconstruction).

In the best scenario, the ASD is closed and the right ventricular outflow tract is reconstructed, the RV is near normal size, and the coronary arteries are normal. Long-term survival in this scenario is 95% or greater. In all other scenarios, long-term survival will not be as good.

CARDIOVASCULAR SHOCK

Cardiovascular collapse or shock from any cause can be associated with cyanosis. The cyanosis in shock is the result of two mechanisms: (i) Increased transit time of blood through the skin vasculature, resulting in increased extraction of oxygen and (ii) right-to-left intra-pulmonary shunting of the blood. Treatment should be directed at the underlying cause of shock and at providing appropriate support to the cardiovascular system with pharmacologic agents.

SELECTED REFERENCES

Ackerman MJ, Wylam ME, Feldt RH, et al. Pulmonary atresia with ventricular septal defect and persistent airway hyperresponsiveness. *J Thorac Cardiovasc Surg*. 2001;122(1):169–177.

Alboliras E, Julsruds P, Danielson G, et al. Definitive operation for pulmonary atresia with intact ventricular septum. *J Thorac Cardiovasc Surg*. 1987;93:454–464.

Brown JW, Ruzmetov M, Okada Y, et al. Truncus arteriosus repair: Outcomes, risk factors, reoperation and management. *Eur J Cardiothorac Surg*. 2001;20(2):221–227.

Castaneda A, Trusler G, Paul M, et al. The early results of treatment of simple transposition in the current era. *J Thorac Cardiovasc Surg*. 1988;95:14–28.

Cho JM, Puga FJ, Danielson GK, et al. Early and long-term results of the surgical treatment of tetralogy Fallot with pulmonary atresia, with or without major aortopulmonary collateral arteries. *J Thorac Cardiovasc Surg*. 2002;124(1):70–81.

Danielson G, Fuster V. Surgical repair of Ebstein anomaly. *Ann Surg*. 1982;496:499–503.

Dearani JA, Danielson GK, Puga FJ, et al. Late follow-up of 1095 patients undergoing operation for complex congenital heart disease utilizing pulmonary ventricle to pulmonary artery conduits. *Ann Thorac Surg*. 2003;75(2):399–410, discussion 410–1.

DiDonato R, Fyfe D, Puga F, et al. Fifteen-year experience with surgical repair of truncus arteriosus. *J Thorac Cardiovasc Surg*. 1985;89:414–422.

Fontan F, Baudet E. Surgical repair of tricuspid atresia. *Thorax*. 1971;26:240–248.

Fuster V, McGoon D, Kennedy M, et al. Long-term evaluation (12 to 22 years) of open heart surgery for tetralogy of Fallot. *Am J Cardiol*. 1980;46:635–642.

Fyfe DA, Driscoll DJ, Di Donato RM, et al. Truncus arteriosus with single pulmonary artery: Influence of pulmonary vascular obstructive disease on early and late operative results. *J Am Coll Cardiol*. 1985;5(5):1168–1172.

Goldmuntz E, Clark BJ, Mitchell LE, et al. Frequency of 22q11 deletions in patients with conotruncal defects [see comment]. *J Am Coll Cardiol*. 1998;32(2):492–498.

Humes R, Porter C, Mair D, et al. Intermediate follow-up and predicted survival after the modified Fontan procedure for tricuspid atresia and double-inlet ventricle. *Circulation*. 1987;76(Suppl IV):67–71.

Idriss F, Ilbawi M, DeLeon S, et al. Arterial switch in simple and complex transposition of the great arteries. *J Thorac Cardiovasc Surg*. 1988;95:29–36.

Jatene A, Fontes V, Paulista P, et al. Successful anatomic correction of transposition of the great vessels: A preliminary report. *Arq Bras Cardiol*. 1975;28:461–464.

Karl TR. Neonatal cardiac surgery. Anatomic, physiologic, and technical considerations. *Clin Perinatol*. 1999;28(1):159–185.

Kirklin J, Blackstone E, Pacifico A. Routine primary vs. two-stage repair of tetralogy of Fallot. *Circulation*. 1979;60:373–386.

Kiziltan HT, Theodoro DA, Warnes CA, et al. Late results of bioprosthetic tricuspid valve replacement in Ebstein's anomaly. *Ann Thorac Surg*. 1998;66(5):1539–1545.

Khositseth A, Danielson GK, Dearani JA, et al. Supraventricular tachyarrhythmias in Ebstein anomaly: Management and outcome. *J Thorac Cardiovasc Surg*. 2004;128(6):826–833.

Knott-Craig CJ, Overholt ED, Ward KE, et al. Repair of Ebstein's anomaly in the symptomatic neonate: An evolution of technique with 7-year follow-up. *Ann Thorac Surg*. 2002;73(6):1786–1792, discussion 1792–3.

Lofland GK. Pulmonary atresia, ventricular septal defect, and multiple aorta pulmonary collateral arteries. *Semin Thorac Cardiovasc Surg Pediatr Card Surg Annu*. 2004;7:85–94.

MacLellan-Tobert SG, Driscoll DJ, Mottram CD, et al. Exercise tolerance in patients with Ebstein's anomaly. *J Am Coll Cardiol*. 1997;29(7):1615–1622.

Massin MM. Midterm results of the neonatal arterial switch operation. A review. *J Vasc Surg*. 1999;40(4):517–522.

McElhinney DB, Driscoll DA, Emanuel BS, et al. Chromosome 22q11 deletion in patients with truncus arteriosus. *Pediatr Cardiol*. 2003;24(6):569–573.

Norwood W, Lang P, Hansen D. Physiologic repair of aortic atresia-hypoplastic left heart syndrome. *N Engl j Med*. 1983;308:23–26.

Planche C, Lacour-Gayet F, Serraf A. Arterial switch. *Pediatr Cardiol*. 1998;19(4):297–307.

Rashkind W, Miller W. Creation of an atrial septal defect without thoracotomy: A palliative approach to complete transposition of the great arteries. *AMA*. 1966;196:991–992.

Rastelli G, McGoon D, Wallace R. Anatomic correction of transposition of the great arteries with ventricular septal defect and subpulmonary stenosis. *J Thorac Cardiovasc Surg*. 1969;58:545–552.

Thompson LD, McElhinney DB, Reddy M, et al. Neonatal repair of truncus arteriosus: Continuing improvement in outcomes. *Ann Thorac Surg*. 2001;72(2):391–395.

Ullmann MV, Gorenflo M, Sebening C, et al. Long-term results after repair of truncus arteriosus communis in neonates and infants. *Thorac Cardiovasc Surg*. 2003;51(4):175–179.

Yetman AT, Freedom RM, McCrindle BW. Outcome in cyanotic neonates with Ebstein's anomaly. *Am J Cardiol*. 1998;81(6):749–754.

Portions of the text have been published previously and are reproduced with permission of the publisher:
Driscoll DJ. Evaluation of the cyanotic newborn. *Pediatr Clin North Am* 1990;37(1):1–24.

CHAPTER 11

Obstructive and Regurgitant Lesions

*"One cannot know how to treat a disease until
one understands the natural history of the disease"*

AORTIC STENOSIS AND INSUFFICIENCY

INCIDENCE AND TYPES

There are four types of aortic stenosis. The most common is aortic valve stenosis (see Fig. 11.1), which comprises approximately 5% of congenital heart defects. The aortic valve cusps or leaflets are congenitally malformed (Fig. 11.1); they may be thickened and the raphe may be fused. Usually, one of the cusps is quite underdeveloped, resulting in so-called bicuspid aortic valve. Indeed, about 1% to 2% of the general population may have a bicuspid aortic valve, but the valve may not be stenotic or insufficient.

The second type of aortic stenosis is supravalvar aortic stenosis. This involves a narrowing of the ascending aorta just above the sinotubular junction. This narrowing may be quite discreet or diffuse. Supravalvar stenosis can occur sporadically, but there is a familial form that results from a defect in the elastin gene on chromosome 7. Supravalvar stenosis also occurs in Williams syndrome, which is associated with typical facies, mental subnormality, and a defect in the elastin gene.

The third type of aortic stenosis is subvalvar aortic stenosis. In this condition, there is a fibromuscular ridge that causes obstruction a short distance below the valve. In addition, turbulence of blood flow caused by the obstruction can damage the valve leaflets, resulting in aortic valve insufficiency. Also, the leaflets of the valve can be fused to the membrane, which can cause leakage of the valve. If instead of a ridge, there is a longer area of obstructive tissue, it is called *tunnel subaortic stenosis*.

The fourth type of aortic stenosis is muscular subaortic stenosis. This is actually a type of hypertrophic cardiomyopathy and is referred to as *hypertrophic obstructive cardiomyopathy* or *hypertrophic subaortic stenosis* (see Chapter 13). This lesion is not discussed in this chapter but will be dealt with in the section dealing with cardiomyopathy.

Aortic insufficiency frequently occurs in conjunction with aortic valve stenosis, especially if the valve is bicuspid. However, aortic insufficiency can occur because of a bicuspid aortic valve even in the absence of aortic stenosis. Aortic insufficiency is frequently a complication of balloon valvuloplasty or surgical aortic valvotomy and may result from endocarditis on

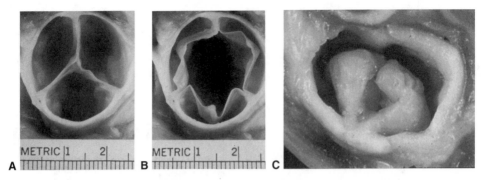

FIGURE 11.1 ● **A:** A normal aortic valve in the closed position. **B:** The normal valve is open. Note the thinness of the leaflets. They are not much thicker than tissue paper. **C:** Stenotic valve. Note the thickened leaflets with only one raphe apparent.

a previously stenotic valve. Aortic insufficiency also is associated with tetralogy of Fallot, pulmonary atresia, Marfan syndrome, and other connective tissue disorders.

CLINICAL PRESENTATION

Aortic valve stenosis is more common in men than in women.

The clinical presentation of aortic valve stenosis depends on the severity of the obstruction. The measure of severity is based on the pressure drop across the valve during systole. Normally, when the left ventricle contracts, the pressure in the ventricle is the same as that in the aorta (see Fig. 11.2); that is, there is no pressure drop or gradient across the aortic valve. In *trivial* aortic stenosis, the pressure difference is 0 to 25 mm Hg, in *mild* stenosis it is 26 to 50 mm Hg, in *moderate* stenosis it is 51 to 79 mm Hg, and in *severe* stenosis it is >80 mm Hg. This classification of severity assumes that cardiac output is normal. If cardiac output is reduced, this classification is unreliable, a situation that may occur in infants with severe aortic stenosis.

Most patients with aortic stenosis are asymptomatic and are diagnosed because of the presence of a cardiac murmur. Rarely, syncope is the presenting sign of aortic stenosis. Some infants with severe aortic stenosis can present with low cardiac output, severely reduced ejection fraction, shock, and/or congestive heart failure. This is referred to as *critical aortic stenosis*. If an infant has poor left ventricular function and aortic stenosis (but without a very high transaortic gradient), aortic valve stenosis still is the likely cause of the poor left ventricular function and must be relieved.

Aortic insufficiency usually presents with a murmur. Severe or progressive aortic insufficiency may present with fatigue, shortness of breath, exercise intolerance, orthopnea, and/or paroxysmal nocturnal dyspnea.

PHYSICAL EXAMINATION

In children and adolescents with aortic stenosis, the peripheral pulses and pulse volumes are normal, and there is no cyanosis.

In patients with mild or moderately severe aortic stenosis, the precordial impulses may be normal. In patients with moderate or severe stenosis, the apical impulse may be increased. There may be a thrill palpable at the base of the heart and over the carotid arteries.

The first and the second heart sounds are normal. With aortic valve stenosis (but not with supravalvar or subvalvar stenosis), an ejection click will be heard immediately after the first

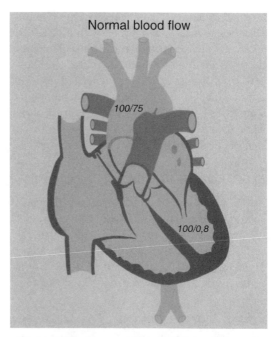

Normal blood flow

100/75

100/0,8

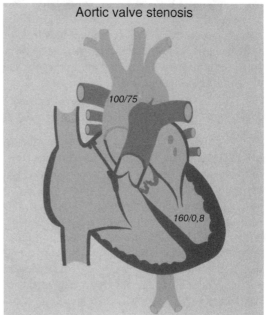

Aortic valve stenosis

100/75

160/0,8

FIGURE 11.2 ● Diagrammatic representation of aortic stenosis (bottom panel). Note that normally the left ventricular pressure is the same as the aortic pressure. In aortic stenosis, the left ventricular pressure is greater than the aortic pressure.

heart sound. This is best heard with the diaphragm of the stethoscope over the apex of the heart or the mid-left sternal border. It is a high-frequency sound. The absence of an aortic ejection click in the presence of other findings consistent with aortic stenosis suggests the presence of subvalvar or supravalvar aortic stenosis.

The murmur of aortic stenosis is systolic and crescendo–decrescendo or "diamond shaped." It is best heard along the left sternal border and radiates to the right upper sternal border. The correlation between the intensity of the murmur and severity of aortic stenosis is not good. However, it is unusual for a murmur of grade 2/6 or less to be associated with severe stenosis. Some patients with aortic stenosis have associated aortic insufficiency, in which case a decrescendo diastolic murmur will be audible.

Aortic insufficiency is characterized by a decrescendo murmur that begins immediately after S_2. The pulse pressure is wide, resulting in "bounding" or "collapsing" pulses. Because there is left ventricular volume overload, the apical impulse may be prominent. Because aortic insufficiency frequently occurs with aortic valve stenosis, the clinical findings of aortic stenosis also may be present.

ELECTROCARDIOGRAPHIC FEATURES

Aortic stenosis and insufficiency are associated with electrocardiographic features of left ventricular hypertrophy (LVH), but the association is inconsistent. The correlation between the presence and/or absence of LVH on the electrocardiogram (ECG) and the severity of aortic stenosis or aortic insufficiency is not good. If there is flattening or inversion of the T waves in leads V_5 and V_6, then it is likely that the aortic stenosis is severe. With severe aortic insufficiency, there may be evidence of myocardial ischemia.

CHEST X-RAY

With aortic stenosis, the heart size usually is normal. Because poststenotic dilation of the aorta occurs with aortic stenosis, the ascending aorta may appear prominent on the chest x-ray. The chest x-ray is not particularly helpful in determining the severity of aortic stenosis.

In contrast to aortic stenosis, the chest x-ray is helpful in determining the severity of aortic insufficiency. Increasing cardiomegaly suggests progressive aortic insufficiency and is helpful in deciding the timing of operation.

ECHOCARDIOGRAPHY AND CARDIAC CATHETERIZATION

The severity of aortic stenosis is based on the pressure gradient across the abnormal aortic valve. Historically, these gradients were measured directly at the time of cardiac catheterization. Indeed, before the era of echocardiography, essentially all patients with aortic stenosis had cardiac catheterization to confirm the diagnosis and to determine the severity of aortic stenosis. Using echocardiography/Doppler techniques it is now possible, noninvasively, to *estimate* the transaortic pressure gradient. One must keep in mind, however, that this is only an estimate. The Doppler assessment of aortic stenosis will provide maximum instantaneous, as well as a mean, transaortic gradient. Most people think that the peak-to-peak gradient that is measured at the time of cardiac catheterization is somewhere between the mean and maximum instantaneous Doppler gradient. Using echocardiography, one can assess left ventricular wall thickness, which also is a reflection of severity.

Echocardiography and Doppler can confirm the presence of aortic insufficiency and are useful in determining the severity of the leakage. Using these techniques, one can determine the regurgitant fraction, the left ventricular systolic and diastolic dimensions, and the left ventricular ejection fraction.

TREATMENT

Treatment of aortic valve stenosis involves manipulating the valve to reduce the stenosis. This can be accomplished by transvenous balloon dilation of the valve, open surgical valvotomy, or surgical valve replacement. In the absence of significant aortic regurgitation, most cardiologists favor transvenous balloon dilation of the valve as the initial procedure for infants and young children. If there is aortic stenosis and significant aortic regurgitation, open surgical valvotomy and valve repair or replacement is the preferred treatment.

Valve replacement includes several possibilities. The stenotic valve could be replaced with a homograft, porcine, or mechanical valve. The advantage of a homograft or porcine valve is that the patient does not have to take warfarin and hence avoids the potential complications of anticoagulation. The disadvantage of these tissue valves is that they last only 8 to 10 years and must then be replaced. The advantage of a mechanical valve is its superior longevity, but lifelong anticoagulation is necessary.

An additional option is the Ross procedure. In this operation, the patient's pulmonary valve is removed and sewn into the aorta in place of the stenotic aortic valve. A homograft valve is then used in the pulmonary position. Unfortunately, after the Ross procedure, the neoaortic valve and the homograft placed into the pulmonary position may fail.

Patients with mild or moderate stenosis do not need balloon dilation or operation. It is generally agreed that patients with transaortic gradient >80 mm Hg should undergo the balloon dilation or operation to reduce the degree of stenosis. In patients with gradients between 50 and 80 mm Hg, the decision to relieve the stenosis is made after considering a number of factors including the patient's age, the presence of associated aortic insufficiency, and left ventricular wall thickness. There are two situations in which the decision to relieve the stenosis might not be related to the magnitude of the gradient. The first is the case of an infant with critical aortic stenosis and congestive heart failure and/or low cardiac output. Relief of the stenosis is indicated in this situation regardless of the magnitude of the gradient. The second situation is that of a patient with syncope or symptoms that clearly are related to the aortic stenosis.

In the Second Natural History Study of Congenital Heart Defects, the 25-year survival of patients with aortic stenosis was 85.1% as compared to an expected survival of 96.4%. In patients with trivial or mild stenosis, the 25-year survival was 92.4% as compared to 81% for patients with moderate or severe stenosis. The following were associated with poorer survival: Male sex, higher transaortic gradient, cardiac symptoms, and older age. In patients who had surgical aortic valvotomy, there was a 40% chance that a second operation would be necessary over a 25-year period. The incidence of bacterial endocarditis was 27.1 per 10,000 person-years of follow-up.

There are several approaches to the management of the patient with significant aortic insufficiency. The options for valve replacement are the same as those discussed in the preceding text for aortic stenosis. In addition, the surgeon can, in select cases, repair the valve. Unfortunately, repair of an insufficient valve fails relatively early in at least 10% of cases. The long-term outcome of aortic insufficiency depends on the severity of the insufficiency and the type of procedure employed to deal with the leakage.

The treatment of discreet or tunnel subvalvar aortic stenosis is surgical resection of the obstructing tissue. At times, it is necessary for the surgeon to perform a "modified Konno" procedure to enlarge the left ventricular outflow tract. This involves creating a ventricular septal defect (VSD) in the outlet septum just below the aortic valve and then closing this defect with a patch, such that the outflow tract is larger. In the absence of aortic insufficiency, the indications for operation are similar to those for aortic valve stenosis. However, if there is significant aortic valve insufficiency, one would operate for a lower transaortic pressure gradient because discreet subvalvar aortic stenosis can cause progressive aortic valve insufficiency, presumably owing to injury to the valve leaflets caused by the eccentric jet of blood through the subaortic area. In addition, the membrane may be attached to the valve leaflets, contributing to the aortic valve insufficiency.

The treatment of supravalvar aortic stenosis involves patch enlargement of the narrow area of the aorta. The indications for operation are the same as those for aortic valve stenosis.

All patients with any type of aortic stenosis or insufficiency must observe prophylactic measures for infective endocarditis.

COARCTATION OF THE AORTA
INCIDENCE AND ASSOCIATED ANOMALIES

Coarctation of the aorta constitutes 5% of congenital cardiac defects. It consists of a ledge-shaped protrusion of tissue into the aorta at a position immediately opposite the insertion of the ductus or ligamentum arteriosus (see Fig. 11.3 and 11.4). In 50% to 85% of cases, there is an associated bicuspid aortic valve. Less commonly, it can be associated with a VSD or subvalvar aortic stenosis. If coarctation is associated with subaortic stenosis and a parachute mitral valve and supravalvar mitral membrane, the complex is referred to as *Shone syndrome*.

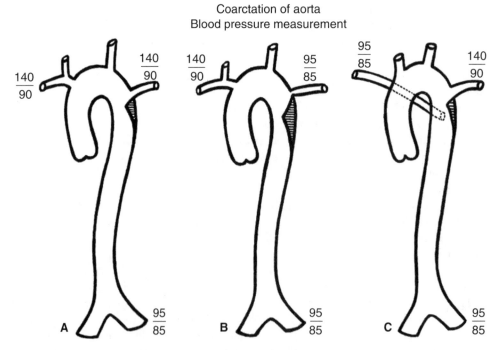

FIGURE 11.3 ● Diagrammatic representation of coarctation of the aorta. Note that the coarctation of the aorta is immediately opposite the site of aortic insertion of the ligamentum arteriosus. The left panel depicts the most common situation in which the subclavian arteries arise normally and there is no narrowing of the left subclavian artery. The center panel shows the arm and leg blood pressures when the origin of the left subclavian artery is stenotic. The right panel indicates the arm and leg blood pressures when the right subclavian artery arises anomalously from the aorta distal to the coarctation.

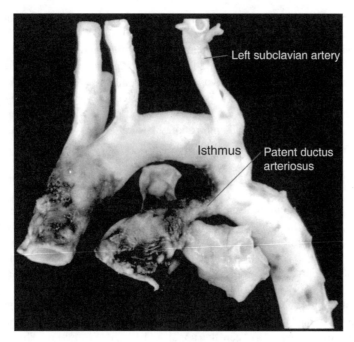

Left subclavian artery

Isthmus

Patent ductus arteriosus

FIGURE 11.4 ● Pathologic specimen of coarctation of the aorta. Note that the coarctation is immediately opposite the site of the insertion of the ductus arteriosus.

Coarctation of the aorta is more common in men than in women and is associated with Turner syndrome.

In some patients, the coarctation can compromise the orifice of the left subclavian artery. In this case, there may be no blood pressure discrepancy between the left arm and the leg. Rather, the discrepancy will be between the right arm and leg (Fig. 11.3, center). Also, if there is aberrant origin of the right subclavian artery from the descending aorta distal to the coarctation of the aorta, then there may be no discrepancy in the blood pressure or pulses between the right arm and the leg (Fig. 11.3, right). Therefore, it is important to measure the blood pressure in both arms and one leg, else one could fail to make the correct diagnosis.

CLINICAL PRESENTATION

The clinical presentation of coarctation of the aorta depends on the severity of the obstruction and the associated anomalies.

Very severe coarctation of the aorta may become apparent within 2 to 5 days of life, when the ductus arteriosus closes. There are two reasons why symptoms of congestive heart failure may occur when the ductus arteriosus closes. If the coarctation is very severe, the blood supply to the descending aorta will be from the right ventricle, through the ductus arteriosus. When the ductus closes, blood supply to the kidney, other abdominal organs, and many muscle groups is compromised. In addition, the blood ejected from the right ventricle that had been traversing the ductus is now additional pulmonary blood flow. The additional pulmonary blood flow in the face of elevated left ventricular end-diastolic pressure leads to pulmonary venous hypertension and pulmonary edema. In less severe cases, before closure of the ductus arteriosus, the flow of blood will be from the aorta through the ductus to the pulmonary artery.

Because some contractile ductal tissue is present in the aortic wall, as the ductus closes, the diameter of the aorta can be reduced and the coarctation made more severe. With increased aortic narrowing, left ventricular work and left ventricular end-diastolic pressure increase, leading to pulmonary edema. Also, blood flow to the kidneys may be compromised.

If the coarctation is not severe enough to cause heart failure in infancy, the patient usually remains asymptomatic. The presence of the defect may be heralded by the detection of a heart murmur or systemic hypertension. Unfortunately, in some instances, the presence of a coarctation is not appreciated until adolescence. Rarely, with previously undetected coarctation of the aorta, a cerebral vascular accident may be the presenting event.

PHYSICAL EXAMINATION

Infants with severe coarctation of the aorta may have the usual signs of congestive heart failure including tachycardia, poor perfusion, grunting, tachypnea, and hepatomegaly. Although low-amplitude or absent pulses in the lower extremities as compared to the upper extremities is the *sine qua non* of coarctation of the aorta, it must be recognized that in infants with coarctation of the aorta and congestive heart failure, low-amplitude or absent pulses may be observed in the upper and the lower extremities as a result of low cardiac output. As the cardiac output improves with treatment, the pulses will return to the upper extremities.

In patients who do not have congestive heart failure, there will be a pulse amplitude and blood pressure discrepancy between the upper and lower extremities. The blood pressure difference results from a lower systolic and mean blood pressure in the lower extremities as compared to the upper extremities. The diastolic blood pressure is not significantly different between the upper and lower extremities (Fig. 11.3).

Because many patients with coarctation of the aorta have an associated bicuspid aortic valve, an aortic ejection click frequently is heard shortly after the first heart sound.

Turbulent blood flow through the area of coarctation produces a systolic ejection murmur that is best heard at the cardiac apex and below the left scapula. Because many patients with coarctation of the aorta have subtle or important abnormalities of the mitral valve, a diastolic murmur may be heard at the apex of the heart.

The formation of collateral vessels can affect the physical findings. Parascapular collateral vessels can produce a continuous murmur in the region of the scapula, and, in some patients, these vessels can be palpated. As collateral vessels form, the pressure gradient across the coarctation decreases, making the arm-to-leg blood pressure gradient an unreliable measure of the severity of coarctation.

ELECTROCARDIOGRAPHIC FEATURES

Although it seems paradoxical, infants with coarctation of the aorta demonstrate voltage criteria for RVH rather than LVH. Older children either have a normal ECG or demonstrate LVH.

CHEST X-RAY

The chest radiographic findings in coarctation of the aorta can be quite varied. Infants with congestive heart failure will have cardiomegaly and increased pulmonary vascular markings. Infants without heart failure or older children may have a normal chest x-ray. If there are significant collateral vessels, rib notching may be apparent. The ascending aorta may be prominent.

ECHOCARDIOGRAPHIC, MAGNETIC RESONANCE IMAGING, AND CARDIAC CATHETERIZATION ISSUES

The presence of coarctation of the aorta is ascertained by clinical examination. Although most coarctations are located opposite the aortic insertion of the ductus or ligamentum arteriosus, the lesion rarely may be located more distally in the aorta. Therefore, echocardiography or some other imaging form is necessary to localize the area of coarctation and to establish the length of the narrow segment. In addition, associated lesions such as aortic stenosis, VSD, or mitral valve disease can be identified and quantified. The severity of the coarctation can be estimated by the degree of LVH, and, in some cases, by measuring the cross-sectional area or the diameter of the coarctation site.

Newer magnetic resonance imaging (MRI) methods are quite good at imaging coarctation of the aorta and assessing its severity. MRI allows detailed imaging of the entire aorta in multiple planes and views. It also allows identification of collateral vessels.

Cardiac catheterization is no longer necessary for the diagnosis of coarctation of the aorta. However, in some cases, it is employed to treat coarctation of the aorta (see the subsequent text).

TREATMENT

The treatment of coarctation of the aorta is to remove or eliminate the obstruction. This can be done surgically or by balloon dilation with or without stent implantation. There are numerous surgical techniques that have evolved over the years. One of the earliest techniques was the Blalock-Park procedure, in which the left subclavian artery was used as a jump graft around the coarctation site. This was abandoned in favor of resecting the site of coarctation and doing an end-to-end anastomosis of the aorta. Subsequently, the technique of applying a patch to the area of coarctation was described. However, this technique is associated with aneurysm of the aorta opposite the site of the patch. Next, the technique of subclavian patch repair became popular and is still used by some surgeons. In this technique, the left subclavian artery is transected and fashioned into an on-lay patch over the site of coarctation. Frequently, this on-lay patch of subclavian artery tissue is not long enough and must be augmented with some type of prosthetic material. Over the last several years, the "extended" and "radically extended" end-to-end anastomosis has been used and is the operation of choice in infants with a hypoplastic isthmus. In this technique, the end of the aorta distal to the area of coarctation is mobilized and anastomosed to the underside of the distal aortic arch. This technique effectively eliminates areas of distal arch and isthmic hypoplasia that frequently accompanies coarctation of the aorta in infants. The choice of surgical technique depends, primarily, on the age of the patient and the presence or absence of isthmic hypoplasia.

Most people agree that balloon dilation is the best method to treat recurrent coarctation of the aorta. For treatment of native coarctation of the aorta, controversy still exists over whether surgical treatment or balloon dilation is better. More recently, balloon dilation combined with percutaneous placement of a stent has been described. This may prove to be a useful technique for patients who are fully or nearly fully grown. The long-term results of stent placement are unknown.

NATURAL HISTORY AND OUTCOME OF TREATMENT

Untreated coarctation of the aorta results in the ravages of sustained long-standing hypertension. These include premature coronary artery disease, intracranial aneurysms, stroke, left ventricular failure, and premature death.

The outcome of repair of coarctation of the aorta is related to the age at the time of repair and the degree of residual or recurrent narrowing at the site of repair. For infants who develop congestive heart failure, operation is indicated despite their very young age. In patients without heart failure, the age of repair must be tempered by the risk of residual or recurrent coarctation of the aorta if operation is performed below 6 months of age and the risk of persistent hypertension if the operation is delayed beyond 4 years of age.

Even with appropriate repair, there seems to be a higher risk of premature vascular disease including heart attack and stroke for patients who have had coarctation of the aorta compared to that for patients without coarctation of the aorta. These patients are also at risk for residual or recurrent coarctation, and other adverse outcomes include aneurysm at the site of repair, intracranial hemorrhage, and endocarditis.

PULMONARY VALVE STENOSIS AND INSUFFICIENCY

INCIDENCE AND TYPES

Pulmonary valve stenosis (with intact ventricular septum) occurs in approximately 4 of 1,000 live births and constitutes 5% to 8% of congenital cardiac defects (see Fig. 11.5). Usually it occurs sporadically. Patients with Noonan syndrome have a greater likelihood of having pulmonary stenosis.

Isolated pulmonary valve insufficiency is rare. It can accompany idiopathic dilation of the pulmonary artery and pulmonary vascular obstructive disease. Most cases of pulmonary insufficiency results from surgical or balloon procedures used to treat pulmonary valve stenosis. Pulmonary insufficiency also can be associated with other conditions such as repaired tetralogy of Fallot.

CLINICAL PRESENTATION

Most patients with pulmonary stenosis or pulmonary insufficiency are asymptomatic and present with a cardiac murmur. The exception to this is the case of an infant with severe pulmonary stenosis (so-called critical pulmonary stenosis) who presents with cyanosis because of right-to-left shunting at the atrial level.

Pulmonary insufficiency as a result of operation or balloon procedures to relieve right ventricular outflow tract obstruction was, at one time, thought to have no significant long-term consequences. It is now becoming clear that in some patients long-standing pulmonary valve insufficiency and right ventricular volume overload may be associated with right ventricular failure and tricuspid regurgitation. In this situation, patients may develop fatigue, exercise intolerance, and/or arrhythmias.

PHYSICAL EXAMINATION

With the exception of infants with critical pulmonary stenosis, other patients with pulmonary valve stenosis are acyanotic. Careful palpation at the lower left sternal border will reveal an increased right ventricular impulse. The first sound is normal and is followed by a click, which is best heard at the upper left sternal border. The frequency (pitch) of the click is lower and more difficult to hear than that associated with aortic valve stenosis. The second heart sound may be normal, widely split, or single, depending on the severity of the pulmonary stenosis. In very mild cases, S_2 can be normally split. As the severity increases, S_2 becomes more widely split. With severe stenosis, the second heart sound becomes single (it is still widely split but closure of the pulmonary valve becomes inaudible).

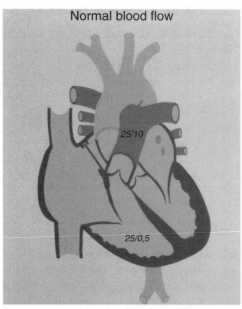

Normal blood flow

25/10

25/0,5

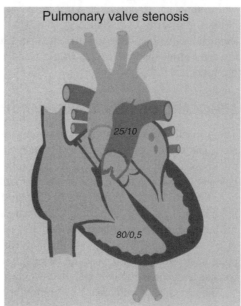

Pulmonary valve stenosis

25/10

80/0,5

FIGURE 11.5 ● Diagrammatic representation of pulmonary valve stenosis. Note that in contrast to normal, the pressure in the right ventricle is greater than the pressure in the pulmonary artery.

The murmur of pulmonary stenosis is an ejection murmur (crescendo–decrescendo or "diamond shaped"), and the peak intensity of the murmur occurs later, as the severity of the stenosis increases. If ventricular failure occurs, a prominent fourth sound may be heard.

Pulmonary insufficiency is characterized by a mid- to high-frequency decrescendo murmur that begins immediately after S_2. In contrast to the murmur of aortic insufficiency, this murmur is louder when the patient is supine than when sitting. With significant pulmonary insufficiency, the right ventricular impulse, felt at the lower left sternal border or in the xiphoid area, may be prominent.

ELECTROCARDIOGRAPHIC FEATURES

The ECG is a fairly reliable measure of the severity of pulmonary valve stenosis. It is characterized by right axis deviation and, as the severity of pulmonary stenosis increases, by increasing evidence of right ventricular hypertrophy (RVH). Nadas and Fyler indicated that the right ventricular pressure could be estimated by multiplying the R-wave voltage in lead V_1 by 3 and by adding 47 to that number. Rudolph suggested that the right ventricular pressure could be estimated by multiplying the R wave in V_{4R} by 5. In the First Natural History Study, a complex equation to predict the right ventricular to pulmonary artery pressure difference was based on the R, S, and T waves in several leads.

Pulmonary insufficiency may be accompanied by electrocardiographic evidence of RVH or subtle signs of right ventricular volume overload (right axis deviation and/or an rSR' pattern in lead V_1).

CHEST X-RAY

With either pulmonary stenosis or insufficiency, the chest x-ray may be normal. With right ventricular enlargement, the apex may be uptilted. Classically, there is a prominent main pulmonary artery segment. In contrast to tetralogy of Fallot, the pulmonary vascular markings are normal. This is because the volume of pulmonary blood flow is normal in patients with pulmonary stenosis but is decreased in patients with tetralogy of Fallot.

As the severity of pulmonary insufficiency increases, the heart size becomes larger. As tricuspid valve insufficiency increases as a result of increasing right ventricular dilatation, the right atrial shadow (i.e., the right-sided border of the cardiac silhouette) becomes more prominent.

ECHOCARDIOGRAPHIC AND CARDIAC CATHETERIZATION ISSUES

The presence and severity of pulmonary stenosis can be assessed using echocardiography. The valve morphology can be determined (i.e., bicuspid or tricuspid valves and the thickness and dysplasia, as well as the mobility, of the cusps). Using the maximum instantaneous Doppler gradient, the right ventricular to pulmonary artery pressure gradient can be estimated. Right ventricular pressure can be estimated using the velocity of the tricuspid regurgitation jet. The severity of pulmonary stenosis in the newborn can be underestimated in the presence of pulmonary hypertension. Elevation of pulmonary resistance can result in a low right ventricular to pulmonary artery gradient even in the presence of severe pulmonary stenosis. Because of this, the severity should be reassessed after pulmonary resistance declines.

The presence of pulmonary regurgitation can be confirmed by echocardiography, and the severity can be ascertained by observing the degree of right ventricular and atrial enlargement, right ventricular function, and the degree of tricuspid regurgitation.

TREATMENT

The currently accepted best method of treatment of significant pulmonary valve stenosis is balloon pulmonary valvuloplasty. Most people agree that valvuloplasty should be performed if the transpulmonary gradient exceeds 50 mm Hg or if there is evidence of RVH on the ECG. In infants, the gradient is less useful, and if the patient has critical pulmonary stenosis (evidenced by poor right ventricular function and/or right-to-left shunting of blood at the atrial level), valvotomy or valvuloplasty is indicted regardless of gradient.

The timing and optimum treatment for pulmonary insufficiency is less well defined than that for pulmonary stenosis. It is generally thought that operation to restore a competent valve in the pulmonary position should be done if there is progressive right ventricular enlargement and/or tricuspid regurgitation, especially in the setting of ventricular arrhythmias and/or progressive exercise intolerance. Unfortunately, the treatment for pulmonary insufficiency is valve replacement, and none of the current implantable valves last for an extended time. Also, it is unclear whether the patient is best served by insertion of a mechanical or tissue valve.

NATURAL HISTORY AND OUTCOME OF TREATMENT

The outcome of untreated trivial or mild pulmonary stenosis, as well as moderate and severe forms that have been treated surgically or by balloon valvuloplasty, is excellent. In the Second Natural History Study, the probability of 25-year survival was 95.7%, no different from a normal population. Repeat operation rarely was necessary. The incidence of bacterial endocarditis was low (0.94 per 10,000 person-years of follow-up).

It is likely that the long-term outcome for most patients with pulmonary insufficiency is excellent even without operation. However, it is becoming clear that some patients with pulmonary insufficiency will develop progressive right ventricular dysfunction. Currently, it appears that patients with congenital heart disease who underwent a Brock procedure (closed surgical valvotomy) at the dawn of cardiac surgery are most likely to develop problems. Also, patients who had repair of tetralogy of Fallot and persistently hypoplastic or stenotic pulmonary arteries are at risk for right ventricular dysfunction.

MITRAL VALVE STENOSIS AND INSUFFICIENCY
INCIDENCE AND TYPES

Isolated congenital mitral stenosis is quite rare. It can result from a supravalvar mitral ring, hypoplastic mitral annulus, dysplastic leaflets, and/or abnormal valve support apparatus. Congenital mitral stenosis occurs most commonly in association with other congenital cardiac anomalies such as coarctation of the aorta, aortic stenosis, and VSD.

In third world countries, by far the most common cause of mitral stenosis and insufficiency is rheumatic fever; this is currently an unusual cause in the United States.

Congenital mitral insufficiency can occur with a congenitally dysplastic or prolapsing mitral valve. It can occur with connective tissue disorders such as Ehlers-Danlos and Marfan syndromes, as well as Hunter and Hurler syndromes. It can be associated with other congenital heart defects that include abnormal formation of the mitral valve such as partial and complete atrioventricular septal defects. Mitral insufficiency can accompany dilated (congestive), restrictive, and hypertrophic cardiomyopathies. Mitral insufficiency may be the presenting feature of anomalous origin of the left coronary artery from the pulmonary artery. This is a result of myocardial infarction secondary to the coronary anomaly.

CLINICAL PRESENTATION

Patients with mild mitral stenosis and/or insufficiency are asymptomatic. As the degree of severity increases, the patient can develop shortness of breath, exercise intolerance, cough, orthopnea, paroxysmal nocturnal dyspnea, hemoptysis, and arrhythmias.

PHYSICAL EXAMINATION

Mitral stenosis produces a middiastolic murmur best heard at the cardiac apex with the patient in the left lateral decubitus position. If the degree of mitral stenosis is severe enough to produce pulmonary hypertension, S_2 may be increased in intensity. With severe stenosis, there may be pulmonary rales.

Mitral insufficiency is associated with a mid- to high-frequency holosystolic murmur, best heard at the cardiac apex with the patient in the left lateral decubitus position. Occasionally, a thrill can be palpated at the cardiac apex. A middiastolic murmur of "relative" mitral stenosis is common because of the increased volume of blood traversing the mitral valve during diastole. As with mitral stenosis, there may be evidence of pulmonary edema and pulmonary hypertension.

ELECTROCARDIOGRAPHIC FEATURES

Both mitral stenosis and insufficiency can be associated with a prolonged P wave that is biphasic or predominantly negative in lead V_1. In severe mitral stenosis or insufficiency, there may be evidence of RVH and, in the case of mitral insufficiency, left ventricular enlargement.

CHEST X-RAY

Because both mitral stenosis and insufficiency are associated with increased left atrial and pulmonary venous hypertension, enlargement of the left atrium and a prominent pulmonary venous pattern may be evident on the chest x-ray. In addition, an enlarged pulmonary artery segment may be present. Because mitral insufficiency, but not mitral stenosis, is associated with left ventricular volume overload, cardiac enlargement may be apparent, with mitral insufficiency.

ECHOCARDIOGRAPHIC AND CARDIAC CATHETERIZATION ISSUES

The presence of mitral stenosis and/or insufficiency can be confirmed by echocardiography. The anatomic features of the valve can be ascertained. The severity of the lesions can be estimated by assessing the size of the left atrium and ventricle, estimating the pressure gradient across the valve, measuring the Doppler flow patterns across the valve, estimating pulmonary artery pressure, and defining associated lesions.

TREATMENT AND OUTCOME OF TREATMENT

Before considering treatment, the severity of the lesion must be determined. It is important to weigh all the various indicators of severity and not to rely solely on one diagnostic test such as echocardiography. The history and physical examination are critically important in assessing severity. Certainly, the patient who has symptoms clearly attributable to mitral stenosis or insufficiency has significant disease. In the asymptomatic patient, one must be cautious to not overestimate the severity on the basis of echocardiographic features alone. For example, if a patient with mitral insufficiency has no diastolic flow murmur, a normal P_2, and a normal chest x-ray and ECG but an "enlarged" left atrium by echocardiography, I would be reluctant to make a diagnosis of severe mitral insufficiency. Similarly, if a patient with mitral stenosis has a normal P_2, chest x-ray, and ECG, I would not make a diagnosis of severe mitral stenosis solely on the basis of the Doppler gradient across the mitral valve.

The treatment and results of treatment of mitral stenosis depend on the specific abnormality of the valve that is contributing to the obstruction. If, for example, the obstruction results primarily from a supravalvar mitral ring, the ring can be resected, leading to an excellent long-term result. On the other hand, if the mitral annulus is small and there is a parachute mitral valve (one papillary muscle to which all the chordae tendinae are attached), then it is difficult, if not impossible, to completely relieve the obstruction.

The repair of mitral insufficiency also depends on the exact reason for the mitral insufficiency. If it results from a congenital cleft in the septal leaflet of the mitral valve, the cleft usually can be closed with a few sutures and the long-term result will be good. If the valve annulus is dilated but left ventricular function is well preserved, an annuloplasty can be done and the results are generally quite good. If there is a flail mitral valve leaflet, artificial chordae can be inserted and a plastic procedure can be performed on the leaflet.

It is clear, for both mitral stenosis and insufficiency, that the greater the complexity of the cause of the valve dysfunction, the less good the long-term result will be. In either case, replacement of the valve has its own long-term consequences. If a valve is replaced in a small child, the valve will be outgrown and reoperation will eventually be necessary. However, in this case, the annulus into which the new valve needs to be placed will be small and cannot be enlarged because it is surrounded by the circumflex coronary artery. In this scenario, the surgeon may have to position the new valve in the left atrium itself. Use of mechanical valve will necessitate long-term anticoagulation with associated risks.

SELECTED REFERENCES

Al-Hroob A, Husayni TS, Freter A, et al. Aortic aneurysm after patch aortoplasty for coarctation: Analysis of patch size and wall growth. *Pediatr Cardiol*. 2003;24(1):10–16.

Alexiou C, Galogavrou M, Chen Q, et al. Mitral valve replacement with mechanical prostheses in children: Improved operative risk and survival. *Eur J Cardiothorac Surg*. 2001;20(1):105–113.

Banerjee A, Kohl T, Silverman NH Echocardiographic evaluation of congenital mitral valve anomalies in children. *Am J Cardiol*. 1995;76(17):1284–1291.

Bergersen LJ, Perry SB, Lock JE Effect of cutting balloon angioplasty on resistant pulmonary artery stenosis. *Am J Cardiol*. 2003;91(2):185–189.

Brown JW, Ruzmetov M, Vijay P, et al. Surgery for aortic stenosis in children: A 40-year experience. *Ann Thorac Surg*. 2003;76(5):1398–1411.

Daou L, Sidi D, Mauriat P, et al. Mitral valve replacement with mechanical valves in children under two years of age. *J Thorac Cardiovasc Surg*. 2001;121(5):994–996.

Driscoll DJ, Michels VV, Gersony WM, et al. Occurrence risk for congenital heart defects in relatives of patients with aortic stenosis, pulmonary stenosis, or ventricular septal defect. *Circulation*. 1993;87(Suppl 2):I114–I120.

Driscoll DJ, Wolfe RR, Gersony WM, et al. Cardiorespiratory responses to exercise of patients with aortic stenosis, pulmonary stenosis, and ventricular septal defect. *Circulation*. 1993;87(Suppl 2):I102–I113.

Elkins RC, Lane MM, McCue C Ross operation in children: Late results. *J Heart Valve Dis*. 2001;10(6):736–741.

Fawzy ME, Awad M, Hassan W, et al. Long-term outcome (up to 15 years) of balloon angioplasty of discrete native coarctation of the aorta in adolescents and adults. *J Am Coll Cardiol*. 2004;43(6):1062–1067.

Gersony WM, Driscoll DJ, Hayes CJ, et al. Second natural history study of congenital heart defects. Quality of life of patients with aortic stenosis, pulmonary stenosis, or ventricular septal defect. *Circulation*. 1993; 87(Suppl 2):I52–I65.

Gersony WM, Driscoll DJ, Hayes CJ, et al. Bacterial endocarditis in patients with aortic stenosis, pulmonary stenosis, or ventricular septal defect. *Circulation*. 1993;87(Suppl 2):I121–I126.

Hayes CJ, Driscoll DJ, Gersony WM, et al. Second natural history study of congenital heart defects. Results of treatment of patients with pulmonary valvar stenosis. *Circulation*. 1993;87(Suppl 2):I28–I37.

Keane JF, Driscoll DJ, Gersony WM, et al. Second natural history study of congenital heart defects. Results of treatment of patients with aortic valvar stenosis. *Circulation*. 1993;87(Suppl 2):I16–I27.

Krishnamoorthy KM, Tharakan JA Balloon mitral valvulotomy in children aged < or = 12 years. *J Heart Valve Dis*. 2003;12(4):461–468.

Lambert V, et al. Long-term results after valvotomy for congenital aortic valvar stenosis in children. *Cardiol Young*. 2000;10(6):590–596.

Latiff HA, Sholler GF, Cooper S Balloon dilatation of aortic stenosis in infants younger than 6 months of age: Intermediate outcome. *Pediatr Cardiol*. 2003;24(1):17–26.

Lorier G, Kalil RA, Barcellos C, et al. Valve repair in children with congenital mitral lesions: Late clinical results. *Pediatr Cardiol*. 2001;22(1):44–52.

Nadas A, Fyler D. *Pediatr Cardiol*. Philadelphia, PA: WB Saunders; 1972.

Ohye RG, Gomez CA, Ohye BJ, et al. The Ross/Konno procedure in neonates and infants: Intermediate-term survival and autograft function. *Ann Thorac Surg*. 2001;72(3):823–830.

Peterson C, Schilthuis JJ, Dodge-Khatami A, et al. Comparative long-term results of surgery versus balloon valvuloplasty for pulmonary valve stenosis in infants and children. *Ann Thorac Surg*. 2003;76(4):1078–1082, discussion 1082–1083.

Poon LK, Menahem S Pulmonary regurgitation after percutaneous balloon valvoplasty for isolated pulmonary valvar stenosis in childhood. *Cardiol Young*. 2003;13(5):444–450.

Prifti E, Vanini V, Bonacchi M, et al. Repair of congenital malformations of the mitral valve: Early and midterm results. *Ann Thorac Surg*. 2002;73(2):614–621.

Puchalski MD, Williams RV, Hawkins JA, et al. Follow-up of aortic coarctation repair in neonates. *J Am Coll Cardiol*. 2004;44(1):188–191.

Qureshi SA, Zubrzycka M, Brzezinska-Rajszys G, et al. Use of covered Cheatham-Platinum stents in aortic coarctation and recoarctation. *Cardiol Young*. 2004;14(1):50–54.

Rao PS, Long-term follow-up results after balloon dilatation of pulmonic stenosis, aortic stenosis, and coarctation of the aorta: A review. *Prog Cardiovasc Dis*. 1999;42(1):59–74.

Rao PS, Jureidini SB, Balfour IC et al. Severe aortic coarctation in infants less than 3 months: Successful palliation by balloon angioplasty. *J Invasive Cardiol*. 2003;15(4):202–208.

Rudolph A, *Congenital diseases of the heart*. Chicago: Year-Book Medical Publishers; 1974.

Sharieff S, Shah-e-Zaman K, Faruqui AM Short- and intermediate-term follow-up results of percutaneous transluminal balloon valvuloplasty in adolescents and young adults with congenital pulmonary valve stenosis. *J Invasive Cardiol*. 2003;15(9):484–487.

Toro-Salazar OH, Steinberger J, Thomas W, et al. Long-term follow-up of patients after coarctation of the aorta repair. *Am J Cardiol*. 2002;89(5):541–547.

Tweddell JS, Pelech AN, Frommelt PC, et al. Complex aortic valve repair as a durable and effective alternative to valve replacement in children with aortic valve disease. *J Thorac Cardiovasc Surg*. 2005;129(3):551–558.

Wolfe RR, Driscoll DJ, Gersony WM, et al. Arrhythmias in patients with valvar aortic stenosis, valvar pulmonary stenosis, and ventricular septal defect. Results of 24-hour ECG monitoring. *Circulation*. 1993; 87(Suppl 2):I89–I101.

CHAPTER 12

Acquired Heart Diseases

"Don't attempt to make a patient better
faster than it took the patient to become ill"

RHEUMATIC FEVER

Acute rheumatic fever is a multisystem inflammatory disorder resulting from an earlier group A β-hemolytic streptococcal infection. Except for its cardiac effects, acute rheumatic fever is a self-limiting, relatively benign disorder. Unfortunately, the cardiac effects of this condition are serious and may be chronic and life threatening.

EPIDEMIOLOGY

The incidence of acute rheumatic fever varies with geographic location and the population studied but, in general, ranges from 3 to 61 per 100,000 school children. The highest incidence occurs in children aged 5 to 14 years. This condition is rare in children younger than 4 years but does occur. Acute rheumatic fever is most common during winter and spring, a seasonal variation similar to that of streptococcal pharyngitis.

The incidence of initial attacks of acute rheumatic fever is increased in disadvantaged populations, presumably because of crowded living conditions that facilitate the spread of streptococcal infection.

STREPTOCOCCUS

Streptococcus is composed of a core of cytoplasm surrounded by a cytoplasmic membrane and a cell wall, which in turn is surrounded by a capsule that constitutes the external surface of the organism. The capsule is composed of hyaluronate, which is nonantigenic. The cell wall is composed of three layers: The outermost protein layer, the middle carbohydrate layer, and the innermost mucopeptide protoplast layer.

The protein layer contains the proteins designated M, T, and R. The M protein is the most important because it determines the virulence of the organism, stimulates the formation of opsonizing and precipitating antibodies, and may impede phagocytosis. Lancefield classified group A β-hemolytic streptococci into serologic types on the basis of the M protein. Acute rheumatic fever can result from infection by any of the serotypes of group A β-hemolytic streptococci, unlike glomerulonephritis, which is associated with only a limited number of the serotypes. Antibodies produced against the M protein antigen can impart long-lasting immunity against reinfection by that specific serotype. The middle layer of the cell wall, the carbohydrate layer, provides the group specification of the *Streptococcus*. N-Acetylglucosamine is the group-specific carbohydrate for group A β-hemolytic streptococci. The mucopeptide innermost layer of the cell wall forms the skeletal component of the cell and is responsible for the shape of the cell. The cytoplasmic membrane is an antigenic lipoprotein, which cross-reacts with several mammalian tissue antigens, including human glomerular basement membrane.

The *Streptococcus* produces a number of extracellular products, some of which are involved in the disease-causing effects of the microorganism. Erythrogenic toxin is pyrogenic and is responsible for the rash of scarlet fever. Streptolysin O is cardiotoxic and leukotoxic and is responsible for the hemolysis of erythrocytes. Streptolysin O elicits an antibody response (producing antistreptolysin O) in 70% to 85% of infected individuals, and this forms the basis of a useful assay of invasive streptococcal infection. Early and effective antibiotic treatment of streptococcal infections can suppress this antibody response. The antigenicity of streptolysin O is inhibited by lipid extracts (probably cholesterol) of rabbit skin, and this property may be responsible for the lack of association between streptococcal skin infections and acute rheumatic fever. Free cholesterol neutralizes streptolysin O, but serum cholesterol, not in a free state, is a poor inhibitor of streptolysin O. Streptolysin S produces the hemolysis characteristic of β-hemolytic streptococci when cultured on sheep blood agar. Extracellular proteinase can cause myocardial necrosis. Streptokinase activates plasma proteins and converts plasminogen to plasmin. Diphosphopyridine nucleotidase elicits an antibody response (producing anti–diphosphopyridine nucleotidase) in 87% of patients with acute rheumatic fever and is a useful adjunct to the antistreptolysin O titer in identifying patients with invasive streptococcal disease. There are four deoxyribonucleases (I, II, III, and IV), all of which are antigenic. Deoxyribonuclease II is produced in the largest quantities in response to group A β-hemolytic streptococcal infection and is the most consistent of the deoxyribonucleases. Antideoxyribonuclease antibodies are useful indicators of invasive streptococcal disease.

PATHOGENESIS

Although it is clear that invasive group A β-hemolytic streptococcal infection is causally related to acute rheumatic fever, the pathogenesis of this relationship is unclear. Most likely, acute rheumatic fever is an autoimmune disease in which invasive streptococcal infection evokes an antibody response from the host, and this antibody attacks antigenically similar host tissues. Four streptococcal–host cross-reactive antigen–antibody systems have been identified: (i) Cardiac myofiber smooth muscle antigen cross-reacting with streptococcal cell wall and cell membrane antigen, (ii) heart valve fibroblast antigen cross-reacting with streptococcal cell membrane antigen, (iii) subthalamic and caudate nuclei antigen cross-reacting with streptococcal cell membrane antigen, and (iv) heart valve and connective tissue antigen cross-reacting with streptococcal group A carbohydrate antigen. Although heart-reactive antibody can be identified in patients with acute rheumatic fever, these antibodies can at times also be identified in patients with streptococcal infection but without acute rheumatic fever.

It is possible that streptococcal extracellular products play a role in the pathogenesis of acute rheumatic fever. Although some of these products are cardiotoxic, the effects of these toxins *in vitro* do not mimic the chronic granulomatous lesions seen in acute rheumatic fever.

CLINICAL MANIFESTATIONS

Fever and arthritis are the two most common initial presenting features of acute rheumatic fever. Three fourths of patients with acute rheumatic fever have joint pain. Classically, the large joints, such as knees, ankles, elbows, and wrists, are involved and are tender, swollen, and erythematous. The pain migrates from one joint to another, each joint being involved for approximately 1 to 5 days. The arthritis persists for 2 to 4 weeks. In general, the severity of the joint symptoms is inversely proportional to the severity of cardiac involvement.

Carditis occurs in 40% to 50% of patients with the first attack of acute rheumatic fever. It may be the presenting feature but more commonly occurs after the onset of arthritis. The endocardium, myocardium, and pericardium may be involved. Carditis may be recognized by the appearance of a new significant cardiac murmur, such as mitral regurgitation or aortic regurgitation, cardiomegaly, or signs and symptoms of congestive heart failure or pericarditis. Congestive heart failure may present initially as fatigue, anorexia, unexplained shortness of breath, or cough. Chest pain may be the first manifestation of pericarditis. Carditis may be insidious and be apparent only by the presence of tachycardia that is disproportionate to the fever during sleep. Also, arrhythmia may be the first manifestation of carditis.

Chorea is a late manifestation of acute rheumatic fever, but the latter condition must be considered in the differential diagnosis of patients with chorea, particularly those aged between 7 and 14 years. Rheumatic chorea is more common in girls than boys and is a rare manifestation of acute rheumatic fever after puberty.

Erythema marginatum is an unusual manifestation of acute rheumatic fever but, if present, is helpful in establishing the diagnosis, particularly in association with other manifestations of the disorder. Erythema marginatum is not pathognomonic for acute rheumatic fever because it can also occur as a manifestation of drug reactions. Erythema marginatum occurs predominantly on the trunk and medial aspect of the proximal parts of the extremities. The eruption begins as pink-colored, slightly raised nonpruritic macules. The borders of the lesions migrate peripherally as the central areas assume normal skin appearance. Heat applied to the skin can accentuate the appearance of erythema marginatum.

Subcutaneous nodules occur in 7% to 20% of patients with acute rheumatic fever. They occur on extensor surfaces, over the spine, and on the scalp. They are nontender, nonpruritic, firm, painless masses. Usually, the diagnosis of acute rheumatic fever would already have been established by the time the subcutaneous nodules appear. In general, subcutaneous nodules occur in patients with relatively severe carditis.

Acute rheumatic fever also may present with abdominal pain, epistaxis, or pneumonia. There have been cases where patients with unsuspected acute rheumatic fever have undergone laparotomy because of an incorrect diagnosis of acute appendicitis.

Many conditions share the clinical manifestations of acute rheumatic fever (see Table 12.1). Many of these conditions are acute self-limiting processes that do not require long-term prophylaxis and are unassociated with an increased risk of cardiac dysfunction. Although it is important to identify a person with acute rheumatic fever, it is equally important not to mislabel patients who do not have acute rheumatic fever. To assist in this distinction, the Jones criteria were developed in the 1940s. The diagnosis of acute rheumatic fever can be made if the patient exhibits two of the major manifestations or one major manifestation and two minor manifestations *and* has evidence of previous streptococcal infection (see Table 12.2).

It must be stressed that evidence of a streptococcal infection must be present *in addition to* the major and minor manifestations. The one exception is the diagnosis of acute rheumatic fever on the basis of an otherwise unexplained chorea. In this case, evidence of

TABLE 12.1

Differential Diagnosis of Rheumatic Fever

Juvenile rheumatoid arthritis
Acute transient synovitis
Innocent murmur with febrile illness
Viral myocarditis
Bacterial arthritis
Sickle cell anemia
Periarteritis nodosa
Kawasaki disease
Lupus erythematous
Dermatomyositis
Henoch-Schönlein purpura
Legg-Calvé-Perthes disease
Slipped capital femoral epiphysis
Leukemia
Habit spasms (tics)
Lyme disease

current or prior streptococcal infection is not necessary. A throat culture and appropriate antistreptococcal enzyme assays should be performed on all patients with suspected acute rheumatic fever to detect any evidence of streptococcal infection. The antistreptolysin O antibody titer is abnormally elevated or an increase or decrease of more than two tube dilutions can be documented in 70% to 85% of patients with acute rheumatic fever. A single value of 500 U is considered indicative of streptococcal infection, and a value of 333 U is of borderline significance. If the antistreptolysin O titer is 333 U or less, additional antistreptococcal antibody assays should be performed. These include antideoxyribonuclease II, anti–nicotinamide adenine dinucleotidase, antihyaluronidase, and antistreptokinase. When the levels of three different streptococcal antibodies are measured, >95% of patients with acute rheumatic fever will have abnormal elevation of at least one. The streptozyme test includes an assay for antibodies against five extracellular antigens of group A β-hemolytic streptococci (streptolysin O, hyaluronidase, streptokinase, deoxyribonuclease II, and nicotinamide adenine dinucleotidase). Unfortunately, false-positive streptozyme test results are common, and the streptozyme test should not be used as a screening test. The streptozyme test is useful in conjunction with a negative or borderline antistreptolysin O titer. A negative result of the streptozyme test and a negative or borderline antistreptolysin O titer indicate that streptococcal infection is unlikely.

TREATMENT

The treatment of patients with acute rheumatic fever depends, to some degree, on the specific manifestations of the rheumatic fever. All patients, regardless of their manifestations, should

TABLE 12.2

Diagnosis of Rheumatic Fever

Jones Criteria	Modified Jones Criteria
Major	**Major**
Carditis	Carditis
Arthralgia	Polyarthritis
Chorea	Chorea
Subcutaneous nodules	Subcutaneous nodules
Recurrence of acute rheumatic fever	Erythema marginatum
Minor	**Minor**
Rash	Prior acute rheumatic fever
Anemia	Arthralgia
Fever	Fever
Elevated erythrocyte sedimentation rate	Elevated erythrocyte sedimentation rate, serum C-reactive
Leukocytosis	protein level
Epistaxis	Leukocytosis
Abdominal pain	Prolonged PR interval on ECG
Precordial pain	**Plus**
Rheumatic pulmonary disease	Evidence of prior streptococcal infection (throat culture,
Plus	scarlet fever, increased antistreptococcal antibodies)
Evidence of prior streptococcal infection (throat culture, scarlet fever, increased antistreptococcal antibodies)	

ECG, electrocardiogram.

have a therapeutic course of antibiotics tailored to eradicate any streptococcal infection. This should be initiated after a throat culture has been obtained to determine whether streptococci are present, but the antibiotics should be administered even in the absence of a positive throat culture. One intramuscular injection of benzathine penicillin G (600,000 to 1,200,000 U) or a 10-day course of penicillin G (200,000 to 250,000 U four times a day) is recommended. Patients who are allergic to penicillin should receive another appropriate antibiotic for 10 days.

As early as 1876 aspirin was recommended for the treatment of acute rheumatic fever. Although salicylates reduce fever and arthritis, there is no evidence that they prevent carditis or permanent damage to the heart. Hench et al., who discovered cortisone, were the first to use steroids in the treatment of patients with acute rheumatic fever. There have been several studies in which the incidence of cardiac disease seemed to be reduced with the use of steroids. However, there were methodologic problems with these studies, and the results probably are inconclusive. In 1955, the results of a combined UK and US study indicated no significant differences among patients treated with aspirin, cortisone, or adrenocorticotropic hormone (ACTH) and the incidence of rheumatic heart disease. The incidence of residual heart disease was related directly to the initial severity of the cardiac disease. Therefore, although aspirin and steroids remain the mainstay of the treatment of patients with acute rheumatic fever, there has been no consistent demonstration that cardiac damage is prevented or minimized by either salicylates or steroids.

Aspirin is the only anti-inflammatory agent that is recommended for the treatment of acute rheumatic fever characterized by arthritis alone or associated with minimal carditis. Minimal carditis includes the presence of minimal cardiomegaly or prolonged PR interval on the electrocardiogram alone or a grade 1/6 to 2/6 apical systolic murmur. The dosage of aspirin is 90 to 120 mg/kg/day or enough to maintain a serum salicylate level of 15 to 25 mg per dL. One to 2 weeks of aspirin treatment is recommended when arthritis alone is present, and 2 to 4 weeks of treatment is recommended when minimal carditis is present in addition to arthritis.

If carditis is severe or moderately severe, the patient should be treated with prednisone (2 mg/kg/day, not to exceed 60 mg per day) for 1 to 4 weeks. Shortly after or simultaneous with stopping steroid therapy, aspirin (90 to 120 mg/kg/day) should be begun and continued for 1.5 to 6 months. Aspirin probably should be continued until active inflammation subsides (until the erythrocyte sedimentation rate is normal). Congestive heart failure may be treated with a digitalis preparation and diuretic drugs. If congestive heart failure is severe, oxygen inhalation may be helpful. Occasionally, operative repair or replacement of a severely compromised cardiac valve may be necessary during acute rheumatic fever if signs and symptoms of severe congestive heart failure are unresponsive to medical therapy.

The importance of bed rest in the treatment of acute rheumatic fever is based on clinical observation and a little scientific investigation. In general, patients with chorea will prefer bed rest because of ataxia and those with arthritis will prefer bed rest because of joint pain. Bed rest for patients with carditis should be tempered by the severity of the carditis, congestive heart failure, and arrhythmia.

Rheumatic chorea is treated by maintaining the patient in a quiet environment. If choreiform movements are severe, the patient's bed rails may have to be cushioned to prevent inadvertent injury. Pharmacologic therapy to control the chorea until it resolves may be helpful.

SEQUELAE

The only serious sequela of acute rheumatic fever is cardiac damage, particularly cardiac valve damage. The mitral and aortic valves are affected most frequently. In general, the severity of chronic rheumatic cardiac disease is proportional to the severity of the initial carditis during an episode of acute rheumatic fever. The clinical features of chronic rheumatic valvular disease depend on the valve affected and the severity of the valvular dysfunction. Also, specific treatment for chronic rheumatic valvular disease is dependent on the severity of the valve dysfunction. Although valvular heart disease is the most common cardiac manifestation of acute rheumatic fever, certain forms of congestive cardiomyopathy may be a late sequela of acute rheumatic fever.

PREVENTION

There are three aspects to the prevention of acute rheumatic fever and its sequelae: (i) Prevention of acute rheumatic fever by accurate and prompt recognition and treatment of streptococcal pharyngitis, (ii) prevention of recurrent acute rheumatic fever through compulsive ongoing prophylaxis against streptococcal infection, and (iii) prevention of bacterial endocarditis in individuals with chronic rheumatic cardiac valve disease.

It is difficult to distinguish clinically between streptococcal pharyngitis and viral pharyngitis. However, an abrupt onset of tender cervical lymphadenopathy, tonsillopharyngeal exudate, headache, anorexia, abdominal pain, and vomiting suggests the possibility of streptococcal pharyngitis. Streptococcal pharyngitis can still be present without these signs and symptoms. The presence of upper respiratory tract symptoms such as rhinitis and conjunctivitis suggests a viral cause for the pharyngitis, but streptococcal infection can cause nasopharyngitis or can be associated with a concomitant viral respiratory tract infection. A throat culture is necessary for an accurate diagnosis of streptococcal pharyngitis. The culture should be obtained by vigorously swabbing both tonsillar pillars and posterior pharynx. The presence of streptococci in the throat of a patient with pharyngitis does not, however, indicate that the organism and the pharyngitis are causally related. Streptococci are not responsible for the disease process in as many as 50% of patients from whom these organisms are isolated from the pharynx and who may be the carriers of the same. Whether a patient is a carrier or the pharyngitis is caused by a new streptococcal infection can be ascertained by an abnormal increase in the level of antistreptococcal antibodies. However, by the time this assessment has been completed, it would be too late to provide adequate treatment with appropriate antibiotics to prevent acute rheumatic fever. Therefore, from a practical standpoint, one must treat all patients with pharyngitis in whom the throat culture is positive for streptococci, recognizing that chronic carriers of streptococci may be treated unnecessarily.

Antibiotic therapy for streptococcal pharyngitis will effectively prevent acute rheumatic fever if the treatment is begun within 7 to 8 days of the onset of pharyngitis. The antibiotic therapy can be delayed until the result of the throat culture is available. However, antibiotic therapy should be started immediately for patients with symptoms of pharyngitis and prior acute rheumatic fever and for those who are at increased risk of spreading streptococcal infection, such as medical personnel and teachers. Antibiotics can then be discontinued in these patients if the throat culture does not reveal streptococcal infection. Patients should not be treated with tetracycline because some strains of streptococci are resistant to this antibiotic. Also, sulfonamide drugs should not be used because these drugs may suppress but not eradicate the streptococcal infection.

Siblings and other household contacts of a patient with acute rheumatic fever should have a throat culture and, if the culture is positive for streptococci, should be treated with appropriate antibiotics although asymptomatic. Household contacts of an index patient with streptococcal pharyngitis who have recently had symptoms suggestive of streptococcal disease should have a throat culture and, if the result is positive, should be treated with appropriate antibiotics. Except during specific outbreaks of streptococcal disease, culturing specimens from asymptomatic household contacts of patients with streptococcal pharyngitis is thought to be unnecessary.

It is essential to prevent recurrent attacks of rheumatic fever. A high risk of recurrence is associated with (i) symptoms of pharyngitis, (ii) young age, (iii) a brief time since the last episode of acute rheumatic fever, (iv) existing rheumatic heart disease, (v) the number of prior attacks of acute rheumatic fever, and (vi) oral rather than parenteral prophylaxis. Prophylaxis should be begun during the initial episode of rheumatic fever. Parenteral administration of 600,000 to 1.2 million U of benzathine penicillin G every 4 weeks is the most effective prophylactic regimen. Reliable patients who have a history of excellent compliance in the use of drugs can receive oral prophylaxis with sulfadiazine (1 g per day for patients weighing >27 kg and 0.5 g per day for those weighing <27 kg), penicillin G (200,000 to 250,000 U by mouth twice a day), or erythromycin (250 mg by mouth twice a day). Because of possible poor compliance with drug regimens, most children and adolescents should receive intramuscular prophylaxis.

The duration of prophylaxis against secondary rheumatic fever is controversial, but the following guidelines may be helpful. Patients who had rheumatic fever without carditis should receive prophylaxis for 5 years or up to 21 years, which ever is longer. Patients who had rheumatic fever with healed carditis but no valvular disease should receive prophylaxis for 10 years or well into adulthood, whichever is longer. Patients with residual carditis (persistent valvular disease) should receive prophylaxis until at least 40 years of age, for at least 10 years after the last episode, or perhaps for life.

Patients with rheumatic cardiac valve disease require prophylaxis against endocarditis. They should receive appropriate prophylaxis against infectious endocarditis (IE) while undergoing invasive procedures that involve nonsterile areas. Some of these include dental cleaning, dental extraction, dental implant, placement of orthodontic bands, tonsillectomy, surgery of the mucosa, rigid bronchoscopy, sclerotherapy for varices, stricture dilation, endoscopic retrograde cholangiopancreatography, cystoscopy, and urethral dilation. The specific guidelines for prophylaxis are periodically updated by the American Heart Association, and the reader should refer to the most recent recommendations.

The penicillin regimen designed for prophylaxis against recurrent rheumatic fever is inadequate for that against bacterial endocarditis because of the emergence of penicillin-resistant oral streptococci in patients receiving penicillin for prophylaxis against rheumatic fever. Therefore, for patients receiving monthly or daily penicillin prophylaxis for acute rheumatic fever, erythromycin or another appropriate antibiotic should be used for prophylaxis against bacterial endocarditis.

KAWASAKI DISEASE

Kawasaki disease is a generalized, acute, self-limited vasculitis of unknown cause. The peak incidence is between 1 and 2 years of age, and 85% of cases occur in children younger than 5 years. The incidence ranges from 9 to 33 per 100,000 in children <5 years old depending upon ethnicity. It is most common in Japanese and other Asian and Pacific children. Although the inflammatory component is self-limited, the disease can produce coronary artery and other systemic artery aneurysms, thromboses, and obstructions. Coronary artery involvement occurs in 15% to 25% of untreated children. It is the most important sequela of Kawasaki disease and can result in myocardial infarction and death.

There is no specific laboratory test for Kawasaki disease. The diagnosis is based on clinical features (see Table 12.3). In general, fever that persists for at least 5 days and at least four of the five principal clinical findings listed in Table 12.3 are necessary to establish the diagnosis. For patients with fever and four or more of the diagnostic criteria, the diagnosis can be made on day 4 of illness. For patients with at least 5 days of fever and fewer than four of the principal clinical features, the diagnosis can be made if there are typical coronary artery abnormalities.

However, there are "incomplete or atypical cases" of Kawasaki disease with classic coronary artery aneurysms or evidence of coronary arteritis (ectasia, perivascular brightness) but fewer than four of the clinical findings listed in Table 12.3. One should consider doing an echocardiogram in infants with persistent unexplained fever to detect coronary changes indicating the presence of Kawasaki disease.

Evidence of myocardial inflammation can be found in approximately 25% of patients with Kawasaki disease. Coronary aneurysms or ectasia develop in 15% to 25% of cases of Kawasaki disease, but they resolve in at least 50% of the cases. The following are risk factors for the development of coronary aneurysms: Male gender, age <1 year, hematocrit <35%, white blood cell count >12,000 × 10^9/L, platelet count <350,000 × 10^9/L, albumin

TABLE 12.3

Clinical Features of Kawasaki Disease

Fever for at least 5 d

Five principal features

1. Peripheral extremity changes: erythema and edema of hands and feet, membranous desquamation of fingertips
2. Polymorphous exanthem
3. Bilateral nonexudative, painless bulbar conjunctival infection
4. Erythema and cracking of lips, strawberry tongue, diffuse infection of oral and pharyngeal mucosa
5. Acute, nonpurulent cervical lymphadenopathy

level <3.5 g per dL, and elevated C-reactive protein level. The most important risk factor for the development of coronary artery obstruction is giant (>8 mm in diameter) coronary aneurysms.

The goals of treatment are to prevent the development of coronary artery aneurysms and to reduce discomfort from the acute inflammatory illness. There has been debate over whether aspirin treatment reduces the incidence of coronary artery aneurysms, but despite this debate, aspirin is used because it relieves symptoms. "High-dosage" aspirin (80 to 100 mg/kg/day in four divided doses) should be started as soon as the diagnosis is made. It is not clear how long high-dosage aspirin should be continued before reducing it to "low dosage" (3 to 5 mg/kg/day). Some experts change the dosage after the child has been afebrile for 48 to 72 hours and others continue high-dosage aspirin until day 14 of illness.

There is good evidence that intravenous gamma globulin (IVIG), particularly when given early in the course of the illness, reduces the incidence of coronary artery aneurysms. This treatment is now standard. IVIG should be administered at a dose of 2 g per kg in a single infusion as soon as the diagnosis is established. Approximately 10% of patients will continue to have fever or have an early recrudescence of fever after treatment with IVIG and aspirin. These patients should be treated with a second dose of IVIG.

The role of steroids in the treatment of Kawasaki disease has been controversial. In one of the earliest reports on the treatment of Kawasaki disease, patients in one arm of the study who received steroids appeared to have a higher incidence of coronary aneurysm than those in other arms of the study. Because of this study, for many years it was thought that steroids were contraindicated in Kawasaki disease. However, this study had relatively few patients and lacked the statistical power to really draw such a conclusion. There is recent evidence that steroids may, in fact, be beneficial in the treatment of Kawasaki disease. Currently, it is suggested that steroids be reserved for patients who continue to have fever and evidence of ongoing inflammation after two or more courses of IVIG. Large-scale randomized studies of the effectiveness of steroids are ongoing, and the results of these trials, no doubt, will clarify the role of steroids in the treatment of this disease.

Treatment after the acute phase of Kawasaki disease (more than 6 weeks after onset) is not well defined. The American Heart Association published guidelines for the long-term management of patients with Kawasaki disease. In patients without coronary artery aneurysms, low-dosage aspirin (3 to 5 mg/kg/day) is discontinued 6 weeks after the onset of illness if the patient is afebrile, there is no evidence of continued inflammation, and the coronary arteries are normal. For patients with coronary artery aneurysms, low-dosage aspirin is continued at least until all aneurysms have resolved. For patients with giant aneurysms, dipyridamole (3 to 6 mg/kg/day) or warfarin can be used in conjunction with low-dosage aspirin until the coronary arteries are normal.

The long-term fate of patients with persistent but nonobstructive coronary aneurysms and of those in whom the aneurysms have resolved is unclear. Presumably, these patients should have continued medical surveillance.

INFECTIOUS ENDOCARDITIS

IE is a microbial infection of the endothelial lining of the heart. Infectious *endarteritis* is a similar disease affecting the endothelium of arteries outside the heart. In this chapter, IE is used to refer to both conditions. IE most commonly is associated with congenital heart defects. The highest incidence occurs in patients with cyanotic heart disease who have had a systemic-to-pulmonary artery shunt operation. IE accounts for 1 of 1,280 pediatric hospital admissions. Its incidence is increasing probably as a result of improved survival of patients with congenital heart disease, increased survival of sick neonates, and extensive use of prosthetic valves, patches, and conduits in the repair of heart defects.

Denuded endothelium provides a nidus for platelet–fibrin clumps that, in turn, provide a substrate for bacterial colonization and development of IE. The most common microbiologic etiologic agents causing IE change over time. However, in general, *Streptococcus viridans* is the most common bacteria causing IE. This is followed by *Staphylococcus aureus*, coagulase-negative *Staphylococcus, Streptococcus pneumoniae*, and "HACEK" organisms (*Haemophilus* species, *Actinobacillus [Haemophilus] actinomycetemcomitans, Cardiobacterium hominis, Eikenella* species, and *Kingella kingae*). In addition to these bacteria, the most common fungal form of IE is caused by *Candida albicans*. This type of IE is frequently associated with indwelling catheters and frequently occurs on the right side of the heart. In 5% to 7% of cases an organism cannot be cultured.

Historically, IE was considered a disease of the left side of the heart and circulation. However, with the increased use of indwelling systemic venous and right atrial catheters, as well as the increased incidence of intravenous drug abuse, right-sided endocarditis has become relatively common.

PRESENTING SIGNS AND SYMPTOMS

The *presentation* of IE can be subtle and nonspecific. Symptoms may include fatigue, weight loss, and intermittent fever. Other presenting symptoms can include weakness, arthralgias, myalgias, weight loss, rigors, and manifestations of septic emboli such as stroke, brain abscess, mycotic aneurysm, and pneumonia or digit pain. Therefore, IE always must be considered for any patient with congenital heart disease and fever of uncertain etiology. IE is one of the great mimics of other diseases.

PHYSICAL FINDINGS

The *physical findings* can be completely normal. However, the patient may exhibit fever, a new or changing cardiac murmur, splinter hemorrhages apparent on the nail beds, conjunctival petechiae, tender subcutaneous nodules on the digits ("Osler nodes"), nontender erythematous lesions on the palms and sides of the feet ("Janeway lesions"), and splenomegaly. Neurologic findings can occur if there have been emboli to the brain. Neonates may exhibit hypotension and/or evidence of congestive heart failure.

DIAGNOSIS

The diagnosis of IE may be difficult if blood cultures are negative for bacteria ("culture-negative IE"). Also, it is important not to mistakenly make a diagnosis of IE when there is only a transient bacteremia but no endothelial or endocardial infection. Because of these issues, the "Duke Criteria" are useful for the diagnosis of IE and should be adhered to (see Tables 12.4 and 12.5).

When the diagnosis is suspected, one should obtain three blood cultures in the first 24 hours and two blood cultures in the next 24 hours. The yield from blood cultures is not improved if the blood is obtained from an artery rather than a vein or if the specimen is obtained before, during, or after a fever spike.

Echocardiography is useful in the diagnosis and management of patients with IE. It is used to detect vegetations and abscesses and assess valve function. In most cases, transthoracic echocardiography is sufficient to detect these, but if the result of this study is negative, a transesophageal echocardiogram should be performed.

TREATMENT

Antibiotics are the mainstay of treatment of IE. The choice of antibiotics, the dose and route of administration, and the duration of treatment depends primarily on the causative organism and whether the IE involves a prosthetic material present in the heart or vascular system. The recommended antibiotics change over time, and the reader should refer to a current reference source for the most recent recommendations. However, at the time this textbook was written, the following recommendations were reasonable.

For penicillin-susceptible *Streptococcus* or *Enterococcus*:

- Penicillin G 200,000 U/kg/day × 4 weeks *or*
- Ceftriaxone 100 mg/kg/day × 4 weeks *or*
- Penicillin or Ceftriaxone *plus* gentamicin 3 mg/kg/day × 2 weeks

For relative Penicillin-resistant *Streptococcus* or *Enterococcus*:

- Penicillin G 300,000 U/kg/day × 4 weeks *or*
- Ceftriaxone 100 mg/kg/day × 4 weeks *plus*
- Gentamicin 3 mg/kg/day × 2 weeks

For highly penicillin-resistant *Streptococcus* or *Enterococcus*:

- Penicillin G 300,000 U/kg/day × 4 to 6 weeks *plus*
- Gentamicin 3 mg/kg/day × 4 to 6 weeks

For treating staphylococcal IE:

- Native valve

  – Nafcillin 200 mg/kg/day × 6 weeks *or*
  – Cefazolin 100 mg/kg/day × 6 weeks *or*
  – Vancomycin 40 mg/kg/day × 6 weeks

TABLE 12.4

Duke Criteria for Diagnosis of Infective Endocarditis

Major Criteria	Minor Criteria

1. Blood culture positive for IE
 	
  A. Typical microorganism consistent with IE from two separate blood cultures, as noted in the following list:
    i. *Viridans streptococci,*[a] *Streptococcus bovis,* or HACEK group of organisms or
    ii. Community-acquired *Staphylococcus aureus* or *Enterococcus* in the absence of a primary focus
  or
  B. Microorganisms consistent with IE from persistently positive blood cultures defined as
    i. Cultures of two blood samples drawn 12 h apart positive for microorganisms or
    ii. All three or a majority of four separate cultures of blood (with the first and last sample drawn 1 h apart)
 	
2. Evidence of endocardial involvement
 	
  A. Positive echocardiogram for IE defined as
    i. Oscillating intracardiac mass on valve or supporting structures in the path of regurgitant jets or on implanted material in the absence of an alternative anatomic explanation or
    ii. Abscess or
    iii. New partial dehiscence of prosthetic valve
  or
  B. New valvular regurgitation (worsening or changing of preexisting murmur not sufficient)
	1. Predisposition: Predisposing heart condition or IV drug use
	2. Fever: Temperature $\geq 38.0°C$
	3. Vascular phenomena: Major arterial emboli, septic pulmonary infarcts, mycotic aneurysm, intracranial hemorrhage, conjunctival hemorrhages, and Janeway lesions
	4. Immunologic phenomena: Glomerulonephritis, Osler nodes, Roth spots, and rheumatoid factor
	5. Microbiologic evidence: Blood culture positive for microorganisms but does not meet a major criterion, as noted earlier, or a serologic evidence of active infection with organism consistent with IE
	6. Echocardiographic findings: Consistent with IE but do not meet a major criterion, as noted earlier

[a]Includes nutritionally variant strains (*Abiotrophia* species).
Excludes single positive cultures for coagulase-negative staphylococci and organisms that do not cause endocarditis.
HACEK, *Haemophilus* species, *Actinobacillus* (*Haemophilus*) *actinomycetemcomitans, Cardiobacterium hominis, Eikenella* species, and *Kingella kingae*; IE, infective endocarditis; IV, intravenous.
Reprinted from Durack D, Lukes A, Bright D. New criteria for diagnosis of infective endocarditis: Utilization of specific echocardiographic findings. *Am J Med.* 1994;96:200–209.

TABLE 12.5

Duke Clinical Criteria for Diagnosis of Infective Endocarditis

Definite IE

Pathologic Criteria

- Microorganisms: Demonstrated by culture or histology in a vegetation, a vegetation that has embolized, or an intracardiac abscess

  or
- Pathologic lesions: Presence of vegetation or intracardiac abscess, confirmed by histology showing active endocarditis

Clinical Criteria (as defined in Table 12.4)

Two major criteria *or*
One major criterion and three minor criteria or
Five minor criteria

Possible IE
Findings consistent with IE that fall short of "definite" but not "rejected"

Rejected
Firm alternative diagnosis for manifestations of endocarditis or
Resolution of manifestations of endocarditis with antibiotic therapy for 4 d or
No pathologic evidence of IE at surgery or autopsy after antibiotic therapy for 4 d

---

IE, infective endocarditis.
Reprinted from Durack D, Lukes A, Bright D. New criteria for diagnosis of infective endocarditis: Utilization of specific echocardiographic findings. *Am J Med.* 1994;96:200–209.

- Prosthetic valve

  – Above *plus*
  – Rifampin 20 mg/kg/day *plus*
  – Gentamicin 3 mg/kg/day

Although one would like to avoid cardiac operation during an episode of IE, sometimes it is necessary. Operation is indicated for (i) acute aortic or mitral insufficiency *associated with significant heart failure unresponsive to medical therapy*, (ii) prosthetic valve dehiscence, (iii) new onset of atrioventricular block, or (iv) presence of a large abscess or abscess extension. Some experts recommend operation to remove vegetations if (i) systemic embolization has occurred during the first 2 weeks of therapy, (ii) if there have been two or more embolic events during or after therapy, or (iii) if there is a mitral valve vegetation that is >10 mm subsequent to an embolic event. Operation also may be indicated for (i) cases in which the bloodstream is not sterilized despite an appropriate course of antibiotics, (ii) relapse of IE, and/or (iii) certain organisms refractory to antibiotic therapy such as *Pseudomonas aeruginosa, Brucella, Coxiella burnetii,* and *Candida* and other fungi.

Treatment of IE involving a prosthetic valve or material may be particularly problematic. It is frequently necessary to remove the prosthetic valve or material to cure the patient. Unfortunately, a different valve or prosthetic material usually needs to be inserted at the time of operation into the infected area.

Patients who have had a recent neurologic complication of IE appear to be at particularly high risk for postoperative complications and death after valve surgery during the acute phases of IE.

COMPLICATIONS

Complications of IE include congestive heart failure (usually resulting from aortic or mitral valve insufficiency), embolic events (involving the brain, lungs, kidney, and coronary artery), perivalve abscess, atrioventricular block, prosthetic valve dehiscence, and metastatic infection (including mycotic aneurysms and glomerulonephritis with or without renal failure).

PROPHYLAXIS

Antibiotic prophylaxis against IE is indicated for the following situations: Prosthetic, bioprosthetic, and homograft valves; prior episode of endocarditis; cyanotic heart disease; surgically constructed systemic-to-pulmonary artery shunts and conduits; most congenital heart defects (see in the subsequent text for exceptions to this); acquired valve dysfunction; hypertrophic cardiomyopathy; and mitral valve prolapse with insufficiency or thickened leaflets. Patients with these conditions should receive appropriate prophylaxis against IE while undergoing invasive procedures that involve nonsterile areas. Some of these include dental cleaning, dental extraction, implant, placement of orthodontic bands, tonsillectomy, surgery of the mucosa, rigid bronchoscopy, sclerotherapy for varices, stricture dilation, ERCP, cystoscopy, and urethral dilation. The specific guidelines for prophylaxis are periodically updated by the American Heart Association, and the reader should refer to the most recent recommendations.

Prophylaxis is *not* necessary for the following situations: Isolated *secundum* atrial septal defect, surgically repaired (without residual hole) ventricular septal defect (>6 months postoperatively), or repaired ductus arteriosus without residual shunt. Prophylaxis also is not required in case of prior coronary artery bypass grafting, mitral valve prolapse without mitral regurgitation or thickened leaflets, innocent heart murmurs, prior Kawasaki disease or rheumatic fever without valve dysfunction, presence of pacemakers, or implanted defibrillators or stents.

SELECTED REFERENCES

Bisno AL, Group A streptococcal infections and acute rheumatic fever. *N Engl J Med*. 1991;325:783–793.

Dajani A, Taubert K, Wilson W, et al. Prevention of bacterial endocarditis: Recommendations by the American Heart Association. *JAMA*. 1997;277:1794–1801.

Dajani A, Taubert K, Ferrieri P, et al. Treatment of acute streptococcal pharyngitis and prevention of rheumatic fever: A statement for health professionals by the Committee on Rheumatic Fever, Endocarditis, and Kawasaki Disease of the Council on Cardiovascular Disease in the Young, The American Heart Association. *Pediatrics*. 1995;96:758–764.

Dajani A, Taubert KA, Takahashi M, et al. Guidelines for long-term management of patients with Kawasaki disease: Report from the Committee on Rheumatic Fever, Endocarditis, and Kawasaki Disease in the Young, American Heart Association. *Circulation*. 1994;89:916–922.

Dochez AR, Avery OT, Lancefield RC. Studies on the biology of streptococcus. I. Antigenic relationships between strains of streptococcus haemolyticus. *J Exp Med*. 1919;30:179–213.

Durack D, Lukes A, Bright D. New criteria for diagnosis of infective endocarditis: Utilization of specific echocardiographic findings. *Am J Med*. 1994;96:200–209.

Ferrieri P, Gewitz M, Gerber M, et al. AHA Scientific Statement, Unique Features of Infective Endocarditis in Childhood. *Circulation*. 2002;105:2115–2127.

Gersony WM. Diagnosis and management of Kawasaki disease. *JAMA*. 1991;265:2699–2703.

Gordis L, Lilienfeld A, Rodriguez R. Studies in the epidemiology and preventability of rheumatic fever − II: Socioeconomic factors and the incidence of acute attacks. *J Chronic Dis*. 1969;21:655–666.

Kaplan EL. Acute rheumatic fever. *Pediatr Clin North Am*. 1978;25:817–829.

Kaplan MH. Rheumatic fever, rheumatic heart disease, and the streptococcal connection: The role of streptococcal antigens cross reactive with heart tissue. *Rev Infect Dis*. 1979;1:988–996.

Kaplan MH, Frengley JD. Autoimmunity to the heart in cardiac disease: Current concepts of the relation of autoimmunity to rheumatic fever, postcardiotomy and postinfarction syndromes and cardiomyopathies. *Am J Cardiol*. 1969;24:459–473.

Kaplan EL, Top FH, Dudding BA Jr, et al. Diagnosis of streptococcal pharyngitis: Differentiation of active infection from the carrier state in the symptomatic child. *J Infect Dis*. 1971;123:490–501.

Kawasaki T. Kawasaki disease. *Cardiol Young*. 1991;1:184–191.

Lancefield RC. Specific relationship of cell composition to biological activity of hemolytic streptococci. *Harvey Lect*. 1941;36:251–290.

Markowitz M, Kuttner AG. Rheumatic fever: Diagnosis, management and prevention. *Major Probl Clin Pediatr*. 1965;2:1–242.

McCrindle B, ed. Advances in Kawasaki Disease. *Prog Pediatr Cardiol*. 2004;19:91–206.

Mylonakis E, Calderwoodl S. Infective endocarditis in adults. *N Engl J Med*. 2001;345:1318–1330.

Newburger JW, Takahashi M, Beiser AS, et al. A single intravenous infusion of gamma globulin as compared with four infusions in the treatment of acute Kawasaki syndrome. *N Engl J Med*. 1991;324:1633–1639.

Newburger J, Takahashi M, Gerber M, et al. Treatment, and long-term management of Kawasaki disease. *Circulation*. 2004;110:2747–2771.

Spagnuoto M, Pasternack B, Taranta A. Risk of rheumatic-fever recurrences after streptococcal infections: Prospective study of clinical and social factors. *N Engl J Med*. 1971;285:641–647.

Stollerman GH. *Rheumatic fever and streptococcal infection*. New York: Grune & Stratton; 1975.

Stollerman GH, Lewis AJ, Schultz I, et al. Relationship of immune response to group A streptococci to the course of acute, chronic and recurrent rheumatic fever. *Am J Med*. 1956;20:163–169.

Wannamaker LW. The differentiation of three distinct desoxyribonucleases of group A streptococci. *J Exp Med*. 1958;107:797–812.

Wannamaker LW. Characterization of a fourth desoxyribonuclease of group A streptococci (abstract). *Fed Proc*. 1962;21:231.

Wannamaker LW. Perplexity and precision in the diagnosis of streptococcal pharyngitis. *Am J Dis Child*. 1972;124:352–358.

Zabriskie JB. Rheumatic fever: A streptococcal-induced autoimmune disease? *Pediatr Ann*. 1982;11:383–396.

Portions of the text have been published previously and are reproduced with permission of the publisher:

Driscoll DJ, Acute rheumatic fever. In: Brandenburg R, Fuster V, Giuliani E, et al., eds. *Cardiology: Fundamentals and practice*. Mosby–Year Book 1987:1380–1385.

Driscoll DJ. Acute rheumatic fever. In: Giuliani E, Fuster V, Gersh, B, et al., eds. *Cardiology: Fundamentals and practice*. Mosby–Year Book; 1991:1610–1616.

Driscoll D. Rheumatic fever and Kawasaki disease. In: Giuliani E, Gersh B, McGoon M, et al., eds. *Mayo clinic practice of cardiology*, 3rd ed, Mosby–Year Book; 1996:1642–1648.

CHAPTER 13

Cardiomyopathy

"If it takes more than 10 minutes of discussion to decide if a patient needs an operation, it is best not to operate"

There are three distinct cardiomyopathies: Hypertrophic, dilated or congestive, and restrictive. Recently, a fourth type, "ventricular noncompaction" has been described.

HYPERTROPHIC CARDIOMYOPATHY

Hypertrophic cardiomyopathy (HC) is a condition in which myocardial thickness is increased. In general, the septal thickness is more marked than that of the posterior wall (see Fig. 13.1). There may or may not be left ventricular (and in some cases, right ventricular) outflow tract obstruction. If there is left ventricular outflow tract obstruction, the condition is termed *hypertrophic obstructive cardiomyopathy* (HOCM). If there is no left ventricular outflow tract obstruction, it is termed *hypertrophic nonobstructive cardiomyopathy*. When there is left ventricular outflow tract obstruction usually there is systolic anterior motion of the mitral valve apparent on echocardiography. Mitral insufficiency frequently can be associated with HC. HC can be associated with chest pain, shortness of breath, exercise intolerance, syncope, and sudden death. It is the most common identifiable nontraumatic cause of death on the athletic field.

ETIOLOGY AND GENETICS

Left ventricular septal and posterior wall hypertrophy can result from numerous causes. However the terms *obstructive* and *nonobstructive HC* usually imply an autosomal dominant condition that results from mutations in one of the following genes that encode proteins of the cardiac sarcomere: β-Myosin heavy chain, cardiac troponin T, α-tropomyosin, and myosin-binding protein C genes, as well as in two genes encoding the myosin light chains. As more causative genes are discovered, the taxonomy for what might now be considered the "wastebasket" term "HC" will change completely. This will be necessary because knowledge of the specific gene defect will allow better definition of the natural history of the disease.

Therefore, when faced with a patient who is known (usually because of an echocardiogram) to have abnormally thick left ventricular walls one must ascertain the cause of

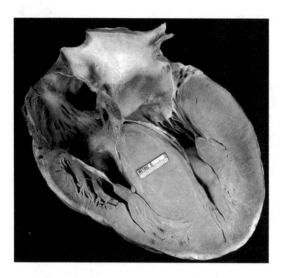

FIGURE 13.1 ● Pathologic specimen of hypertrophic cardiomyopathy. Note the markedly thickened septum and left ventricular posterior wall.

the ventricular hypertrophy. This is particularly important for infants and young children because some believe that in these age-groups one is more likely to find underlying causes for the hypertrophy than in older age-groups.

In the newborn period, it is well-recognized that infants born to mothers with diabetes can have a transient form of HC. Other conditions that can be associated with increased left ventricular wall thickness are glycogen storage diseases, mitochondrial disorders, disorders of oxidative metabolism, carnitine deficiency, β-oxidation defects, Noonan syndrome, Costello syndrome, Friedreich's ataxia, nonspecific causes of cardiac inflammation, and steroid administration among others. Once all of these causes have been eliminated, one is left with a diagnosis of HC presumably resulting from sarcomere mutations, which, with the current state of knowledge, are lumped together for purposes of ascertaining the natural history and the results of treatment.

Once a diagnosis of a presumed sarcomeric form of HC is made, first-degree relatives of the index cases should undergo echocardiograms to screen for familial cases. For first-degree relatives with normal echocardiograms, the interval between subsequent screenings is unclear. Some investigators have suggested yearly screening for children and adolescents on the assumption that HC is more likely to become apparent during the years of rapid growth. Other investigators think that screening echocardiograms every 2 to 5 years is reasonable. Gene testing to identify affected family members is becoming available. Initially, one needs to identify the gene mutation in the patient and then screen the family members for that gene.

HISTORY

Patients with HC usually come to medical attention in one or more of the following ways: Detection of a murmur, an abnormal electrocardiogram, from family screening or a positive family history, from evaluation of syncope, chest pain, palpitations, or out of hospital cardiac arrest.

PHYSICAL EXAMINATION

The physical findings can be variable. For patients with nonobstructive forms of HC, there is no characteristic murmur. There may or may not be a prominent apical impulse, and an S_4.

In some patients, obstruction can be unmasked and a murmur will appear with maneuvers to lower systemic vascular resistance such as inhalation of amyl nitrate or assuming a standing position.

Patients with obstructive HC will have systolic ejection murmur. Unfortunately, in subtle cases one can mistake this murmur for an innocent flow murmur. There may be a bifid pulse.

ELECTROCARDIOGRAM

The classic electrocardiogram shows evidence of left and frequently biventricular hypertrophy. For patients with HC and restrictive left ventricular filling, there can be evidence of atrial enlargement.

CHEST X-RAY

The chest x-ray is not diagnostic.

ECHOCARDIOGRAPHY

The echocardiogram is most important in making the diagnosis of HC. Classically, there will be asymmetric septal hypertrophy and systolic anterior motion of the mitral valve. Echocardiography and Doppler sonography will allow assessment of the absence, presence, and degree of left and right ventricular outflow tract obstruction. Echocardiography allows quantification of the thickness of the ventricular walls.

NATURAL HISTORY AND TREATMENT

Although HC can be associated with symptoms of fatigue, shortness of breath, chest pain, and palpitations, the most important concern is the increased risk of sudden death. The exact magnitude of the risk of sudden death is still being clarified. In the past, it was thought that the risk of sudden death was 3% per year. However, more recent population-based studies indicate that the risk is closer to 1% per year. Several years ago, it was thought that one could predict patients who were at high risk of death by the specific gene defect causing the HC. Unfortunately, this has not proved to be correct. However, as more genes are identified and larger cohorts of patients with specific gene mutations are identified, this may yet be the case.

The ability to identify patients at high risk for sudden death is still crude but the following features may be associated with higher risk for sudden death: Diagnosis in childhood, septal thickness exceeding 30 mm, nonsustained ventricular tachycardia, failure of normal increase of systolic blood pressure during exercise, family history of premature death associated with HC, significant left ventricular outflow tract obstruction, and prior cardiac arrest.

The current paradigm for treating HC is to identify those patients at high risk for sudden death and implant an automatic internal cardiac defibrillator (AICD). There is reasonably good data that this strategy prolongs life. However, it is not clear which patients are at high enough risk to have this rather expensive treatment.

For symptomatic patients who are not at high risk for sudden death and do not qualify for implantation of an AICD, treatment with a β-blocker or amiodarone can be considered.

For patients with significant left ventricular outflow tract obstruction, surgical myotomy/ myectomy, or alcohol ablation can be done. There is increasing evidence that elimination of the obstruction prolongs life and relieves symptoms.

Patients with HC should be restricted from competitive athletics.

DILATED OR CONGESTIVE CARDIOMYOPATHY

Dilated or congestive cardiomyopathy is a descriptive diagnosis implying that the left ventricle is dilated with reduced systolic function (see Fig. 13.2). Normal left ventricular ejection fraction is 50% to 60%. Anything <50% is abnormal and could indicate the presence of dilated cardiomyopathy.

ETIOLOGY AND GENETICS

Dilated cardiomyopathy can result from a variety of specific disorders. If no specific disorder is identified, it is termed *idiopathic dilated cardiomyopathy*. Some of the specific disorders include: Carnitine deficiency, β-oxidation defects, selenium deficiency, mitochondrial defects, myocarditis, coronary artery anomalies (anomalous origin of the left coronary artery from the pulmonary artery), thyrotoxicosis, storage diseases, amyloidosis, and postpartum cardiomyopathy among many others. Dilated cardiomyopathy can be induced by alcohol, tachycardia, or drugs (i.e., doxorubicin [Adriamycin], cocaine). It is generally thought that in the absence of any explanation for the cardiomyopathy, a prior unrecognized viral myocarditis may be the culprit. Several gene defects have been described as causing dilated cardiomyopathy (see Table 13.1). Additional genes will be described in the future.

The genetic aspects of dilated cardiomyopathy depend on the underlying cause. However, for idiopathic dilated cardiomyopathy 20% to 30% of index cases will have family members with abnormal ventricular function. Currently, it is unclear if conditions such as alcoholic-associated cardiomyopathy and postpartum cardiomyopathy are distinct disorders or simply "second hits" that result in the clinical expression of dilated cardiomyopathy in patients with a familial predisposition to develop cardiomyopathy.

HISTORY

Infants and young children may present with a murmur of mitral valve insufficiency or signs and symptoms of congestive heart failure. These may include tachypnea, poor feeding, poor

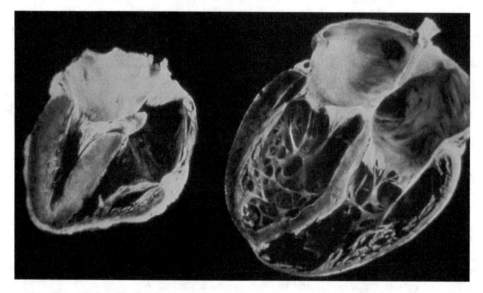

FIGURE 13.2 ● Normal heart on the left compared to dilated cardiomyopathy on the right.

TABLE 13.1

Mutations Associated with Dilated Cardiomyopathy

Cardiac actin	Metavinculin	α-Myosin heavy chain
Desmin	Myosin-binding protein C	SUR2A
δ-Sarcoglycan	Muscle LIM protein	Lamin A/C
β-Myosin heavy chain	α-Actin-2	Dystrophin
Cardiac troponin T	Phospholamban	Tafazzin
α-Tropomyosin	Cypher/LIM binding domain 3	Cardiac troponin I
Titin		

weight gain, tachycardia, fussiness, and/or chest congestion. Older patients may present with fatigue, shortness of breath, exercise intolerance, syncope, and/or arrhythmia. Obviously, it is important to obtain a history of prior infectious illness, and alcohol and drug use.

PHYSICAL EXAMINATION

It is possible for a patient to have dilated cardiomyopathy and yet have a perfectly normal physical examination. However, most patients will have an abnormal physical examination. In infants, there may be tachypnea, intercostal and/or subcostal retractions, tachycardia, sweating, and evidence of poor weight gain. The first sound is usually normal. The second heart sound may be increased if there is associated pulmonary hypertension. There may be a holosystolic midfrequency murmur of mitral regurgitation and a diastolic gallop rhythm at the apex of the heart. Older patients may have auscultatory findings similar to that of the infant. Older patients will be less likely to have retractions but may have pulmonary rales. It is impossible to make a firm diagnosis of dilated cardiomyopathy based on the physical examination alone.

ELECTROCARDIOGRAM

The features of the electrocardiogram depend, to some extent, on the cause of the dilated cardiomyopathy. For example, an infant with cardiomyopathy secondary to anomalous origin of the left coronary artery from the aorta may have evidence of a myocardial infarction and ischemia. This may include left axis deviation, poor precordial R-wave progression, Q waves in the inferior and precordial leads, as well as ST elevation in the precordial leads. A patient with dilated cardiomyopathy secondary to Pompe disease will have a short PR interval and very large QRS voltages especially in the precordial leads. A patient with tachycardia-induced dilated cardiomyopathy may have tachycardia and evidence of an ectopic atrial rhythm or atrial flutter. Beware!!!! It is very easy to overlook an important atrial tachyarrhythmia in this setting. A common mistake is to attribute a higher than normal heart rate, such as 120 to 140 beats per minute, to a heart failure instead of recognizing the fact that the patient has a primary tachycardia causing the heart failure. It is not uncommon for patients to be referred for cardiac transplantation for "idiopathic dilated cardiomyopathy" when in fact they have tachycardia-induced cardiomyopathy, and once recognized and treated appropriately are completely cured.

In cases of idiopathic dilated cardiomyopathy, the electrocardiographic features are non-specific and may include evidence of atrial enlargement and/or ventricular enlargement.

CHEST X-RAY

The chest x-ray usually demonstrates cardiomegaly and may show evidence of pulmonary congestion or pulmonary venous hypertension. Somewhat surprisingly, a few patients with dilated cardiomyopathy will have a normal heart size on the chest x-ray.

ECHOCARDIOGRAM

The echocardiogram is essential to establish a diagnosis of dilated cardiomyopathy. The *sine quo non* is reduced ejection fraction and increased diastolic and/or systolic left ventricular dimensions. One also can determine the ventricular wall thickness that may have important prognostic implications. Some investigators have found that patients with dilated cardiomyopathy and normal or increased left ventricular wall thickness have a better prognosis than those with thin walls.

It is critical, especially in infants, to establish that both coronary arteries originate from the aorta; that is, to absolutely exclude the presence of anomalous origin of the left coronary artery from the pulmonary artery. Even experienced echocardiographers can miss this diagnosis by erroneously interpreting a portion of the transverse sinus as the left coronary artery.

NATURAL HISTORY AND TREATMENT

The natural history of dilated cardiomyopathy depends on the underlying cause. For example, infants with cardiomyopathy secondary to anomalous origin of the left coronary artery from the aorta, generally, will do very well if the condition is diagnosed early and the operation is performed to attach the anomalous coronary artery to the aorta. Patients with cardiomyopathy secondary to carnitine deficiency will do very well if the diagnosis is made early in life and appropriately treated with carnitine replacement. Patients with acute myocarditis can improve as the myocarditis wanes. Patients with tachycardia-induced cardiomyopathy, usually, will improve significantly. Frequently, the cardiomyopathy will resolve completely once the tachycardia is controlled.

For patients with idiopathic dilated cardiomyopathy, the rule of thumb is that one third will have improvement of cardiac function, in one third cardiac function will remain about the same but the patient survives for many years, and one third will continue to get worse and either die or have cardiac transplantation. These ratios have been true for many years and remain true today. Hopefully, with newer drugs to treat myocardial dysfunction the outlook will improve.

Obviously, the underlying cause of the cardiomyopathy, if known, must be treated. The differential diagnosis will differ depending upon the age at presentation. In older patients, myocarditis, tachycardia-induced, or familial, and idiopathic dilated cardiomyopathy are probably the most common causes. For infants, one must exclude metabolic causes. The following are reasonable initial screening tests for metabolic causes of cardiomyopathy: Plasma amino acids, free and total carnitine, lactate and pyruvate, ammonia, fasting glucose, selenium, as well as urine organic acids, screening for inborn errors of metabolism, and acylcarnitine.

There have been tremendous improvements in the pharmacologic therapy of myocardial dysfunction in the past 15 years. Patients with depressed myocardial function should be treated with appropriate doses of an angiotensin-converting enzyme (ACE) inhibitor, β-blocker, spironolactone, and diuretics. The role of digitalis in this setting continues to be debated. However, this drug was the mainstay of therapy for "dropsy" since Withering described digitalis in the 18th century. Most experienced clinicians continue to use digitalis. One of the major mistakes in treating children with dilated cardiomyopathy is not using appropriate drugs in appropriate doses.

Left ventricular function will improve for most patients when treated with appropriate drugs. Indeed, ventricular function may become normal. The question that then arises is when should the drugs be discontinued? The answer to this question is elusive and probably varies for different patients. Once ventricular function becomes normal, it may be reasonable to wean and discontinue diuretics other than spironolactone. It is difficult to know, among an ACE inhibitor, β-blocker, and spironolactone, which to discontinue; but I prefer to discontinue them in the following order: Spironolactone, β-blocker, and lastly the ACE inhibitor. As one discontinues the drugs one must monitor ventricular function, and if ventricular function declines the drug regimen must be augmented.

Unfortunately, children who have recovery of ventricular function, even when it is sustained for many years, can experience a deterioration many years later. For this reason, these patients require lifelong surveillance.

Because 25% to 30% of patients with idiopathic dilated cardiomyopathy will have affected family members, echocardiographic screening of first-degree relatives is recommended.

RESTRICTIVE CARDIOMYOPATHY

Restrictive cardiomyopathy is a relatively rare form of cardiomyopathy in which diastolic function is abnormal. The ventricles are "stiff." This results in elevated atrial and end-diastolic pressures and dilated atria. In adults, amyloidosis is the most common cause of restrictive cardiomyopathy. In children, the cause of primary restrictive cardiomyopathy is unknown. The prognosis for restrictive cardiomyopathy in infants and children is very poor and cardiac transplantation is recommended soon after the diagnosis is made.

VENTRICULAR NONCOMPACTION

For many years, clinicians have been aware of hearts in which the myocardium appeared "feathery" and "embryonic." More recently, this has been thought to represent embryonic arrest in the normal development of the myocardium. As the left ventricular myocardium forms, it "compacts" eliminating deep crevices. Therefore, the appearance of left ventricle noncompaction is one of deep crevices in the left ventricle, particularly at the apex. There have been a number of studies suggesting that this is a unique form of cardiomyopathy that can be associated with arrhythmias and sudden death. The diagnosis is made by the echocardiographic appearance of the left ventricular myocardium. Unfortunately, the distinction between what is normal and what is abnormal is not perfectly clear. The diagnostic criteria and the best manner of treating this condition continue to evolve.

SELECTED REFERENCES

Akagi T, Benson L, Lightfoot NE, et al. Natural history of dilated cardiomyopathy in children. *Am Heart J*. 1991;121(5):1502–1506.

Berger S, Dhala A, Friedberg DZ. Sudden cardiac death in infants, children, and adolescents. *Pediatr Clin North Am*. 1999;46(2):221–234.

Bruno E, Maisuls H, Juaneda E, et al. Clinical features of hypertrophic cardiomyopathy in the young. *Cardiol Young*. 2002;12(2):147–152.

Bryant RM. Hypertrophic cardiomyopathy in children. *Cardiol Rev*. 1999;7(2):92–100.

Burch M, Siddiqi SA, Celermajer DS, et al. Dilated cardiomyopathy in children: Determinants of outcome. *Br Heart J*. 1994;72(3):246–250.

Cetta F, et al. Idiopathic restrictive cardiomyopathy in childhood: Diagnostic features and clinical course. *Mayo Clin Proc*. 1995;70(7):634–640.

Chen SC, Balfour IC, Jureidini S. Clinical spectrum of restrictive cardiomyopathy in children. *J Heart Lung Transplant*. 2001;20(1):90–92.

Denfield SW. Sudden death in children with restrictive cardiomyopathy. *Card Electrophysiol Rev*. 2002;6(1–2):163–167.

Gajarski RJ, Towbin JA. Recent advances in the etiology, diagnosis, and treatment of myocarditis and cardiomyopathies in children. *Curr Opin Pediatr*. 1995;7(5):587–594.

Holmgren D, Wahlander H, Eriksson BO, et al. Cardiomyopathy in children with mitochondrial disease; clinical course and cardiological findings [see comment]. *Eur Heart J*. 2003;24(3):280–288.

Lakkis N. New treatment methods for patients with hypertrophic obstructive cardiomyopathy. *Curr Opin Cardiol*. 2000;15(3):172–177.

Lemire EG. Noonan syndrome or new autosomal dominant condition with coarctation of the aorta, hypertrophic cardiomyopathy, and minor anomalies. *Am J Med Genet*. 2002;113(3):286–290.

Maron BJ. Hypertrophic cardiomyopathy: A systematic review. *JAMA*. 2002;287(10):1308–1320.

Maron BJ, Isner JM, McKenna WJ. 26th Bethesda conference: Recommendations for determining eligibility for competition in athletes with cardiovascular abnormalities. Task Force 3: Hypertrophic cardiomyopathy, myocarditis and other myopericardial diseases and mitral valve prolapse. *Med Sci Sports Exerc*. 1994;26(Suppl 10):S261–S267.

Maron BJ, McKenna WJ, Danielson GK, et al. American College of Cardiology/European Society of Cardiology clinical expert consensus document on hypertrophic cardiomyopathy. A report of the American College of Cardiology Foundation Task Force on Clinical Expert Consensus Documents and the European Society of Cardiology Committee for Practice Guidelines. *J Am Coll Cardiol*. 2003;42(9):1687–1713.

McMahon AM, van Doorn C, Burch M, et al. Improved early outcome for end-stage dilated cardiomyopathy in children [erratum appears in *J Thorac Cardiovasc Surg*. 2004;127(2):616]. *J Thorac Cardiovasc Surg*. 2003;126(6):1781–1787.

Mestroni L, et al. Guidelines for the study of familial dilated cardiomyopathies. Collaborative Research Group of the European Human and Capital Mobility Project on Familial Dilated Cardiomyopathy. *Eur Heart J*. 1999;20(2):93–102.

Nield LE, McCrindle BW, Bohn DJ, et al. Outcomes for children with cardiomyopathy awaiting transplantation. *Cardiol Young*. 2000;10(4):358–366.

Rusconi P, Gomez-Marin O, Rossique-Gonzalez M, et al. Carvedilol in children with cardiomyopathy: 3-year experience at a single institution. *J Heart Lung Transplant*. 2004;23(7):832–838.

Schowengerdt KO Jr, Towbin JA. Genetic basis of inherited cardiomyopathies. *Curr Opin Cardiol*. 1995;10(3):312–321.

Shaddy RE. Cardiomyopathies in adolescents: Dilated, hypertrophic, and restrictive. *Adoles Med State Art Rev*. 2001;12(1):35–45.

Taliercio CP, Seward JB, Driscoll DJ, et al. Idiopathic dilated cardiomyopathy in the young: Clinical profile and natural history. *J Am Coll Cardiol*. 1985;6(5):1126–1131.

Towbin JA. Molecular genetic basis of sudden cardiac death. *Pediatr Clin North Am*. 2004;51(5):1229–1255.

CHAPTER 14

Coronary Artery Anomalies

"The worst enemy of good is better"

NORMAL CORONARY ARTERY ANATOMY

There are two major coronary arteries—left and right. The left main coronary artery divides into the left anterior descending and the circumflex coronary arteries (see Fig. 14.1). Branches of the left anterior descending coronary artery include the left conus, septal, and diagonal arteries. Branches of the circumflex coronary artery may include the sinus node artery, Kugel's artery, marginal arteries, and the left atrial circumflex artery. Branches of the right coronary artery include the conal branch, the sinus node artery, an atrial branch, the right ventricular muscle branches (including the acute marginal branch), the posterior descending coronary artery, the atrioventricular node artery, and septal branches. The "dominant coronary artery" is the one giving rise to the posterior descending coronary artery. It originates from the right coronary artery in 80% of individuals and from the left coronary artery in 20% (see Fig. 14.2).

ANOMALOUS ORIGIN OF THE LEFT CORONARY ARTERY FROM THE PULMONARY ARTERY

Anomalous origin of the left coronary artery from the pulmonary artery (ALCAPA) may be the most important coronary anomaly that pediatricians and pediatric cardiologists must deal with (see Fig. 14.3). Usually, the anomalous coronary artery arises from the left sinus of the pulmonary artery. A patient with ALCAPA may present with signs and symptoms of myocardial infarction and congestive heart failure in infancy, or the condition may be unassociated with myocardial infarction or symptoms of heart disease until detected serendipitously in adulthood or at autopsy. The age at presentation depends on the amount of collateral circulation between the right and left coronary artery systems. Patients with well-developed collateral connections may not develop myocardial infarction and may do well. Patients with poor collateral circulation can have a myocardial infarction, which is apparent at an early age.

In the immediate newborn period, pulmonary artery resistance and pressure are elevated, flow through the anomalously arising left coronary artery is antegrade from the pulmonary artery, and myocardial perfusion is adequate. As pulmonary artery resistance and pulmonary pressure decrease, antegrade flow of blood from the pulmonary artery through the left

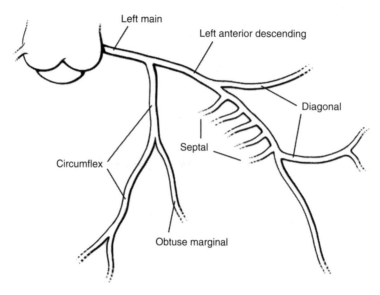

FIGURE 14.1 ● Normal left coronary artery system.

coronary artery decreases. If there is inadequate collateral circulation between the right and left coronary arteries, myocardial infarction will occur. If collateral circulation exists, myocardial infarction may or may not occur, depending on the degree of retrograde flow from the right coronary system through the collateral circulation.

Clinical features of ALCAPA in infancy are similar to those of myocarditis and cardiomyopathy, and the diagnosis of ALCAPA must be considered in the differential diagnoses of

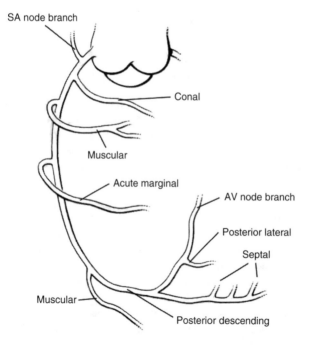

FIGURE 14.2 ● Normal right coronary artery system. SA, sinoatrial; AV, atrioventricular.

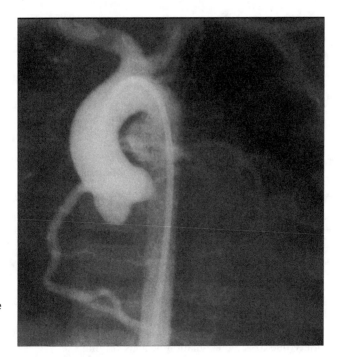

FIGURE 14.3 ● An angiogram showing the origin of the left coronary artery from the pulmonary artery. Note that the contrast was injected into the aortic root. The right coronary artery clearly originates from the aorta. However, the left coronary artery fills late and contrast is seen exiting the left coronary artery into the main pulmonary artery.

unexplained congestive heart failure and poor left ventricular function, or mitral regurgitation in infancy. In teenagers and adults, the presence of ALCAPA may be suspected if there is unexplained cardiomegaly, mitral insufficiency, or a continuous cardiac murmur. Angina may occur secondary to coronary steal. A carefully performed and accurately interpreted echocardiogram will provide the diagnosis. However, the echocardiographer must be careful not to confuse the transverse sinus with the left coronary artery.

The ideal treatment of ALCAPA is to detect the presence of the anomaly before myocardial infarction occurs and to establish a coronary system that prevents myocardial infarction. All cases in infancy, however, come to medical attention only after myocardial ischemia and infarction have occurred. Infants with ALCAPA and poor left ventricular function (ejection fraction <20%) have a poorer outcome than patients with an ejection fraction >20%.

Attempts to establish a two–coronary-artery system for patients with ALCAPA is indicated when the condition is diagnosed. There are several surgical procedures that have been described to establish the origin of both the coronary arteries from the aorta. It is unclear as to which procedure is superior, and the surgeon should use the technique with which he or she is most comfortable. Patients with ALCAPA and evidence of congestive heart failure benefit from treatment with digitalis and diuretics until surgery can be performed. Infants with evidence of acute myocardial infarction should be treated with oxygen, sedation, rest, and diuretics until surgery can be performed.

ANOMALOUS ORIGIN OF THE LEFT CORONARY ARTERY FROM THE RIGHT SINUS OF VALSALVA

Anomalous origin of the left coronary artery from the right sinus of Valsalva is a rare but important malformation because it is associated with a significant risk of sudden death (see Fig 14.4). Patients in whom the aberrantly arising left coronary artery passes between

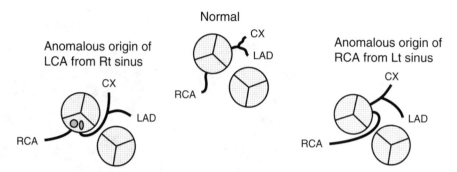

FIGURE 14.4 ● Origin of the left coronary artery (LCA) from the right aortic sinus of Valsalva (left figure). When the left coronary artery passes between the aorta and the pulmonary artery, there is a risk of sudden death. Origin of right coronary artery (RCA) from left sinus of Valsalva (right figure). Lt, left; Rt, right; CX, circumflex coronary artery; LAD, left anterior descending coronary artery; RCA, right coronary artery.

the aorta and the pulmonary artery appear to be at the greatest risk for sudden death. Sudden death is presumably due to myocardial ischemia as a result of compression of the left coronary artery between the aorta and the pulmonary artery, an elliptical rather than a circular os of the left coronary artery, and compromise of the lumen of the left coronary artery due to acute angulation near its origin.

Patients are usually asymptomatic until sudden death occurs, although some patients may have symptoms of angina or coronary insufficiency, which may include syncope or light-headedness associated with exercise. This diagnosis must be considered in children and adolescents with angina-like chest pain and exercise-associated syncope or presyncope. If this condition is suspected, exercise testing may reveal electrocardiographic evidence of ischemia, but a normal exercise study does not exclude the diagnosis. A carefully performed and properly interpreted echocardiogram will provide the diagnosis. When the left coronary artery passes between the aorta and the pulmonary artery, surgical repair is indicated to prevent sudden death. The decision of whether surgery is needed when the left coronary artery does not pass between the two great arteries is less clear.

ANOMALOUS ORIGIN OF THE RIGHT CORONARY ARTERY FROM THE LEFT SINUS OF VALSALVA

Anomalous origin of the right coronary artery from the left sinus of Valsalva is detected less often than anomalous origin of the left coronary artery from the right sinus of Valsalva. In an autopsy study, 25% of decedents with this anomaly had died suddenly. The indications for surgical repair of this lesion are less clear than when the left coronary artery arises anomalously from the right sinus of Valsalva. However, if the right coronary artery arises from the left sinus of Valsalva, courses between the aorta and pulmonary artery, and is the dominant coronary artery, most clinicians would recommend repair. Also, surgical repair of this anomaly is indicated if signs and symptoms of myocardial ischemia are present and there are no other apparent causes of myocardial ischemia.

CONGENITAL CORONARY OSTIA WEB

A rare but important cause of coronary insufficiency is the presence of a membrane covering the orifice of a coronary artery. Usually, it involves the left coronary ostia and is frequently associated with a dysplastic or bicuspid aortic valve. This diagnosis must be considered in the differential diagnosis of angina pectoris or exercise-associated syncope.

SINGLE CORONARY ARTERY

A single coronary artery occurs in approximately 2 of every 1,000 patients. It is associated with transposition of the great arteries, coronary artery fistula, and bicuspid aortic valve. The clinical significance of a single coronary artery is unclear. Patients in whom the single coronary artery arises from the right coronary sinus, with a connecting branch that travels between the aorta and the pulmonary artery, and then distributes in the location of a normal left coronary artery may be at risk for sudden death due to acute angulation of the connecting branch. This is similar to the situation in which the left coronary artery originates from the right sinus of Valsalva.

CORONARY ARTERY FISTULA

Coronary artery fistula constitutes 0.2% to 0.4% of congenital cardiac defects. Fistulae originate equally from the right and left coronary arteries. Usually, the fistula connects to the right ventricular cavity. The right atrium is the second most common terminus, and two thirds of fistulae draining into the right atrium originate from the right coronary artery. A fistula can also terminate in the pulmonary artery, left atrium, left ventricle, superior vena cava, or coronary sinus, or a persistent left superior vena cava. The involved coronary artery is usually dilated, and the chamber in which the fistula terminates may be enlarged.

In childhood and adolescence, the fistula usually does not produce symptoms, but signs and symptoms of congestive heart failure can occur secondary to a large left-to-right shunt. The presence of a fistula usually is detected by the finding of a continuous precordial murmur. There may be a precordial thrill, decreased diastolic blood pressure, and widened pulse pressure. Physical findings may be confused with those of patent ductus arteriosus, but usually the murmur of a patent ductus arteriosus is best heard in the left infraclavicular area and that of a coronary artery fistula at the midleft sternal border. Except for a small fistula, coronary artery fistulae should be closed. Fistulae can be closed surgically or using a variety of interventional cardiac catheterization techniques.

CORONARY ARTERY PATTERNS ASSOCIATED WITH CONGENITAL HEART DEFECTS

TETRALOGY OF FALLOT

Although only 4% to 5% of patients with tetralogy of Fallot have associated coronary artery anomalies, these abnormalities must be identified so that damage to the essential coronary arteries is avoided during the repair of tetralogy of Fallot. In 4% of patients with tetralogy of Fallot, the left anterior descending coronary artery originates from the right coronary artery. Single coronary artery is the second most common coronary anomaly associated with tetralogy of Fallot. Forty percent of cases with tetralogy of Fallot have a long and large right conus artery that distributes to a significant mass of myocardium.

d-TRANSPOSITION OF THE GREAT ARTERIES

There are two major coronary artery patterns in d-transposition of the great arteries. Usually, the right coronary artery arises from the posterior aortic sinus, and the left coronary artery arises from the left coronary sinus and divides into a circumflex coronary artery and an anterior descending coronary artery. The right aortic sinus of Valsalva is the noncoronary cusp.

In the second coronary artery pattern, the right coronary artery arises from the posterior aortic sinus and gives rise to the circumflex coronary artery, which passes posterior to the pulmonary artery. The anterior descending coronary artery arises from the left coronary sinus, and the right aortic sinus of Valsalva is the noncoronary sinus.

I-TRANSPOSITION OF THE GREAT ARTERIES

The aorta is anterior and to the left of the pulmonary artery in l-transposition of the great arteries (also known as *corrected transposition of the great arteries* or *ventricular inversion*). One aortic sinus of Valsalva is oriented anteriorly (anterior sinus of Valsalva), one posterior and rightward (right sinus of Valsalva), and one posterior and leftward (left sinus of Valsalva). The right coronary artery originates from the right aortic sinus of Valsalva and divides into an anterior descending branch that follows the course of the interventricular sulcus. The right coronary artery continues to follow a course in the right atrioventricular sulcus. The left coronary artery originates in the left aortic sinus of Valsalva and follows the course of the circumflex coronary artery in the left atrioventricular sulcus. The left (circumflex) coronary artery then produces a marginal branch and continues as the posterior descending coronary artery.

SELECTED REFERENCES

Baltaxe H, Amplatz K, Levin D. *Coronary angiography*. Springfield, IL: Charles C Thomas; 1975.

Baltaxe H, Wixson D. The incidence of congenital anomalies of the coronary arteries in the adult population. *Radiology*. 1977;122:47.

Barth CW III, Roberts WC. Left main coronary artery originating from the right sinus of Valsalva and coursing between the aorta and pulmonary trunk. *J Am Coll Cardiol*. 1986;7(2):366–373.

Barth CW III, Bray M, Roberts WC. Sudden death in infancy associated with origin of both left main and right coronary arteries from a common ostium above the left sinus of Valsalva. *Am J Cardiol*. 1986;57(4):365–366.

Cheitlin M, DeCastro C, McAllister H. Sudden death as a complication of anomalous left coronary origin from the anterior sinus of Valsalva, a not-so-minor congenital anomaly. *Circulation*. 1974;50:780.

Driscoll D, Nihill M, Mullins C, et al. Management of symptomatic infants with anomalous origin of the left coronary artery from the pulmonary artery. *Am J Cardiol*. 1981;47:642.

Elliott L, Amplatz K, Edwards J. Coronary arterial patterns in transposition complexes. *Am J Cardiol*. 1966;17:362.

Fellows K, Freed M, Keane J, et al. Results of routine preoperative coronary angiography in tetralogy of Fallot. *Circulation*. 1975;51:561.

Frommelt PC, Frommelt M, Tweddell J, et al. Prospective echocardiographic diagnosis and surgical repair of anomalous origin of a coronary artery from the opposite sinus with an interarterial course [see comment]. *J Am Coll Cardiol*. 2003;42(1):148–154.

Hurwitz R, Caldwell R, Girod D, et al. Clinical and hemodynamic course of infants and children with anomalous left coronary artery. *Am Heart J*. 1989;118:1176.

Kragel AH, Roberts WC. Anomalous origin of either the right or left main coronary artery from the aorta with subsequent coursing between aorta and pulmonary trunk: Analysis of 32 necropsy cases. *Am J Cardiol*. 1988;62(10 Pt 1):771–777.

Maron BJ, Epstein SE, Roberts WC. Causes of sudden death in competitive athletes. *J Am Coll Cardiol*. 1986;7(1):204–214.

Maron BJ, Shirani J, Poliac LC, et al. Sudden death in young competitive athletes. Clinical, demographic, and pathological profiles [see comment]. *JAMA*. 1996;276(3):199–204.

Roberts W. Major anomalies of coronary arterial origin seen in adulthood. *Am J Cardiol*. 1986;111:941.

Roberts WC, Kragel AH. Anomalous origin of either the right or left main coronary artery from the aorta without coursing of the anomalistically arising artery between aorta and pulmonary trunk. *Am J Cardiol*. 1988;62(17):1263–1267.

Roberts WC, Robinowitz M. Anomalous origin of the left anterior descending coronary artery from the pulmonary trunk with origin of the right and left circumflex coronary arteries from the aorta. *Am J Cardiol*. 1984;54(10):1381–1383.

Roberts WC, Shirani J. The four subtypes of anomalous origin of the left main coronary artery from the right aortic sinus (or from the right coronary artery). *Am J Cardiol*. 1992;70(1):119–121.

Roberts WC, Siegel RJ, Zipes DP. Origin of the right coronary artery from the left sinus of valsalva and its functional consequences: Analysis of 10 necropsy patients. *Am J Cardiol*. 1982;49(4):863–868.

Shirani J, Roberts WC. Origin of the left main coronary artery from the right aortic sinus with retroaortic course of the anomalistically arising artery. *Am Heart J*. 1992;124(4):1077–1078.

Virmani R, Roberts WC. Sudden cardiac death. *Hum Pathol*. 1987;18(5):485–492.

Portions of the text have been published previously and are reproduced with permission of the publisher:

Driscoll DJ. Congenital anomalies of the coronary arteries. In: Garson A, Bricker T, McNamara D, eds. *The science and practice of pediatric cardiology*. Lea & Febiger; 1990:1453–1461.

Driscoll DJ. Congenital coronary artery anomalies. In: Oski F, DeAngelis C, Feigin R, et al. eds. *Principles and practice of pediatrics*. JB Lippincott Co; 1990:1456–1459.

Driscoll DJ. Coronary artery abnormalities. In: Oski F, DeAngelis C, Feigin R, et al. eds. *Principles and practice of pediatrics*, 2nd ed. JB Lippincott Co; 1994:1594–1596.

Index

Page numbers followed by '*f*' indicate figures; those followed by '*t*' indicate tables.

A

Abdominal situs inversus, 28*f*

Abnormal conotruncal septation, 107

Acquired heart diseases, 137–150

    infectious endocarditis (IE), 146–150

    Kawasaki disease, 144–146

    rheumatic fever, 137–144

Acute appendicitis, 139

Acyanotic heart disease, 7

AICD. *See* Automatic internal cardiac defibrillator

    (AICD)

ALCAPA. *See* Anomalous origin of the left coronary

    artery from the pulmonary artery (ALCAPA)

American Heart Association Task Force, 59

Anaerobic threshold, 32

Aneuploidy, 66–67

Aneurysm, 58

Angina, 52

Angiograms, 27

Anomalous coronary artery, 58, 158, 161

Anomalous origin of the left coronary artery from the

    pulmonary artery (ALCAPA), 161–163

    clinical features of, 162

    treatment for, 163

Antistreptolysin O, 140

Aorta, 4, 5, 166

    coarctation of, 8, 39, 126*f*, 126–130

        associated anomalies, 126–127

        Blalock-Park procedure,

            129

        cardiac catheterization issues, 129

        chest x-ray, 128

        clinical presentation of, 127–128

        echocardiographic catheterization issues, 129

        electrocardiographic features of, 128

        history of, 129

        incidence of, 126–127

        magnetic resonance imaging issues, 129

        pathologic specimen of, 127*f*

        physical examination of, 128

        treatment of, 129

        treatment outcome, 129

    origin of pulmonary artery, 87

Aortic insufficiency, 121, 122

Aortic stenosis, 8, 38–39, 46, 61, 123*f*

    cardiac catheterization, 124

    chest x-ray, 124

    clinical presentation of, 122

    echocardiography catheterization, 124

    electrocardiographic features of, 124

    incidence of, 121–122

    murmur of, 123

    physical examination of, 122–124

    recurrence rates for, 62*t*

    subvalvar, 121

    supravalvar, 121

    treatment of, 124–126

    types of, 121–122

Aortic valve, 122*f*

Aortic valve cusps, 121

Aortic valve stenosis, 122

    recurrence risk for, 62*f*

Aorticopulmonary window (AP), 8, 86, 87*f*

Arrhythmia, 19, 20

Arterial switch

    Jatene procedure, 98

Arteries

    d-transposition of, 93*f*

Arteriovenous fistula, 88

ASD. *See* Atrial septal defect (ASD)

Aspirin, 142

Asthma, 51

    exertional, 53

Athletes

    screening of, 58

Atrial hypertrophy, 25

Atrial septal defect (ASD), 5, 7, 25, 75*f*, 76*f*, 73–78,

    96

    cardiac catheterization issues, 77

    chest x-ray, 77

    clinical presentation of, 76

    echocardiographic catheterization issues, 77

    electrocardiographic features of, 77

    embryology of, 74–76

    history of, 78

    incidence of, 74–76

Atrial septal defect (ASD) (*Continued*)
   ostium secundum, 74
   physical examination of, 76–77
   treatment of, 77–78
   treatment outcome, 78
   types of, 74–76
Atrial septostomy
   Rashkind balloon, 100
Atrial switch
   Senning and Mustard operations, 100
Atrioventricular block, 1
   first-degree, 22, 23*f*
   second-degree, 22, 23*f*
     Mobitz II, 23, 23*f*
     types of, 22
   third-degree, 24, 24*f*
Atrioventricular septal defects (AVSDs), 62, 85*f*,
   84–86
   cardiac catheterization issues, 86
   chest x-ray, 86
   clinical presentation of, 85
   echocardiographic catheterization issues, 86
   electrocardiographic features of, 85
   embryology of, 84–85
   Gerbode defect, 85
   history of, 86
   incidence of, 84–85
   physical examination of, 85
   treatment of, 86
   treatment outcome, 86
   types of, 84–85
Atrioventricular sulcus, 166
Automatic internal cardiac defibrillator (AICD),
   155
AVSDs. *See* Atrioventricular septal defects (AVSDs)

B
β-blockers, 1
β-hemolytic streptococcal infection, 137
Bicuspid aortic valve, 58, 165
Biventricular hypertrophy, 83, 155
Blalock-Taussig (subclavian artery), 104
Blood flow, 2–4
Blood oxygen content, 90*t*
Blood oxygen saturation, 73, 91
Blood pressure, 4, 16, 34, 38
   change with increasing work, 35*f*
Blood vessel wall, 4
Bradyarrhythmias, 22
Bronchitis, 52
Brugada syndrome, 55

C
Cardiac arrhythmias, 55
Cardiac auscultation, 14*f*, 12–15
Cardiac catheterization, 8, 27–28, 81
Cardiac cycle, temporal location, 15
Cardiac damage, 142

Cardiac dysfunction, 139
Cardiac enlargement, 25
Cardiac murmur, 80, 122
Cardiac output (CO), 1, 34–35, 38, 90
   determinants of, 1–2
     ejection fraction (EF), 1
     end-diastolic volume (EDV), 1
Cardiac rhythm, 17–24
   left atrial, 18
   low right atrial, 18
Cardiac shock, 92
Cardiac valve damage, 142
Cardio inhibitory syncope, 56
Cardiomegaly, 98
Cardiomyopathy, 8, 153–159
Cardiovascular physiology, 1–5
   cardiac output (CO), 1–2
   compliance, 4–5
   Fick principle, 3*f*, 3–4
   Laplace's law, 4, 4*f*
   Ohm's law, 2
   Poiseuille's law, 2–3
   resistance, 4–5
Cardiovascular shock, 118
Cardiovascular system, 29
   function of, 34
Carditis, 139
Carnitine deficiency, 156
Carotid bruit, 43, 45–46
Carotid pulse volume, 45
CHD. *See* Congenital heart disease (CHD)
Chest cage, 49
Chest pain, 49–53
   cardiac causes of, 52
   causes of, 51–52
     asthma, 51
     cardiac causes, 52
     gastrointestinal diseases, 52
     infection, 52
     pericarditis, 52
     pneumothorax, 52
   distribution of causes of, 50*t*
   medical evaluation of, 52–53
   outcome of, 53
   treatment of, 53
   types of, 49–51
     costochondritis, 49
     hypersensitive xiphoid syndrome, 51
     idiopathic chest pain, 50
     non-specific chest wall pain, 50
     precordial catch syndrome, 51
     sickle cell disease, 51
     slipping rib syndrome, 51
     Tietze syndrome, 50
     trauma and muscle strain, 51
Chest radiography, 25–26, 96
Chest wall, 16, 49
Chest wall pain
   nonspecific, 50

Chest x-ray, 7, 77
CHF. *See* Congestive heart failure (CHF)
Children
    electrocardiographic screening of, 58–59
Chorea, 139
Chronic congestive heart failure, 10
Circumflex coronary artery, 161, 166
Classical vasovagal presyncope, 57
Clubbing, 10
CO. *See* Cardiac output (CO)
Compliance, 4–5
Congenital coronary ostia web, 164
Congenital heart defects (CHDs), 25
    coronary artery patterns associated with, 165–166
    history of, 8–9
    palpation, 10–12
    patient categorization, 7
    physical examination of, 10
        inspection, 10
    physiologic consequences of cyanotic forms, 90
Congenital heart disease, 24
    approach to diagnosis, 95–96
    chest radiography, 96
    chromosomal abnormalities, 66–69
        aneuploidy, 66–67
    cyanotic, 93
    electrocardiogram (ECG), 96
    history of, 95
    Holt-Oram syndrome, 66
    Marfan syndrome, 63–66
    microdeletion syndromes, 67
    multifactorial inheritance of, 61–63
    Noonan syndrome, 66
    physical examination of, 95–96
    principles of inheritance of, 61–69
    single gene defects, 63
Congenital heart disease (CHDs), 61
Congenital mitral insufficiency, 133
Congestive cardiomyopathy, 156–159
Congestive heart failure (CHF), 9, 76, 142
Contractility, 2
Cor triatriatum, 8
Coronary arteriovenous fistulae, 83
Coronary artery
    anatomy of, 161
Coronary artery aneurysms, 144
Coronary artery anomalies, 59, 161–166
Coronary artery fistula, 165
Coronary artery stenoses, 118
Coronary cameral fistulae, 83
Coronary insufficiency, 52, 164
Coronary sinus
    unroofed, 75
Costochondritis, 49–50
Crescendo-decrescendo murmur, 45
Critical aortic stenosis, 8, 122
Critical pulmonary stenosis, 7, 8
Cyanosis, 8, 10, 11*f*, 89, 97
    presence of, 8

pulmonary causes of, 95*t*
Cyanotic heart disease, 7, 8

D
Decompensated metabolic acidosis, threshold for, 36
Decrescendo murmur, 15
Denuded endothelium, 146
Diastolic blood pressure, 34
Diastolic murmurs, 15
Digital clubbing, 11*f*
Dilated cardiomyopathy, 156, 156*f*
    chest x-ray, 158
    echocardiogram, 158
    electrocardiogram, 157
    etiology of, 156
    genetics of, 156
    history of, 156, 158–159
    mutations associated with, 157*t*
    physical examination of, 157
    treatment of, 158–159
Distal arch, 129
Dominant coronary artery, 161
Doppler techniques, and echocardiography, 26, 124
Down syndrome, 66, 84
Ductus arteriosus, 98, 105, 127

E
Ebstein anomaly, 7, 25, 27*f*, 116*f*, 117*f*, 116–117
    treatment outcome, 117
ECG. *See* Electrocardiogram (ECG)
Echocardiography, 26, 59, 134
    Doppler techniques, 26, 77
    use of, 92
Echocardiography screening, 58
EDV. *See* End-diastolic volume (EDV)
EF. *See* Ejection fraction (EF)
Ehlers-Danlos syndrome, 133
Eisenmenger syndrome, 82
Ejection fraction (EF), 1, 2
Electrical cardioversion, 20
Electrocardiogram (ECG), 7, 17, 37–38, 46, 56, 96
Electrocardiographic screening
    of children, 58–59
    issues in, 59
    recommendations in, 59
Electrocardiographic signal, 37
Electrocardiography, 17–25
    cardiac enlargement and hypertrophy, 25
    cardiac rhythm, 17–24
End-diastolic volume (EDV), 1
Endocardial fibroelastosis, 55
Endocarditis prophylaxis, 78, 84
Endoscopic retrograde cholangiopancreatography (ERCP), 144
Energy, 31
ERCP. *See* Endoscopic retrograde cholangiopancreatography (ERCP)

Ergometers, 37
Erythema marginatum, 139
Erythrocythemia, 89
Erythrogenic toxin, 138
Exercise
   cardiac responses to, 32–35
      blood pressure, 34
      cardiac output (CO), 34–35
      heart rate, 32–34
      stroke volume (SV), 34–35
   cardiorespiratory response to, 40
   heat rate, change of, 34*f*
   maximal aerobic power, 30–32
   power, 30–32
   types of, 37
   ventilatory responses to, 35–36
   work, 30–32
Exercise performance, determinants of, 29–30
Exercise testing, 39
   methodology of, 37
Exertional asthma, 53

F
Fascicular rhythm, 19
Fick principle, 3–4
First-degree AV block, 22
Fitness, 36–37
Fossa ovalis, 74

G
Gastroesophageal reflux, 52
Gastrointestinal diseases, 52
Gianturco coils, 84
Glenn anastomosis, 115
Glomerulonephritis, 138
Great arteries
   arterial switch
      Jatene procedure, 98
      Senning and Mustard operations, 100
   atrial enlargement, 98*f*
   d-transposition of, 97*f*, 99*f*, 101*f*, 96–102, 165
      treatment outcome, 102
      with no ventricular septal defect, 98–100
      with ventricular septal defect, 100
      with ventricular septal defect and pulmonary
        stenosis, 100
   l-transposition of, 166

H
HC. *See* Hypertrophic cardiomyopathy (HC)
Head bobbing, 10
Heart attack, 9
Heart murmurs, 15, 43, 76
   frequency of, 15
   intensity of, 15
   location in chest, 16
   loudness of, 15
   pitch of, 15

Heart rate (HR), 1, 32–34, 37–38
   measurement techniques, 37–38
Heart sounds, 15
His bundle, 19
HLHS. *See* Hypoplastic left heart syndrome (HLHS)
HOCM. *See* Hypertrophic obstructive
   cardiomyopathy (HOCM)
Holosystolic murmur, 15
Holt-Oram syndrome, 66
Homograft valve, 125
HR. *See* Heart rate (HR)
Hunter syndrome, 133
Hurler syndrome, 133
Hypercyanotic spells, 104
   treatment of, 105*t*
Hypersensitive xiphoid syndrome, 51
Hypertrophic cardiomyopathy (HC), 52, 55, 66, 154*f*,
   153–155
   chest x-ray, 155
   echocardiography, 155
   electrocardiogram, 155
   etiology of, 153–154
   genetics of, 153–154
   history of, 154–155
   physical examination of, 154
   treatment of, 155
Hypertrophic nonobstructive cardiomyopathy, 153
Hypertrophic obstructive cardiomyopathy (HOCM),
   121, 153
   murmur of, 16
Hypertrophy, 25
Hypoplastic left heart syndrome (HLHS), 113, 115
   treatment outcome, 115
Hypothyroidism, 67
Hypoxemia, 40, 89

I
ICD. *See* Implantable cardiac defibrillator (ICD)
Idiopathic chest pain, 50
Idiopathic dilated cardiomyopathy, 156
Idiopathic hypercalcemia, 68
Idiopathic hypertrophic subaortic stenosis. *See*
   Hypertrophic obstructive cardiomyopathy (HOCM)
IE. *See* Infectious endocarditis (IE)
Implantable cardiac defibrillator (ICD), 19
Increased fitness, 36*t*
Infection, 52
Infectious endocarditis (IE), 144, 146–150
   complications of, 150
   diagnosis of, 147
      Duke criteria, 148, 149*t*
   physical findings in, 146
   prophylaxis, 150
   signs of, 146
   symptoms of, 146
   treatment of, 147–150
Inlet VSD, 79
Innocent murmurs, 43–47
   assessment of, 46–47

carotid bruit, 45–46
  of childhood, 43
  physiologic pulmonary branch stenosis, 46
  pulmonary flow murmur, 43–45
  still's murmur, 45
  venous hum, 45
Intermittent junctional rhythm, 18
Interventricular sulcus, 166
Intravenous gamma globulin (IVIG), 145
Isolated levocardia, 28*f*
Isotonic exercise, 34
Isthmic hypoplasia, 129
IVIG. *See* Intravenous Gamma Globulin (IVIG)

J
JET. *See* Junctional ectopic tachycardia (JET)
Junctional ectopic tachycardia (JET), 20, 21*f*
Junctional rhythm, 18, 19*f*
  treatment for, 18
Junctional tachycardia, 20

K
Kawasaki disease, 144–146
  clinical features of, 145*t*
Kawasaki syndrome, 52
Kugel's artery, 161

L
LAE. *See* Left atrial enlargement (LAE)
Laplace's law, 4
  cardiovascular implications of, 4
Left atrial enlargement (LAE), 25
Left atrial rhythm, 18, 18*f*
Left coronary artery
  anomalous origin from right sinus of Valsalva,
    164*f*, 163–164
  origin from pulmonary artery, 163*f*
Left coronary artery system, 162*f*
Left subclavian artery, 127
Left ventricular hypertrophy (LVH), 25, 69,
  124
Left-to-right shunts, 73–88
  magnitude of, 73
Ligamentum arteriosus, 126
Low right atrial rhythm, 18, 18*f*
LVH. *See* Left ventricular hypertrophy (LVH)
Lymphangiectasia, 66

M
Magnetic resonance angiography (MRA), 8
Magnetic resonance imaging (MRI), 7, 129
MAPCAs. *See* Multiple aorta pulmonary collateral
  arteries (MAPCAs)
Marfan syndrome, 4, 52, 63–66, 133
  cardiac issues in, 63
  causes of death in, 63
  diagnostic criteria for, 64*t*
  differential diagnosis of, 65*t*

Maximal aerobic power, 31
Maximum voluntary ventilation (MVV), 36
Microdeletion syndromes, 67
Mitral insufficiency, 153
  repair of, 135
Mitral stenosis, 8, 16
Mitral valve, 5
Mitral valve prolapse, 52, 58
Mitral valve stenosis, 133–135
  cardiac catheterization issues, 134
  chest x-ray, 134
  clinical presentation of, 133
  echocardiographic catheterization issues, 134
  electrocardiographic features of, 134
  incidence of, 133
  isolated congenital, 133
  physical examination of, 134
  treatment of, 134–135
  treatment outcome, 134–135
  types of, 133
Mobitz I, 22–23
Mobitz II, 22–23
MRA. *See* Magnetic resonance angiography (MRA)
MRI. *See* Magnetic resonance imaging (MRI)
Multiple Aorta Pulmonary Collateral Arteries
  (MAPCAs, 106
Muscle strain, 51
Muscular invagination, 79
Muscular subaortic stenosis, 121
Muscular VSD, 79
MVV. *See* Maximum voluntary ventilation (MVV)
Myocardial infarction, 118, 161
Myocardial inflammation, 144
Myocardial ischemia, 124
Myocardial oxygen consumption, 4
Myocarditis, 8

N
Neonatal cardiac transplantation, 115
Neonate
  pulmonary branch stenosis of, 43
Nontraumatic death, in athletes
  causes of, 58*t*
Noonan syndrome, 66

O
Obstructive hypertrophic cardiomyopathy, 8
Obstructive lesions, 121–135
Ohm's law, 2
Open surgical valvotomy, 125
Ostium primum ASD, 74
Ostium secundum, 74

P
Pallor, 10
Palpation, 10–12
Paroxysmal junctional tachycardia (PJT), 20

Patent ductus arteriosus (PDA), 8, 25, 74, 83*f*, 82–84, 165
    cardiac catheterization issues, 84
    chest x-ray, 84
    clinical presentation of, 82
    echocardiographic catheterization issues, 84
    electrocardiographic features of, 83
    embryology of, 82
    history of, 84
    incidence of, 82
    physical examination of, 83
    treatment of, 84
    treatment outcome, 84
PDA. *See* Patent ductus arteriosus (PDA)
Peak effort, 31
Peak exercise study, 31
Pectus excavatum, 40
Pediatric arrhythmias, 17
Pediatric cardiology
    clinical applications of exercise testing in, 38–40
Pediatric electrophysiology, 17
Pediatric exercise testing, 29–40
    cardiac responses to exercise, 32–35
        blood pressure, 34
        cardiac output and stroke volume, 34–35
        heart rate, 32–34
    clinical applications, in pediatric cardiology, 38–40
        aortic stenosis, 38–39
        coarctation of the aorta, 39
        pectus excavatum, 40
        pulmonary atresia with ventricular septal defect 39–40
        single ventricle, 40
    determinants of exercise performance, 29–30
    fitness, 36–37
    measurement techniques, 37–38
        blood pressure, 38
        cardiac output and stroke volume, 38
        heart rate and electrocardiogram, 37–38
        ventilation, 38
    methodology, 37
    ventilatory responses to exercise, 35–36
    work, power and maximal aerobic power, 30–32
Percussion, 12
Pericardial effusion, 1, 25
Pericarditis, 1, 52
Periodic respiration, 10*f*
Peripheral edema, 12
Peripheral pulmonary artery stenosis, 69
Pharyngitis, 143
Physiologic pulmonary branch stenosis, 46
PJT. *See* Paroxysmal junctional tachycardia (PJT)
Pleurodynia, 52
Pneumonitis, 52
Pneumothorax, 52
Poiseuille's law, 2–3
Polycythemia, 3
Precordial catch syndrome, 51
Precordial impulses, 10

    location of, 13*f*
Precordial murmur, 165
Premature death, 9
Prolonged QT-interval syndrome, 24, 24*f*, 55
    treatment of, 24
Prophylaxis, 144
Prosthetic valve dehiscence, 149
Pulmonary artery, 90
    surgical banding of, 111
Pulmonary artery atresia
    eventual repair of, 106
    with ventricular septal defect, 105–106
        treatment outcome, 106
Pulmonary artery pressure, 2
Pulmonary atresia, 7, 25
    with intact ventricular septum, 117–118
        treatment outcome, 118
    with ventricular septal defect, 39
Pulmonary bed, 2
Pulmonary branch stenosis, 44*f*
Pulmonary edema, 10, 92, 95, 127
Pulmonary flow murmur, 43–45
Pulmonary hypertension, 2, 85
Pulmonary insufficiency, 130
Pulmonary regurgitation, 132
Pulmonary stenosis, 7, 11, 100
    recurrence rates for, 62*t*
Pulmonary valve, 100
Pulmonary valve stenosis, 26, 131*f*, 130–133
    cardiac catheterization of, 132
    chest x-ray, 132
    clinical presentation of, 130
    echocardiographic catheterization of, 132
    electrocardiographic features of, 132
    history of, 133
    incidence of, 130
    physical examination of, 130–131
    treatment of, 132
    treatment outcome, 133
    types of, 130
Pulmonary valvuloplasty, 132
Pulmonary vascular obstructive disease, 2, 107
Pulmonary vasculature, 8
Pulmonary veins, 114
Pulmonary venous hypertension, 127
Pulmonary venous obstruction, 8
Pulmonic stenosis, 8
Pulse oximeter, 8
Pulse volume, 10

R
RAE. *See* Right atrial enlargement (RAE)
Red blood cells, 3
Regurgitant lesions, 121–135
Repetitive sarcomere shortening, 29
Residual heart disease, 141
Resistance, 4–5
Respiratory compensation, 36

Respiratory distress syndrome, 92
Respiratory rate, 10
Restrictive cardiomyopathy, 1, 159
Rheumatic cardiac valve disease, 144
Rheumatic chorea, 142
Rheumatic fever, 137–144
   acute, 137
   clinical manifestations of, 139–140
   diagnosis of, 141*t*
   differential diagnosis of, 140*t*
   epidemiology of, 137
   pathogenesis of, 138
   prevention of, 142–144
   sequelae, 142
   streptococcus, 137–138
   streptozyme test, 140
   treatment of, 140–142
Right atrial enlargement (RAE), 25
Right coronary artery
   anomalous origin from left sinus of Valsalva, 164
Right coronary artery system, 162*f*
Right ventricle (RV), 89
Right ventricular fistulae, 118
Right ventricular hypertrophy (RVH), 25, 132
Right-to-left shunts, 89–118
RV. *See* Right ventricle (RV)
RVH. *See* Right ventricular hypertrophy (RVH)

S

Sarcomere shortening, 29
   repetitive, 29
   skeletal muscle, 29
Scarlet fever, 138
Second-degree AV block, 22
Septic shock, 8
Sequelae, 142
Shone syndrome, 126
Sick sinus syndrome, 1
Sickle cell disease, 51
Single coronary artery, 165
Single gene defects, 63
Single ventricle, 40
   Fontan operation, 40
Sinus bradycardia, 22, 22*f*
Sinus node artery, 161
Sinus of Valsalva, 53, 65, 164, 166
Sinus rhythm, 17*f*
Sinus venosus ASD, 74
Situs inversus totalis, 18
Skeletal muscle sarcomere shortening, 29
Skin edema, 10
Slipping rib syndrome, 51
   hooking maneuver, 51
Stationary cycles, 37
Stenotic valve, 122
Steroids
   role of, 145
Still's murmur, 16, 43, 45
Streptococcal infection, 139

Streptococcal pharyngitis, 137
   antibiotic therapy, 143
Streptococcus, 137–138
Streptolysin O, 138
   antigenicity of, 138
Streptolysin S, 138
Stroke volume (SV), 1, 34–35, 38
Sudden death, 55–59
   in children and adolescents, 57
   prevention of, 58
Sudden infant death syndrome, 57
Sudden unexpected death, 57
Superior vena cava (SVC), 75
Supracristal VSD, 78
Supravalvar aortic stenosis, 68
Supravalvar stenosis, 121
Supraventricular tachycardia (SVT), 20
   electrocardiogram in, 20*f*
   treatment of, 20
SV. *See* Stroke volume (SV)
SVC. *See* Superior vena cava (SVC)
SVT. *See* Supraventricular tachycardia (SVT)
Sweating, 10
Syncope, 55–59
   in children and adolescents, 55–57
   occurrence rates of, 56*f*
Systemic arteriovenous fistula, 8
Systemic venous return, 94
Systolic ejection murmur, 76, 105, 107, 114, 128
Systolic hypertension
   exercise-induced, 39
Systolic pulmonary ejection murmur, 96

T

Tachyarrhythmias, 20
TAPVR. *See* Totally anomalous pulmonary venous return (TAPVR)
Tetralogy of Fallot (TOF), 7, 25, 26*f*, 91, 91*f*, 103*f*, 104*f*, 102–105, 165
   intracardiac repair of, 104
   management of, 103–104
   treatment outcome, 104–105
Tietze syndrome, 50
Tissue oxygenation, 90*t*
TOF. *See* Tetralogy of Fallot (TOF)
Totally anomalous pulmonary venous return (TAPVR), 94*f*, 95, 114–115
   treatment outcome, 115
Transforming growth factor β (TGF β), 63
Trauma, 51
Treadmills, 37
Tricuspid atresia, 7, 109–112
   definitive treatment of, 111
   diagnosis of, 109
   Fontan operation, 111, 112, 113*f*, 113*t*
   with normally related great arteries, 111
   with pulmonary artery atresia, 111
   with transposed great arteries, 111
   treatment outcome, 112

Tricuspid diastolic murmur, 96
Tricuspid insufficiency, 96, 117
Tricuspid regurgitation jet, 132
Tricuspid valve, 5
Tricuspid valve prosthesis, 117
Truncal valve, 107
Truncus arteriosus, 7, 87–88, 109*f*, 107–109
    treatment outcome, 107
Tunnel subaortic stenosis, 121
Tunnel subvalvar aortic stenosis, 125
Turner syndrome, 67

U
Univentricular heart, 112–114
    treatment outcome, 114

V
Valsalva maneuver, 16, 20
Vasodepressor, 56
Vasovagal syncope, 55
Velocardiofacial syndrome, 67
Venous hum, 43, 45, 83
Ventilation
    measurements of, 38
Ventilatory anaerobic threshold, 32
Ventricular hypertrophy, 25, 82, 102, 109, 154
Ventricular noncompaction, 159
Ventricular rhythm, 19
Ventricular septal defect (VSD), 5, 7, 25, 39, 58, 61,
    73, 79*f*, 80*f*, 78–82

cardiac catheterization issues, 81
chest x-ray, 81
clinical presentation, 79–80
echocardiographic catheterization issues, 81
electrocardiographic features of, 81
embryology of, 78–79
history of, 82
incidence of, 78–79
inlet, 79
muscular, 79
physical examination of, 80–81
recurrence rates for, 62*t*
supracristal, 78
treatment of, 81–82
treatment outcome, 82
types of, 78–79
Ventricular septum, 7, 79
Ventricular tachycardia (VT), 19, 22*f*, 55
Viral pharyngitis, 143
VSD. *See* Ventricular septal defect (VSD)
VT. *See* Ventricular tachycardia (VT)

W
Wall tension, 4
Wenckebach, 22
Williams syndrome, 52, 68–69
    Coanda effect, 69
    cocktail party personality, 68
    supravalvar pulmonary stenosis in, 69
Wolff-Parkinson-White (WPW) syndrome, 55, 116

A to Z of
COCKTAILS

A to Z of COCKTAILS

Introduction by John Doxat

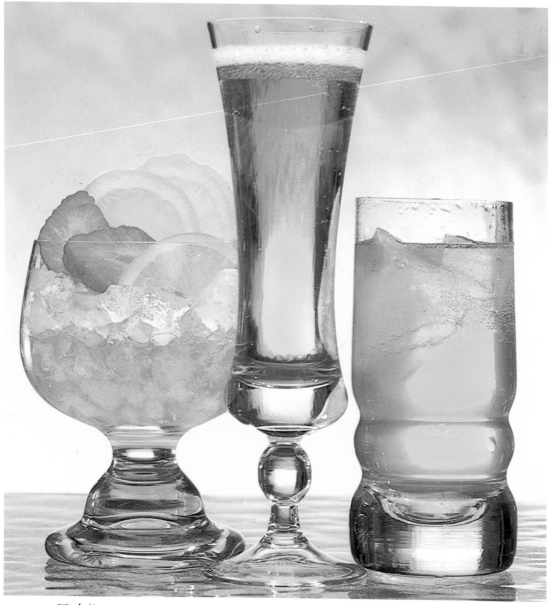

Ward Lock Limited · London

Translation © Ward Lock Limited 1980
Illustrations © Orbis-Verlag für Publizistik 1980

First published in Great Britain in 1980
by Ward Lock Limited, 116 Baker Street,
London W1M 2BB, a Pentos Company.

Filmset in Monophoto Apollo by
Asco Trade Typesetting Ltd, Hong Kong.
Printed and bound in Hong Kong by
South China Printing Co.

British Library Cataloguing in Publication Data

A to Z of cocktails.
  1. Cocktails
  I. Title
  641.8′74   TX951
ISBN 0-7063-5831-7

Introduction

Cocktail is an odd way to describe a drink. Yet it is accepted the world over as covering an enormous range of mixes. A cocktail may be short and strong, or long and weak. It may be bone dry or sugary sweet, fizzy or frothy. Cocktails come in all colours of the rainbow. They are not necessarily even alcoholic. No one can compute how many cocktails have been listed: over 7000 are on the records of the United Kingdom Bartenders' Guild alone, and these are only some in the archives of the 23 professional bartenders' organisations affiliated to the International Bartenders' Association. Hardly a day goes by without some new cocktail being invented, for a competition, to fête some special occasion—or simply for the fun of it.

Yet the origin of the word itself is unknown. In my own researches I have unearthed nine legends as to how 'cocktail' came to be associated with a compound of various potable ingredients. The one I deem most credible comes from 18th century England. It was customary, in the instance of a good horse but not a thoroughbred, to dock the animal's tail, indicating that, though sound, it was of mixed stock. Such a horse was said to be 'cock-tailed', or to be a 'cocktail'. It is

reasonable to assume that a mixed drink would attract the same description.

We rightly think of the USA as the true home of the cocktail, and it was indeed there that the first known definition occurred. In a journal called *The Balance*, a cocktail was said to be 'a stimulating liquor composed of spirits of any sort, sugar, water and bitters'. That was in 1806: so much for any idea that cocktails are strictly modern phenomena.

Cocktails are mentioned in *Tom Brown's Schooldays*, Thackeray's *The Newcomes*—a book that could do with stimulation—and Charles Dickens's *Martin Chuzzlewit*. In those days cocktails were mainly associated with sport or outdoor social occasions when they were bottled up in advance and used for morning refreshment. The fortunes of the now huge American drink and food conglomerate Heublein's were founded on a bottle cocktail issued commercially in 1892.

It was inevitable that with the coming of cocktail bars in the USA, in supplement to the usually simpler 'saloons', cocktails should take a social step upwards. Europeans were behind the Americans in this respect. The first cocktail bar in London was not opened until 1910, and until quite recently it was customary to call such specialised places American Bars.

The Cocktail Age—circa 1922–35—was partly born of Prohibition. Though the Americans had long been inventive in the field of cocktails, absence of legal spirits not only increased their drinking but tested their ingenuity in blending ingredients to cover the taste of hooch. Bootlegged, imported liquor was equally employed to produce established cocktails and indulge the new fashion for exotic ones. By the mid-Twenties, well-to-do folk in many of the world's big cities were drinking cocktails at parties or in smart American Bars.Cocktails were accepted by all except the most staid members of Society.

The craze declined in the later Thirties as the world assumed—at least Europe did—a more serious shape. The classic cocktails survived but social drinking, at home or in bars, returned to less complex drinks. In Britain the rather boring sherry party enjoyed a vogue: it may have been more in keeping with the times but it was not nearly as much fun as the cocktail party. The USA, mercifully 'wet' again, kept the cocktail flag flying, even during the war. She still leads.

There has gradually been, starting in the Sixties, a revival in interest in cocktails. I attribute this not only to wider affluence but also to the broadening effect of holidays abroad. People encounter fresh drinks, find bars where exciting mixes, unknown in their home towns, are made. Undoubtedly we are becoming much more adventurous in our social drinking.

The established classics have taken on a new lease of life; a few, such as *Harvey Wallbanger* and *Tequila Sunrise*, have earned a permanent niche for themselves. Others have proved more ephemeral, as has always been the case. The world of the cocktail is one of constant movement.

There are students of mixology who maintain that the word cocktail is too loosely used—that one should talk of crustas, twists, sours, daisies, flips, and other precise names. We need not bother over much. Although a cocktail is generally understood to be an aperitif containing some alcohol, it has never been strictly defined as such. All we can say is that it is a mixed drink, which means that every recipe in this book may loosely qualify as a cocktail.

The joy of making cocktails is akin to that of cooking. A good recipe may inspire you to cook a dish or mix a drink exactly as described. Or it may set your imagination working to create new variations. I think that is an important point. Do not feel that a drink recipe is immutable: by all means take it as a guideline and give your enterprise full rein. Some now well-established mixes arrived as mutations of previous ones.

First, a word on equipment. Those readers who are already well supplied must bear with me whilst I deal with essentials. Cocktails—other than those mixed directly in the glass from which they will be drunk—are either shaken or stirred. It is usual to shake those recipes which have juices, cordials or liqueurs in them which will not easily mix with spirits without brisk blending.

The professional style of shaker comes in the form of two cones—one of metal, the other of metal or glass. The metal and glass variety is the true Boston shaker. The ingredients, usually including ice, are placed in one cone and the other cone is fitted snugly into this. A protective cloth is wrapped round them and they are shaken vigorously for a few seconds—or longer according to the degree of refrigeration and dilution required. One cone is then removed—not easy for the amateur—and the contents of the remaining cone are strained into the requisite number of glasses. This requires experience and fine judgement. The strainer should be that spring-edged type known as the 'Hawthorn' which can adapt to a fairly wide range of apertures. It is easily taken apart for cleaning or can be simply rinsed when used for different mixes.

Amateur domestic cocktailmen more usually employ three-part shakers—a base for the ingredients, a section containing a strainer, and a lid. If of good quality, well made and close fitting, these are excellent. Inferior models can either jam tight or leak. Always wrap a cloth round the shaker: it will prevent frost-bite and ameliorate disaster should the shaker come apart in your hands.

If a shaker frightens you, a mixing glass will do for all cocktails—and is a prerequisite for many. Mixing glasses come in a variety of guises, but whatever the shape they should not be over decorated. A mixing glass is basically a jug with a small lip. You put in the ingredients following the recipe and stir them together. Then, in most cases, you use a Hawthorn strainer.

Hygiene of equipment is very important: a cocktail tainted by silver polish is most unattractive. A long bar-spoon is useful. As well as being used for stirring and measuring (it has the same capacity as a teaspoon), it can get olives and cherries out of deep bottles.

Not to be forgotten is a sharp knife for slicing fruits and paring citrus peel—and I do mean sharp. You will also need a board to cut on.

If you are setting up a domiciliary cocktail bar, you can go to town on ancillary equipment. But please try to avoid gimmickry: you will win no points with dedicated cocktailmen. Special bitters bottles are good. You transfer a quantity of bitters—Angostura, orange, peach—to these smaller containers, which are fitted with nozzles that make it impossible to shake out more than a drop or two at a time. This is what is meant by a 'dash'—a single quick shake from such a bottle (roughly the equivalent of $\frac{1}{5}$ teaspoon).

You need an ice-bucket. So here is the moment to say something about ice. First, unless your tap water is specially good you cannot make good ice, so you had best make your ice with neutral spa water. Secondly, ice from a domestic refrigerator is not ideal: it is slowly-frozen 'soft ice'. You will do better, for parties, to make your ice in a deep freezer.

Amusing ice can be made by putting a few spots of flavorless food-colouring into water, producing polychromatic cubes. These add some fun to non-alcoholic cocktails—to which years ago I gave the name mocktails—or will enliven other mixtures.

For drinks demanding crushed ice, put the ice blocks in a cloth and smash them with a mallet, or feed smallish pieces into a robust electric blender. A blender is splendid for recipes requiring ingredients to be completely mixed with crushed ice. Such drinks must always be served with straws.

Expert bartenders rarely use measures when making cocktails: they rely on their eye. But in Britain and the United States measures (based on the fluid ounce) are still widely employed in home cocktail-mixing. In Australia, where the move to metrication is complete, measures are hardly ever used.

Widely used in homes everywhere are automatic measuring and pouring devices which fit into spirit bottles. These are efficient enough, but I do feel they give an impression of meanness, and are unprofessional. Pourers to fit into spirit and other bottles ensure easy serving without too much dripping. They should be removed after use and washed; bottles should be kept closed when not in use.

Any glass containing a cocktail is effectively a cocktail glass, although the type most commonly used is a small, stemmed glass with a capacity of about 80 ml (3 fl oz). For longer drinks you will need wine goblets and tumblers both large and small. Flips are traditionally served in a medium-sized, tall, stemmed glass, and layered liqueurs in a small, narrow, 'pousse-café' glass. Coloured glass is best avoided, though cut-glass is permissible. Elegance rather than extravagance: that's the keynote. But these are purely personal preferences.

One thing to avoid is filling the glass too full: awkward to drink from, and dangerous to furniture. Work out roughly the total size of your mix, allowing for melting ice, and use a glass with a content rather larger than the total.

Now for the prime ingredients. A basic stock of spirits would be good dry gin, blended Scotch whisky, sound standard cognac brandy, vodka (not imported), dark and white rum. In wine, standard port, dry sherry, simple red wine, standard dry white wine. Of liqueurs, the only absolute essential is Cointreau, the most famous curaçao. In aperitifs, you need three vermouths: dry, bianco and red; and Campari. In bitters, you will find Angostura essential.

Oranges, lemons—limes if obtainable— should be to hand: sometimes the rind is as important as the juices. Frozen fruit juices are acceptable, but nothing is quite like the real thing, freshly squeezed. Fresh fruit juices must always be strained before being added to a cocktail—unless the whole cocktail is strained at a later stage.

There is only one excellent lime juice cordial—Rose's. Grenadine syrup is in numerous recipes: as this is flavoured with pomegranate, you are unlikely to be able to make it yourself. However, you can make an acceptable plain sugar syrup by boiling 500 g (1 lb) sugar in 600 ml (1 pint) water. (To make sugar syrup for individual recipes, use 1 tablespoon sugar to 2 tablespoons water.) Another syrup, attractive both in colour and taste, mildly alcoholic, is *crème de cassis*, but if you are hard pushed, use straight blackcurrant juice (such as Ribena), not synthetic blackcurrant cordial. You had better have a bottle of genuine maraschino (cocktail) cherries to hand: the liquid can prove useful too. You will also need stoned green olives.

If you see an unusual recipe you like but you do not have, or cannot find, one of the ingredients—and some are fairly rare—think of a possible taste substitute or try changing the recipe into something similar but subtly different. Gradually build up your stocks—spirits like tequila; liqueurs such as Galliano. When travelling, look out for strange and interesting small bottles. Above all use your own ingenuity, making these recipes one of your instruments for successful hospitality and personal enjoyment.

This volume comes out over 100 years since the very first cocktail book, Jerry Thomas's *The Bon Vivant's Guide*, was published in the USA, and it almost coincides with the centenary of the second, Harry Johnson's *Bartenders' Manual*, which contains several mixes included in the following pages. It is a worthy successor to the work of those pioneers.

It is advisable to follow **either** the metric **or** the imperial measures when using this book.

All cocktails serve one person, unless indicated otherwise.

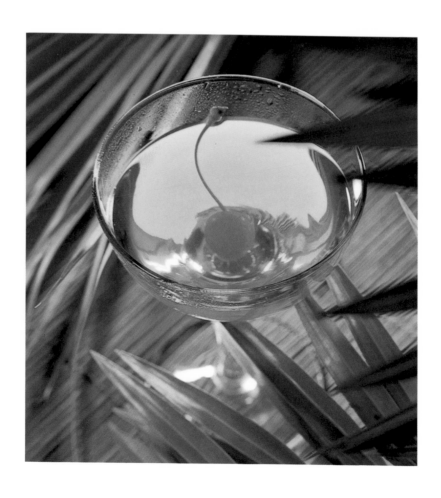

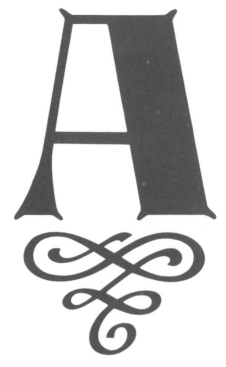

ABC

5 ice cubes
20 ml/¾ oz Armagnac
20 ml/¾ oz Bénédictine
1 dash Angostura bitters
champagne
1 lemon slice
2 orange segments
3 cocktail cherries

Crack two ice cubes and put in a shaker with Armagnac, Bénédictine and bitters. Shake. Crush remaining ice and put in a goblet. Strain in contents of shaker and top up with champagne. Decorate with lemon slice, orange segments and cocktail cherries. Serve with a straw.

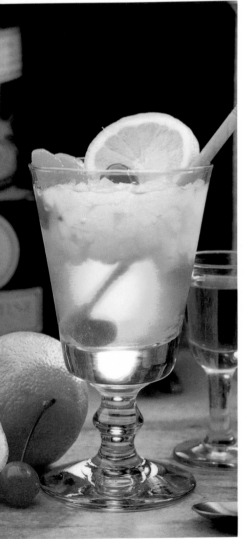

ABC

Acapulco

4 ice cubes
50 ml/2 oz tequila
25 ml/1 oz crème de cassis
1 teaspoon sugar syrup
1 lemon slice
soda water

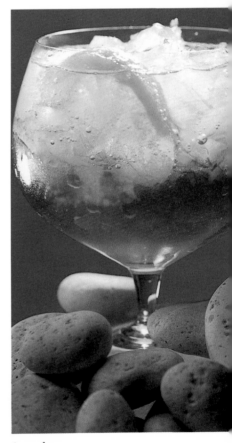

Acapulco

Crush ice and put in a balloon glass. Add tequila, crème de cassis and sugar syrup, and stir well. Add lemon slice and top up with soda water.

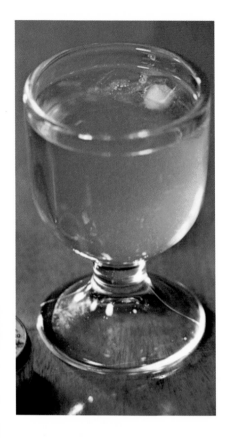

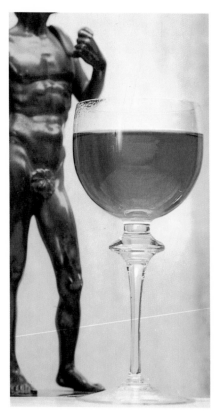

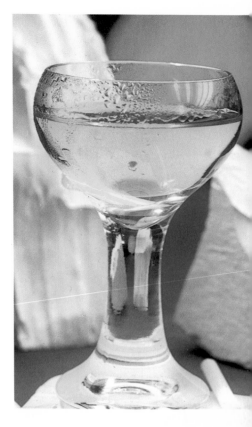

Adam and Eve

2–3 ice cubes
20 ml/¾ oz brandy
20 ml/¾ oz gin
20 ml/¾ oz Cointreau

Crack ice and put in a shaker with other ingredients. Shake well and strain into a cocktail glass.

Admiral's Highball

4 ice cubes
40 ml/1½ oz tokay
20 ml/¾ oz whisky
1 teaspoon pineapple juice
1 teaspoon lemon juice
soda water

Put three ice cubes in a mixing glass with tokay, whisky, pineapple juice and lemon juice. Stir and strain into a cocktail glass. Top up with soda water and add remaining ice cube.

From left to right: Admiral's Highball, Adonis, Alaska

Adonis

3 ice cubes
25 ml/1 oz sherry
20 ml/¾ oz red vermouth
1 dash Angostura bitters

Put ice in a mixing glass with other ingredients. Stir and strain into a cocktail glass.

Afterwards

4 ice cubes
15 ml/½ oz brandy
15 ml/½ oz kirsch
15 ml/½ oz crème de menthe
2 teaspoons grenadine

Crush ice and put in a tall champagne glass. Add other ingredients and stir well. Serve with a straw.

Agadir

3 ice cubes
25 ml/1 oz coffee liqueur
25 ml/1 oz orange juice
Coca-Cola or sparkling wine
1 orange slice

Put ice in a tall tumbler with coffee liqueur and orange juice. Stir, and top up with Coca-Cola or sparkling wine. Float orange slice on top or fix on rim of glass. Serve with a straw.

Alaska

2–3 ice cubes
40 ml/1½ oz gin
15 ml/½ oz yellow Chartreuse

Crack ice and put in a shaker with other ingredients. Shake well and strain into a cocktail glass.

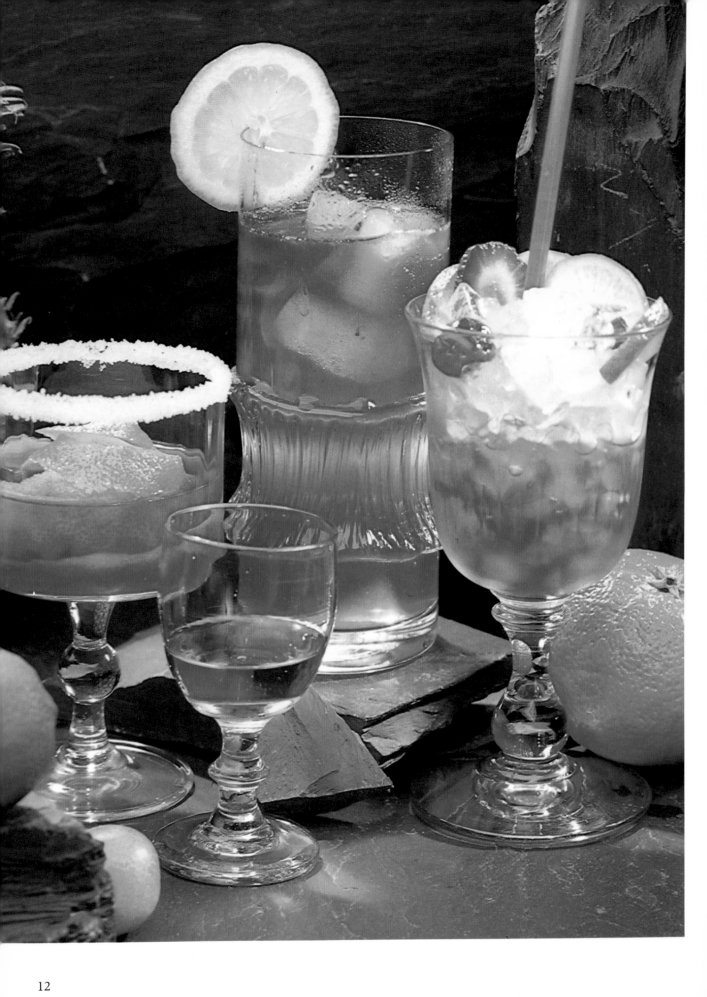

Alexander

2–3 ice cubes
20 ml/$\frac{3}{4}$ oz brandy
20 ml/$\frac{3}{4}$ oz crème de cacao
20 ml/$\frac{3}{4}$ oz cream

Crack ice and put in a shaker with other ingredients. Shake well and strain into a cocktail glass.

American Beauty

50 ml/2 oz dry vermouth
50 ml/2 oz orange juice
25 ml/1 oz brandy
20 ml/$\frac{3}{4}$ oz grenadine
4 ice cubes
1 cocktail cherry
2 lemon slices
2 apple or orange slices
1 strawberry
1 teaspoon port

Put vermouth, orange juice, brandy and grenadine in a mixing glass and stir well. Crush ice and put in a goblet, add contents of mixing glass and decorate with cherry and slices of fruit. Trickle port over top and serve with a straw and a spoon.

American Cooler

3 ice cubes
100 ml/4 oz red wine
25 ml/1 oz rum
15 ml/$\frac{1}{2}$ oz sugar syrup
1 teaspoon orange juice
1 teaspoon lemon juice
soda water
1 lemon slice

Put ice in a tall tumbler with wine, rum, sugar syrup, orange juice and lemon juice. Stir well and top up with soda water. Fix lemon slice on rim of glass.

From left to right: Amour Crusta, American Cooler, American Beauty

American Glory

4 ice cubes
25 ml/1 oz orange juice
2 teaspoons grenadine
sparkling wine
1 orange slice

Crush ice and put in a tall champagne glass. Add orange juice and grenadine and top up with sparkling wine. Decorate with orange slice and serve with a straw.

Americano

3 ice cubes
25 ml/1 oz red vermouth
25 ml/1 oz Campari
soda water
piece of lemon rind

Put ice in a tumbler with vermouth and Campari. Stir and top up with soda water. Decorate with piece of lemon rind and serve with a straw.

Amour Crusta

15 ml/$\frac{1}{2}$ oz lemon juice
1 tablespoon castor sugar
2–3 ice cubes
50 ml/2 oz tawny port
1 teaspoon Cointreau
1 teaspoon maraschino
2 dashes peach bitters
2 dashes lime juice
spiral of lemon peel

Dip rim of a cocktail glass first in lemon juice, shaking off excess, then in sugar. Allow frosting to dry. Crack ice and put in a shaker with remaining ingredients except lemon peel. Shake well and strain into glass. Decorate with lemon peel.

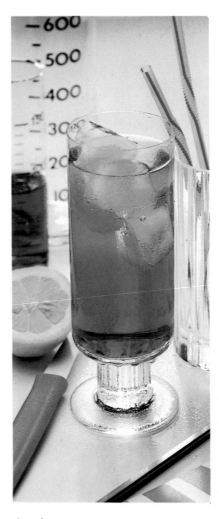

Americano

Angel's Face

2–3 ice cubes
20 ml/$\frac{3}{4}$ oz gin
20 ml/$\frac{3}{4}$ oz apricot brandy
2 teaspoons calvados

Crack ice and put in a shaker with other ingredients. Shake well and strain into a cocktail glass.

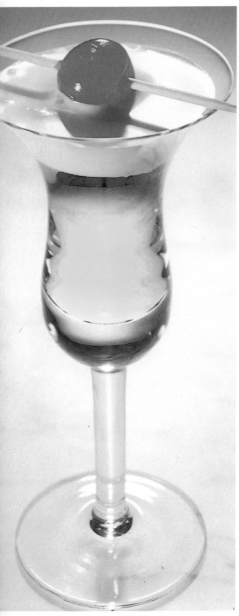

Angel's Kiss

Angel's Lips

50 ml/2 oz Bénédictine
20 ml/¾ oz cream

Pour Bénédictine into a pousse-café glass. Add cream, pouring it gently over back of a spoon so that it floats on surface.

Anisette Cocktail

2–3 ice cubes
20 ml/¾ oz gin
20 ml/¾ oz Pernod
20 ml/¾ oz anisette
1 dash Angostura bitters

Crack ice and put in a shaker with gin, Pernod and anisette. Shake well. Strain into a cocktail glass and add bitters. A glass of iced water may be offered with this cocktail.

Annabelle

3 ice cubes
25 ml/1 oz Grand Marnier
25 ml/1 oz kirsch
25 ml/1 oz orange juice
1 orange slice
spiral of orange peel

Crush ice and put in a shaker. Add Grand Marnier, kirsch and orange juice and shake well. Put orange slice in a large cocktail glass and add contents of shaker. Spear orange peel on a cocktail stick and use to decorate.

Applejack Rabbit

2–3 ice cubes
25 ml/1 oz applejack or calvados
20 ml/¾ oz orange juice
2 teaspoons lemon juice
1 teaspoon sugar syrup
1 dash orange bitters

Crack ice and put in a shaker with other ingredients. Shake well and strain into a cocktail glass.

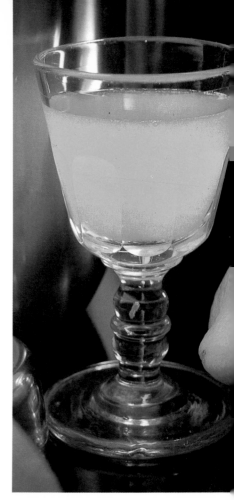

Applejack Rabbit

Apricot Blossom

2–3 ice cubes
25 ml/1 oz plum brandy
25 ml/1 oz orange juice
20 ml/¾ oz apricot brandy

Crack ice and put in a shaker with other ingredients. Shake well and strain into a large cocktail glass.

Apricot Brandy Daisy

2–3 ice cubes
25 ml/1 oz apricot brandy
25 ml/1 oz lemon juice
1 teaspoon brandy
sparkling wine

Crack ice and put in a shaker with apricot brandy, lemon juice and brandy. Shake well and strain into a tall champagne glass. Top up with sparkling wine.

Angel's Kiss

40 ml/1½ oz apricot brandy
15 ml/½ oz cream
1 cocktail cherry

Pour apricot brandy into a pousse-café glass. Add cream, pouring it gently over back of a spoon so that it floats on surface. Spear cherry on a cocktail stick and use to decorate.

14

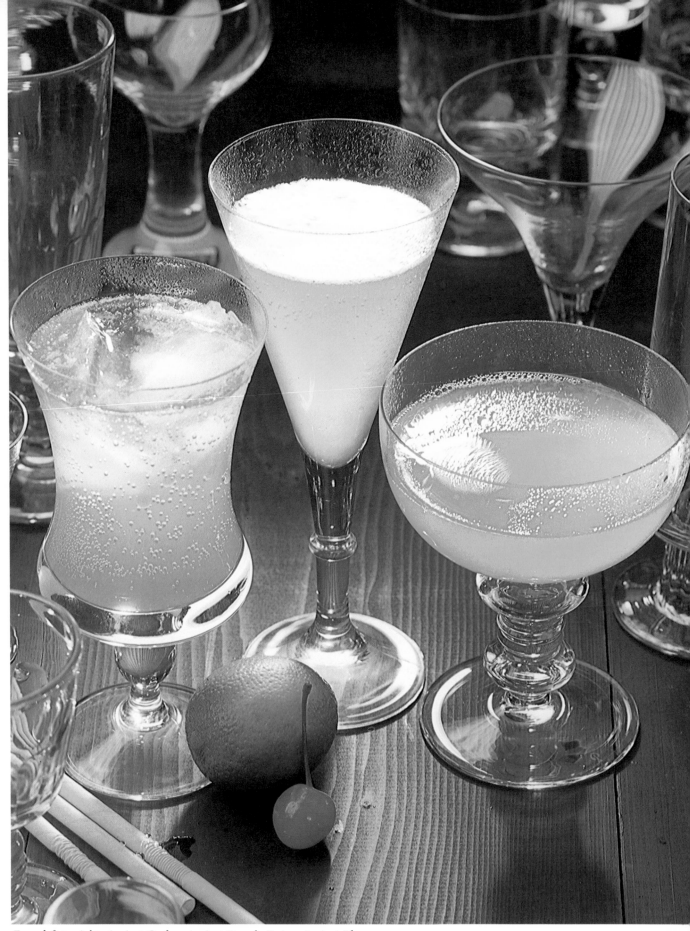

From left to right: Apricot Cooler, Apricot Brandy Daisy, Apricot Blossom

Apricot Cooler

(picture on page 15)

3 ice cubes
25 ml/1 oz apricot brandy
25 ml/1 oz orange juice
25 ml/1 oz lemon juice
1 teaspoon grenadine
soda water

Put ice in a goblet with apricot brandy, orange juice, lemon juice and grenadine. Stir well and top up with soda water.

April Shower

2 ice cubes
25 ml/1 oz brandy
25 ml/1 oz Bénédictine
50 ml/2 oz orange juice
soda water

Put ice in a tall goblet with brandy and Bénédictine. Stir well and add orange juice. Top up with soda water and serve with a straw.

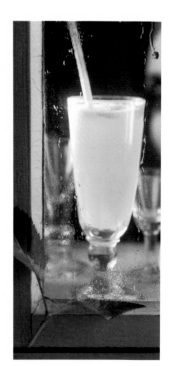

April Shower

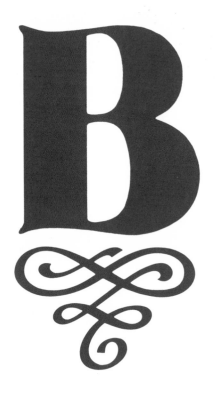

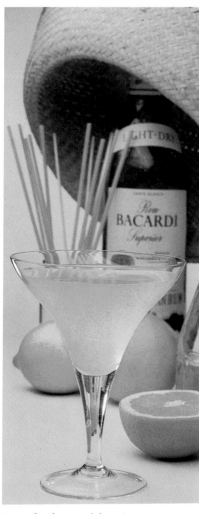

Bacardi Blossom (above)
Bacardi Highball (right)

Bacardi Blossom

2–3 ice cubes
40 ml/1½ oz white rum
2 teaspoons orange juice
2 teaspoons lemon juice
1 teaspoon sugar syrup

Crack ice and put in a shaker with other ingredients. Shake well and strain into a cocktail glass.

Bacardi Highball

3 ice cubes
25 ml/1 oz white rum
25 ml/1 oz Cointreau
1 teaspoon lemon juice
soda water

Crack two ice cubes and put in a shaker. Add rum, Cointreau and lemon juice. Shake well and strain into a goblet or glass mug. Add remaining ice cube and a shot of soda water. Serve with a straw.

Balalaika

2–3 ice cubes
40 ml/1½ oz vodka
15 ml/½ oz Cointreau
15 ml/½ oz lemon juice
spiral of orange peel

Crack ice and put in a shaker with vodka, Cointreau and lemon juice. Shake well and strain into a large cocktail glass. Decorate with spiral of orange peel.

16

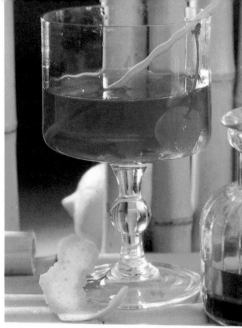

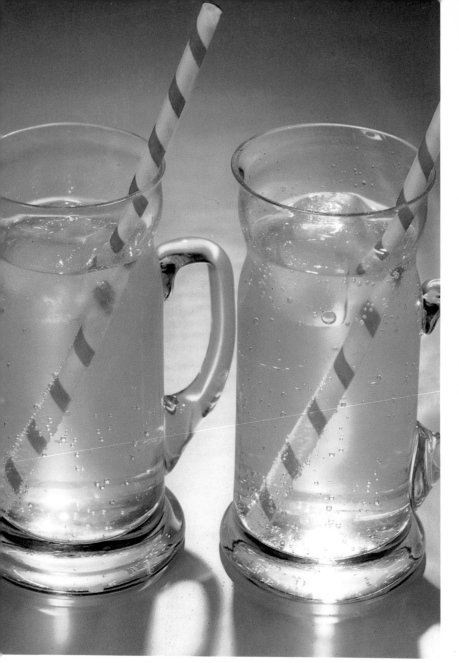

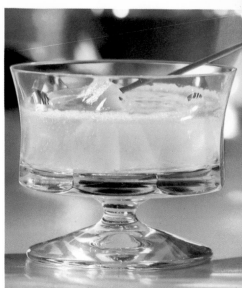

Bamboo (top)
Barfly's Dream (above)

Bamboo

2 ice cubes
25 ml/1 oz dry vermouth
25 ml/1 oz sherry
2 dashes Angostura bitters
1 dash orange bitters
1 cocktail cherry
piece of lemon peel

Put ice, vermouth, sherry, Angostura and orange bitters in a mixing glass. Stir well. Strain into a cocktail glass and decorate with cherry. Squeeze lemon peel over top and serve with a straw.

Barbarians' Tracks

2–3 ice cubes
25 ml/1 oz Scotch whisky
2 teaspoons gin
2 teaspoons rum
2 teaspoons crème de cacao
2 teaspoons cream
piece of lemon peel

Crack ice and put in a shaker with all other ingredients except lemon peel. Shake well and strain into a cocktail glass. Squeeze lemon peel over top.

Barfly's Dream

2–3 ice cubes
15 ml/½ oz gin
15 ml/½ oz white rum
15 ml/½ oz pineapple juice
4–5 pineapple chunks

Crack ice and put in a shaker with gin, rum and pineapple juice. Shake well and strain into a cocktail glass. Decorate with pineapple chunks and serve with a cocktail stick.

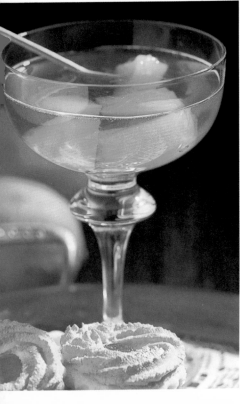

Bazooka

2–3 ice cubes
25 ml/1 oz green Chartreuse
2 teaspoons brandy
2 teaspoons cherry brandy
2 teaspoons gin
4–5 pineapple chunks

Crack ice and put in a shaker with Chartreuse, brandy, cherry brandy and gin. Shake well and strain into a cocktail glass. Decorate with pineapple chunks and serve with a cocktail stick.

Beau Rivage

2–3 ice cubes
15 ml/½ oz white rum
15 ml/½ oz gin
1 teaspoon dry vermouth
1 teaspoon red vermouth
1 teaspoon grenadine
1 teaspoon orange juice

Crack ice and put in a shaker with other ingredients. Shake well and strain into a cocktail glass.

Beautiful

2–3 ice cubes
15 ml/½ oz dry vermouth
2 teaspoons white rum
2 teaspoons gin
2 teaspoons grenadine
2 teaspoons orange juice
1 orange slice

Crack ice and put in a shaker with all other ingredients except orange slice. Shake well and strain into a cocktail glass. Fix orange slice on rim of glass.

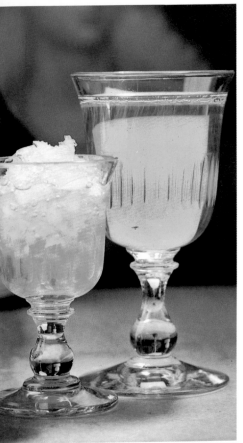

Bazooka (top left), Bénédictine Frappé (far left), Bénédictine Pick-me-up (left)

Bel Ami

20 ml/¾ oz brandy
20 ml/¾ oz apricot brandy
20 ml/¾ oz cream
2 tablespoons vanilla ice cream

Put all ingredients in an electric blender, mix, and serve in a wine goblet with ice cream wafers.

Bénédictine Frappé

3 ice cubes
25 ml/1 oz Bénédictine

Crush ice and put in a cocktail glass. Pour Bénédictine over ice and serve with a straw.

Bénédictine Pick-me-up

2–3 ice cubes
40 ml/1½ oz Bénédictine
2 dashes Angostura bitters
sparkling wine

Crack ice and put in a shaker with Bénédictine and bitters. Shake and strain into a champagne glass. Top up with sparkling wine.

Berlin

3 ice cubes
20 ml/¾ oz gin
20 ml/¾ oz Madeira
20 ml/¾ oz orange juice
1 dash Angostura bitters

Crush ice and put in a shaker with other ingredients. Shake well and pour into a cocktail glass. Serve with a straw.

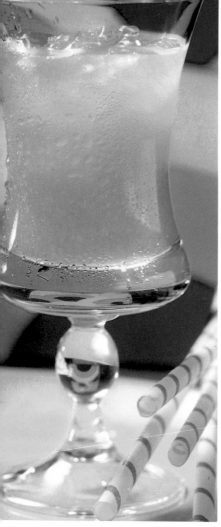

Berlin

Betsy Ross

2–3 ice cubes
25 ml/1 oz brandy
25 ml/1 oz port
2 dashes Cointreau
1 dash Angostura bitters

Crack ice and put in a shaker with other ingredients. Shake well and strain into a cocktail glass.

Between the Sheets

2–3 ice cubes
20 ml/$\frac{3}{4}$ oz brandy
20 ml/$\frac{3}{4}$ oz white rum
20 ml/$\frac{3}{4}$ oz Cointreau
15 ml/$\frac{1}{2}$ oz orange juice

Crack ice and put in a shaker with other ingredients. Shake well and strain into a large cocktail glass.

Bijou

2 ice cubes
15 ml/$\frac{1}{2}$ oz gin
15 ml/$\frac{1}{2}$ oz green Chartreuse
15 ml/$\frac{1}{2}$ oz red vermouth
1 dash orange bitters
1 olive
piece of lemon peel

Put ice in a mixing glass with gin, Chartreuse, vermouth and bitters. Stir well and strain into a cocktail glass. Spear olive on a cocktail stick and use to decorate. Squeeze lemon peel over top.

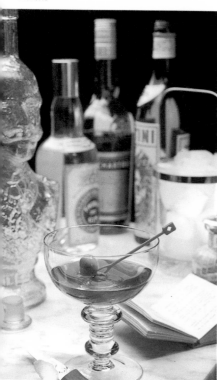

Bijou

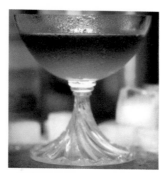

Black Russian

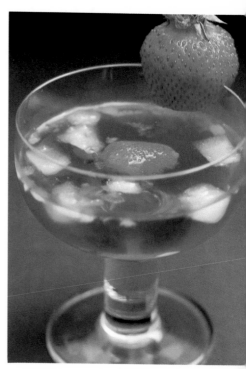

Bloodhound

Black Russian

2–3 ice cubes
40 ml/1$\frac{1}{2}$ oz vodka
15 ml/$\frac{1}{2}$ oz coffee liqueur

Put ice in a mixing glass with vodka and coffee liqueur. Stir well and strain into a cocktail glass.

Bloodhound

4 ice cubes
15 ml/$\frac{1}{2}$ oz gin
15 ml/$\frac{1}{2}$ oz dry vermouth
15 ml/$\frac{1}{2}$ oz red vermouth
2–3 dashes strawberry liqueur
4 strawberries

Crack ice. Put half cracked ice in an electric blender with gin, vermouths, strawberry liqueur and two strawberries. Blend briefly and strain into a cocktail glass. Add remaining cracked ice and decorate with remaining strawberries. Serve with a straw and a spoon.

Bloody Mary

25 ml/1 oz vodka
50 ml/2 oz tomato juice
15 ml/½ oz lemon juice
2 dashes Worcestershire sauce
1 ice cube (optional)

Put vodka, tomato juice, lemon juice and Worcestershire sauce in a tumbler and stir. Crush ice, if using, and add to cocktail.

Blue Day

2–3 ice cubes
40 ml/1½ oz vodka
20 ml/¾ oz blue curaçao
peel ½ lemon
1 lemon slice

Crack ice and put in a shaker with vodka and curaçao. Shake well. Squeeze lemon peel over a cocktail glass. Strain in contents of shaker and fix lemon slice on rim of glass.

Blue Lady

2–3 ice cubes
25 ml/1 oz gin
15 ml/½ oz blue curaçao
15 ml/½ oz lemon juice
1 cocktail cherry

Crack ice and put in a shaker with gin, curaçao and lemon juice. Shake well and strain into a cocktail glass. Decorate with cherry.

Blue Monday Nightcap (1)

2–3 ice cubes
25 ml/1 oz vodka
15 ml/½ oz blue curaçao
15 ml/½ oz Cointreau

Crack ice and put in a shaker with other ingredients. Shake well and strain into a tall glass.

Blue Monday Nightcap (2)

3 ice cubes
40 ml/1½ oz vodka
15 ml/½ oz Cointreau

Put ice in a mixing glass with vodka and Cointreau. Stir well and pour into a large cocktail glass.

Boniface the Good

2–3 ice cubes
2 egg yolks
1 tablespoon castor sugar
50 ml/2 oz Cointreau
50 ml/2 oz orange juice
sparkling wine

Crack ice and put in a shaker with egg yolks, sugar, Cointreau and orange juice. Shake well and strain into a goblet. Top up with sparkling wine and serve with a straw.

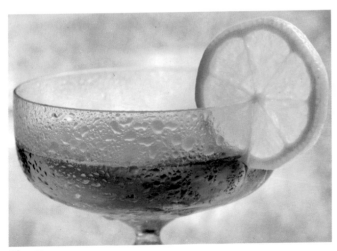

Blue Day

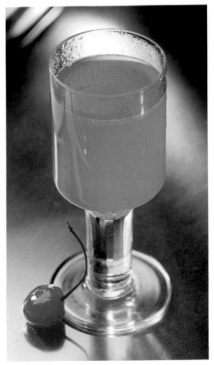

Blue Lady

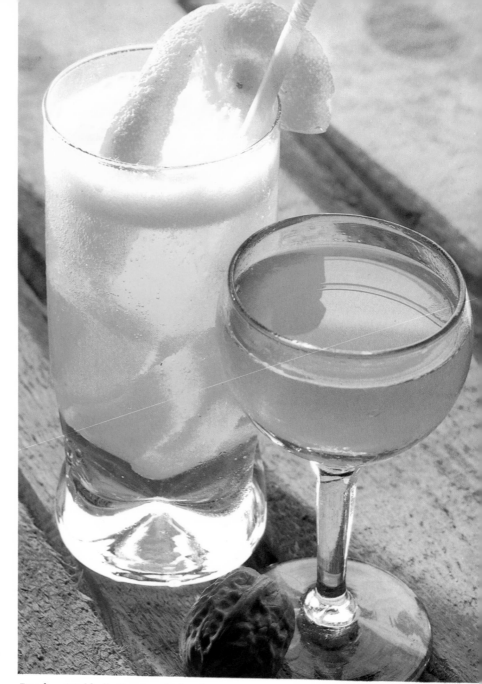

Bourbon Highball, Bourbon Cocktail

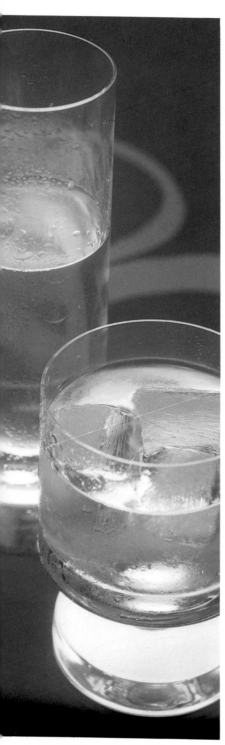

Blue Monday Nightcaps (1 and 2)

Bourbon Cocktail

2–3 ice cubes
25 ml/1 oz Bourbon whisky
2 teaspoons Bénédictine
2 teaspoons Cointreau
2 teaspoons lemon juice
1 dash Angostura bitters

Crack ice and put in a shaker with other ingredients. Shake well and strain into a cocktail glass.

Bourbon Highball

4 ice cubes
25 ml/1 oz Bourbon whisky
soda water or ginger ale
spiral of lemon peel

Put ice and whisky in a tumbler. Add soda water or ginger ale to taste. Decorate with spiral of lemon peel and serve with a straw.

21

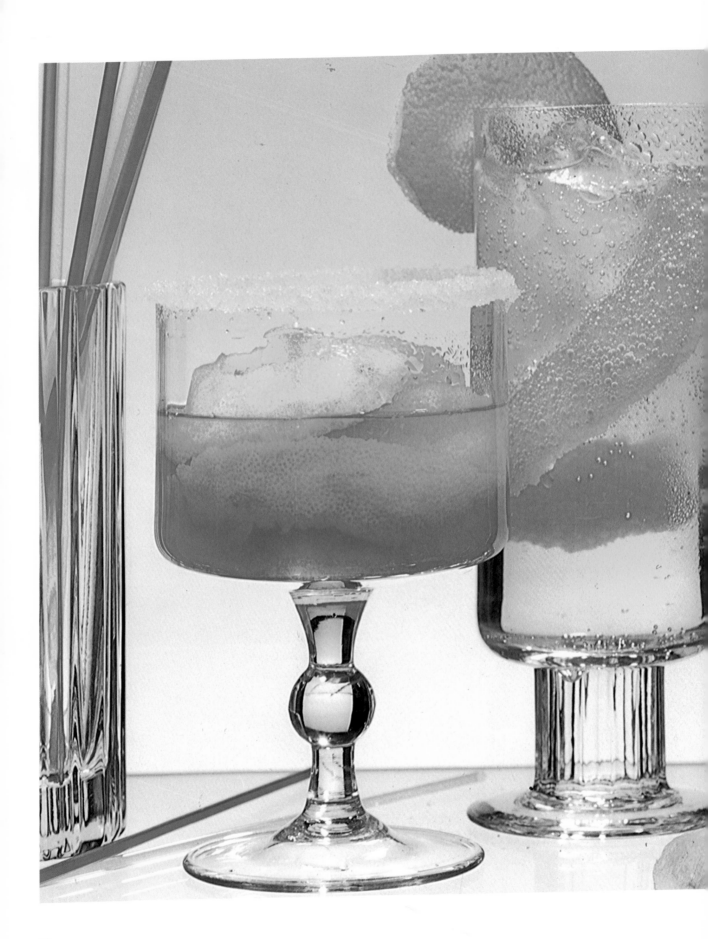

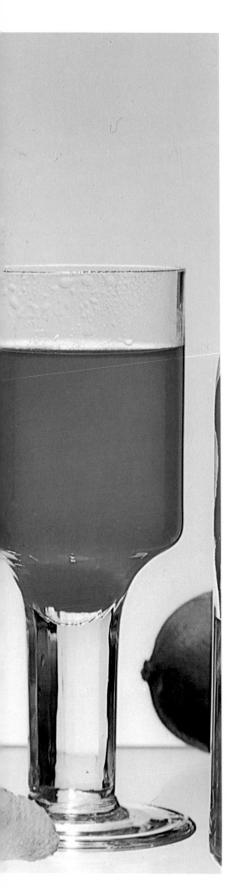

Brandy Cocktail

1−2 ice cubes
40 ml/1½ oz brandy
20 ml/¾ oz red vermouth
2 dashes Angostura bitters
piece of lemon peel
(optional)

Crack ice and put in a mixing glass. Add brandy, vermouth and bitters. Stir well and strain into a cocktail glass. Add piece of lemon peel, if liked.

Brandy Cooler

3−4 ice cubes
50 ml/2 oz brandy
soda water
spiral of orange peel

Put ice and brandy in a tall glass. Top up with soda water and decorate with spiral of orange peel.

Brandy Crusta

15 ml/½ oz lemon juice
1 tablespoon castor sugar
2−3 ice cubes
50 ml/2 oz brandy
1 teaspoon sugar syrup
3 dashes maraschino
2 dashes Angostura bitters
spiral of lemon peel

Dip rim of a large cocktail glass first in lemon juice, shaking off excess, then in sugar. Allow frosting to dry. Crack ice and put in a shaker with brandy, sugar syrup, maraschino and bitters. Shake well and strain into glass. Decorate with spiral of lemon peel.

From left to right: Brandy Crusta, Brandy Cooler, Brandy Cocktail

Brandy Daisy

2−3 ice cubes
25 ml/1 oz brandy
15 ml/½ oz lemon juice
2 teaspoons grenadine
soda water
3−4 cocktail cherries

Crack ice and put in a shaker with brandy, lemon juice and grenadine. Shake well and strain into a champagne glass. Top up with soda water. Decorate with cherries and serve with a cocktail stick.

Brandy Fix

40 ml/1½ oz brandy
20 ml/¾ oz cherry brandy
15 ml/½ oz lemon juice
1 teaspoon sugar syrup
1 ice cube
1 lemon slice

Put brandy, cherry brandy, lemon juice and sugar syrup in a small goblet. Stir well. Crush ice and add to glass. Lay lemon slice on top. Serve with a straw.

Brandy Flip

2−3 ice cubes
1 egg yolk
2 teaspoons sugar syrup
50 ml/2 oz brandy
nutmeg (optional)

Crack ice and put in a shaker with egg yolk. sugar syrup and brandy. Shake very well and strain into a flip glass. Grate a little nutmeg over top, if liked, and serve with a straw.

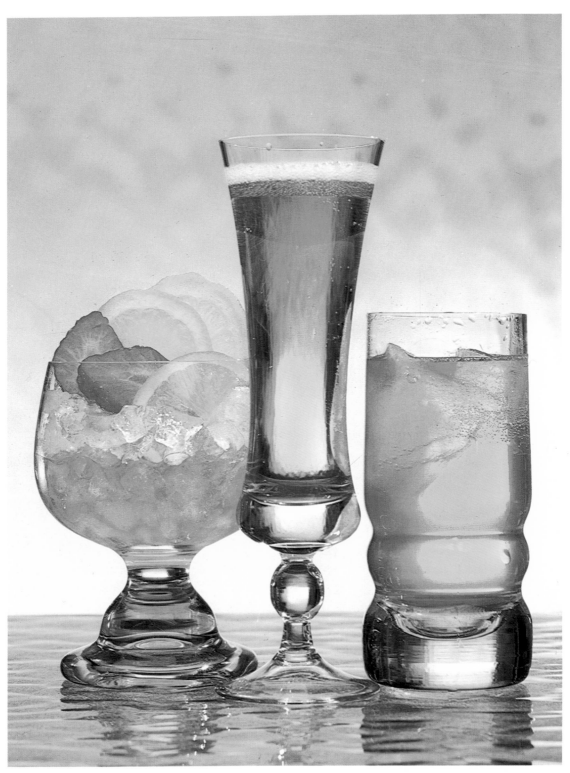

From left to right: Brandy Smash, Brandy Pick-me-up, Brandy Highball

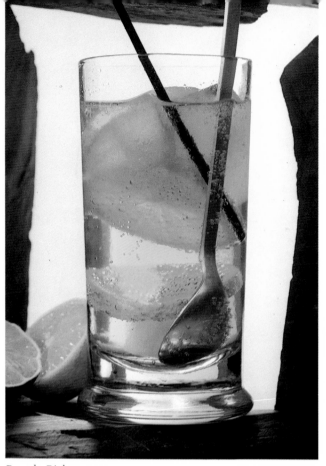

Brandy Rickey

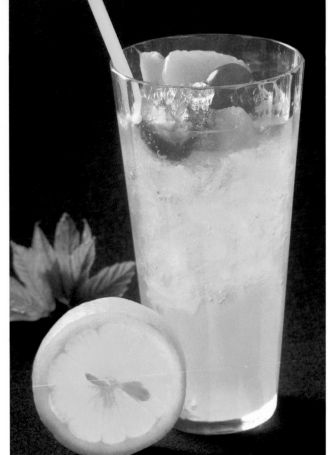

Brandy Tea Punch

Brandy Highball

3 ice cubes
25 ml/1 oz brandy
1 teaspoon lemon juice
1 teaspoon sugar syrup
1 dash orange bitters
soda water

Crack one ice cube and put in shaker. Add brandy, lemon juice, sugar syrup and bitters. Shake well and strain into a tumbler. Add remaining ice and top up with soda water.

Brandy Pick-me-up

2–3 ice cubes
25 ml/1 oz brandy
1 teaspoon sugar syrup
champagne

Crack ice and put in a shaker with brandy and sugar syrup. Shake well and strain into a flip glass. Top up with champagne.

Brandy Rickey

3–4 lemon slices
25 ml/1 oz brandy
2–3 ice cubes
soda water

Put lemon slices in a tumbler and press with a spoon to make juice run. Add brandy and ice and top up with soda water. Serve with a straw and spoon.

Brandy Smash

1 teaspoon castor sugar
1 teaspoon water
3 sprigs of mint
50 ml/2 oz brandy
3–4 ice cubes
3–4 lemon, lime or orange slices
2 strawberries (optional)
1–2 grapes (optional)

Put sugar in a shaker with water. Add mint, crush well with a spoon and remove. Add brandy and shake well. Crush ice and put in a balloon glass. Strain contents of shaker into glass and decorate with lemon, lime or orange slices and other available fruits. Serve with a straw and spoon.

Brandy Tea Punch

2–3 ice cubes
40 ml/1½ oz brandy
40 ml/1½ oz strong cold tea
20 ml/¾ oz Cointreau
15 ml/½ oz lemon juice
2 teaspoons sugar syrup
2 peach slices
2 cocktail cherries
2 strawberries

Crush ice and put in a tumbler with brandy, tea, Cointreau, lemon juice and sugar syrup. Stir well and decorate with fruits. Serve with a straw and a spoon.

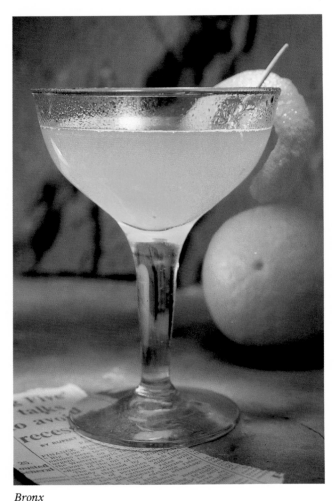

Bronx

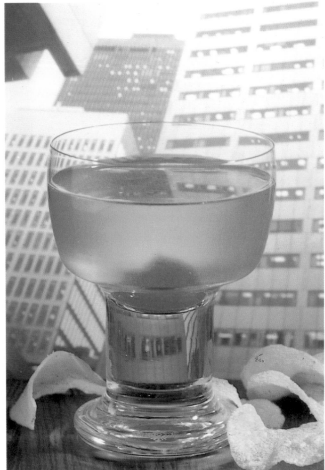

Brooklyn

Bronx

2–3 ice cubes
15 ml/½ oz gin
15 ml/½ oz dry vermouth
15 ml/½ oz red vermouth
15 ml/½ oz orange juice
1 dash Angostura bitters
spiral of orange peel

Crack ice and put in a shaker with gin, vermouths, orange juice and bitters. Shake well and strain into a cocktail glass. Spear orange peel on a cocktail stick and use to decorate.

Brooklyn

2–3 ice cubes
25 ml/1 oz whisky
25 ml/1 oz dry vermouth
2 teaspoons maraschino
3 dashes Amer Picon
1 cocktail cherry

Crack ice and put in a shaker with whisky, vermouth, maraschino and Amer Picon. Shake well and strain into a cocktail glass. Decorate with cherry.

Buck's Fizz

80 ml/3 oz orange juice
champagne

Put orange juice in a tall tumbler and top up with champagne.

Bullshot

2–3 ice cubes
40 ml/1½ oz vodka
50 ml/2 oz strong cold beef
   consommé
salt, pepper

Put ice in a mixing glass with other ingredients. Stir and strain into a large cocktail glass.

Burnt Punch

80 ml/3 oz hot water
50 ml/2 oz red wine
2 cloves
piece of lemon peel
1 grapefruit slice
3 sugar lumps
15 ml/½ oz rum

Put water, wine, cloves and lemon peel in a warmed flameproof punch glass and stir. Lay grapefruit slice on top of glass and place sugar lumps on top. Pour rum over sugar lumps. Stand glass on an asbestos mat and set light to sugar lumps.

Butler's Good Morning Flip

2 ice cubes
1 egg
1 egg yolk
2 teaspoons castor sugar
40 ml/1½ oz sherry
3 dashes Angostura bitters
sparkling wine

Crush ice and put in a shaker with egg, egg yolk, sugar, sherry and bitters. Shake very well and pour into a large cocktail glass. Top up with sparkling wine and serve with a straw.

Butterfly Flip

2–3 ice cubes
1 egg yolk
1 tablespoon castor sugar
25 ml/1 oz brandy
25 ml/1 oz crème de cacao
25 ml/1 oz cream
nutmeg

Crack ice and put in a shaker with egg yolk, sugar, brandy, crème de cacao and cream. Shake very well and strain into a large cocktail glass. Grate a little nutmeg over top and serve with a straw.

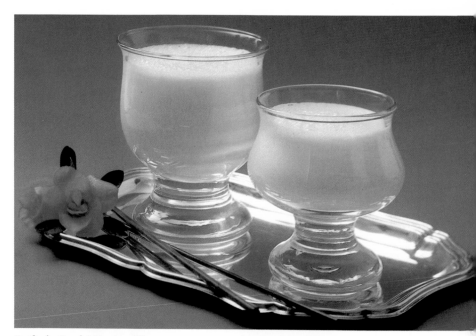

Butler's Good Morning Flip

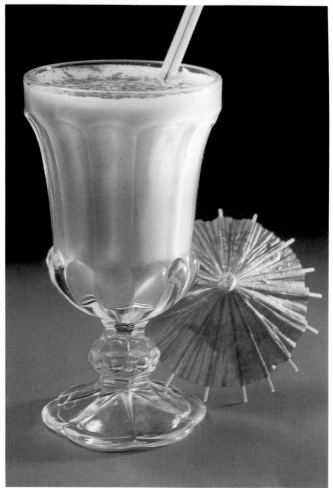

Butterfly Flip

Byrrh Cocktail

2–3 ice cubes
20 ml/¾ oz Byrrh
20 ml/¾ oz rye whisky
20 ml/¾ oz red vermouth

Put ice in a mixing glass with other ingredients and stir. Strain into a cocktail glass.

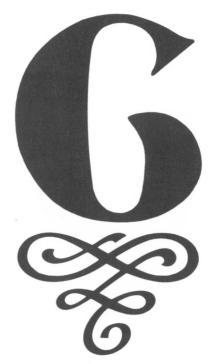

C and S

2 ice cubes
25 ml/1 oz green Chartreuse
25 ml/1 oz Scotch whisky

Put ice in a mixing glass with Chartreuse and whisky. Stir and strain into a cocktail glass.

Cablegram Cooler

3 ice cubes
25 ml/1 oz whisky
15 ml/½ oz lemon juice
1–2 teaspoons sugar syrup
ginger ale
spiral of orange peel

Crack two ice cubes and put in a shaker with whisky, lemon juice and sugar syrup. Shake well and strain into a goblet. Top up with ginger ale and add remaining ice. Decorate with spiral of orange peel and serve with a straw.

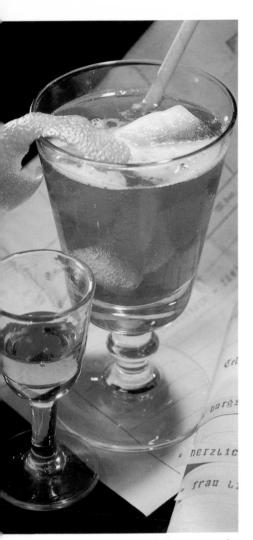

Cablegram Cooler

Cacao Frappé

3 ice cubes
25 ml/1 oz crème de cacao
25 ml/1 oz very strong cold coffee
2–3 cocktail cherries

Crush ice and put in a shallow champagne glass. Add crème de cacao and coffee, and stir. Decorate with cherries and serve with a straw and a spoon.

Calvados Cocktail

2–3 ice cubes
25 ml/1 oz calvados
25 ml/1 oz Cointreau
15 ml/½ oz orange juice
3 dashes orange bitters

Crack ice and put in a shaker with other ingredients. Shake and strain into a cocktail glass.

Calvados Smash

2–3 ice cubes
2 tablespoons mixed fruit
1 teaspoon castor sugar
soda water
3 sprigs of mint
25 ml/1 oz calvados
3 dashes crème de menthe
1 dash Bénédictine
apple juice
1 mint leaf

Crush ice, put in a tall glass and add fruit. Put sugar in a shaker and add a shot of soda water. Add sprigs of mint and crush well with a spoon. Add calvados, crème de menthe and Bénédictine and shake well. Strain into glass and top up with apple juice. Decorate with mint leaf and serve with a straw.

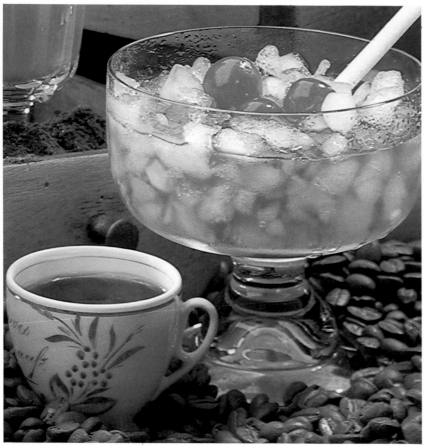

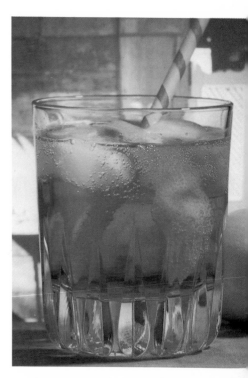

Cacao Frappé

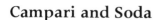

Campari and Soda

2–3 ice cubes
40 ml/1½ oz Campari
soda water
spiral of lemon peel

Put ice in a large tumbler, add Campari and top up with soda water to taste. Decorate with spiral of lemon peel and serve with a straw.

Campino

15 ml/½ oz Campari
15 ml/½ oz dry vermouth
15 ml/½ oz red vermouth
15 ml/½ oz gin
2 dashes crème de cassis
soda water
spiral of orange peel

Put Campari, vermouths, gin and crème de cassis in a mixing glass. Top up with soda water and stir. Pour into a small tumbler and decorate with spiral of orange peel.

Cape Kennedy

2–3 ice cubes
20 ml/¾ oz orange juice
20 ml/¾ oz lemon juice
1 teaspoon whisky
1 teaspoon rum
1 teaspoon Bénédictine
1 teaspoon sugar syrup

Crack ice and put in a shaker with other ingredients. Shake well and strain into a cocktail glass.

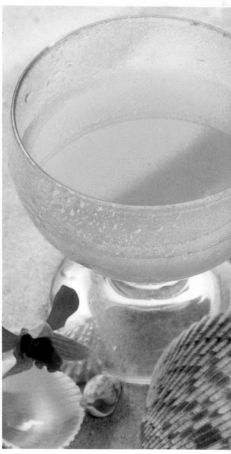

Campari and Soda (top)
Cape Kennedy (above)

29

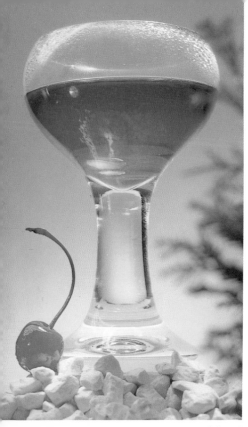

Capri (above)
Carioca (right)

Capri

2–3 ice cubes
40 ml/1½ oz brandy
15 ml/½ oz red vermouth
1 teaspoon Campari
1 cocktail cherry

Put ice in a mixing glass with brandy, vermouth and Campari. Stir and strain into a cocktail glass. Decorate with cherry.

Carioca

2–3 ice cubes
25 ml/1 oz Grand Marnier
20 ml/¾ oz rum
2 teaspoons rosehip syrup
1 teaspoon instant coffee powder
1 dash lemon juice
15 ml/½ oz whipped cream
   (optional)

Crack ice and put in a shaker with all other ingredients except cream. Shake and strain into a cocktail glass. Pipe whipped cream on top, if liked. Serve with a straw.

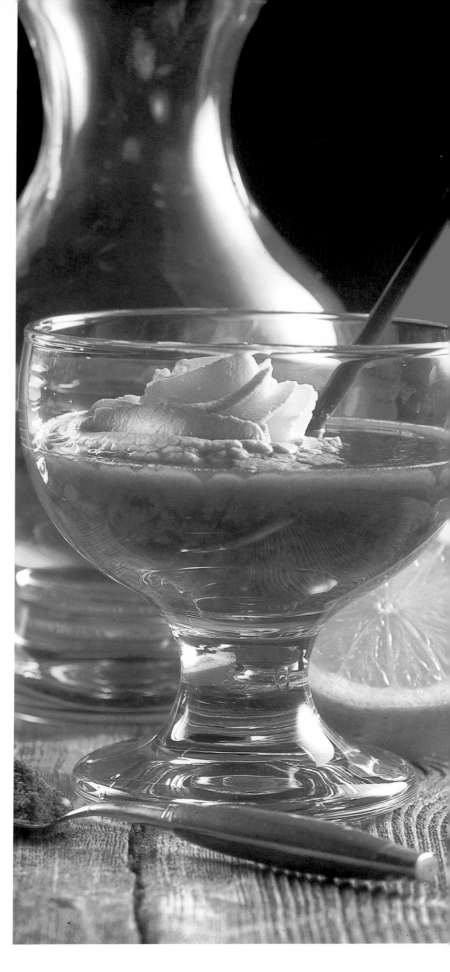

30

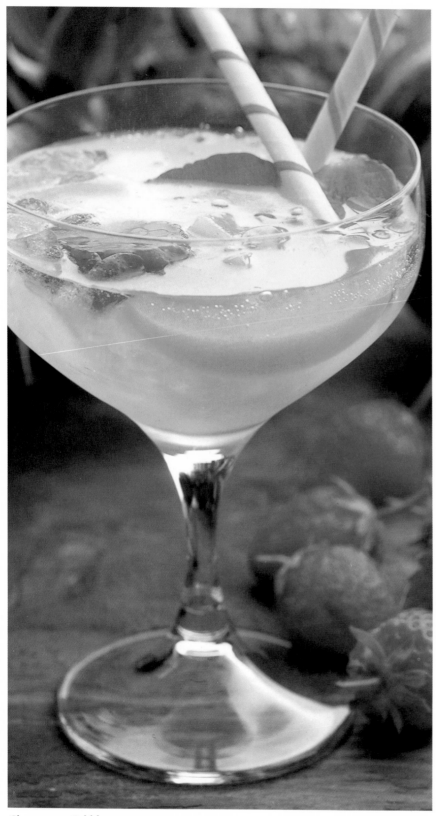

Champagne Cobbler

Champagne Cobbler

3–4 ice cubes
3 strawberries (sliced) or cocktail
   cherries
4 peach slices
3 pineapple chunks
1 teaspoon Cointreau
1 teaspoon maraschino
1 teaspoon lemon juice
champagne

Crush ice and put in a goblet. Smooth top of crushed ice and decorate with fruits. Add Cointreau, maraschino and lemon juice and top up with champagne. Serve with a straw and a spoon.

Champagne Cocktail

(picture on page 327)

1 sugar lump
2 dashes Angostura bitters
1 ice cube
champagne
piece of lemon peel

Put sugar lump in a shallow champagne glass and soak with bitters. Add ice, top up with champagne and squeeze lemon peel over top. Serve with a straw.

Champagne Daisy

2–3 ice cubes
20 ml/$\frac{3}{4}$ oz yellow Chartreuse
20 ml/$\frac{3}{4}$ oz lemon juice
2 teaspoons grenadine
champagne
fruit in season

Crack ice and put in a shaker with Chartreuse, lemon juice and grenadine. Shake well and strain into a shallow champagne glass. Top up with champagne and decorate with pieces of fruit. Serve with a cocktail stick and a straw.

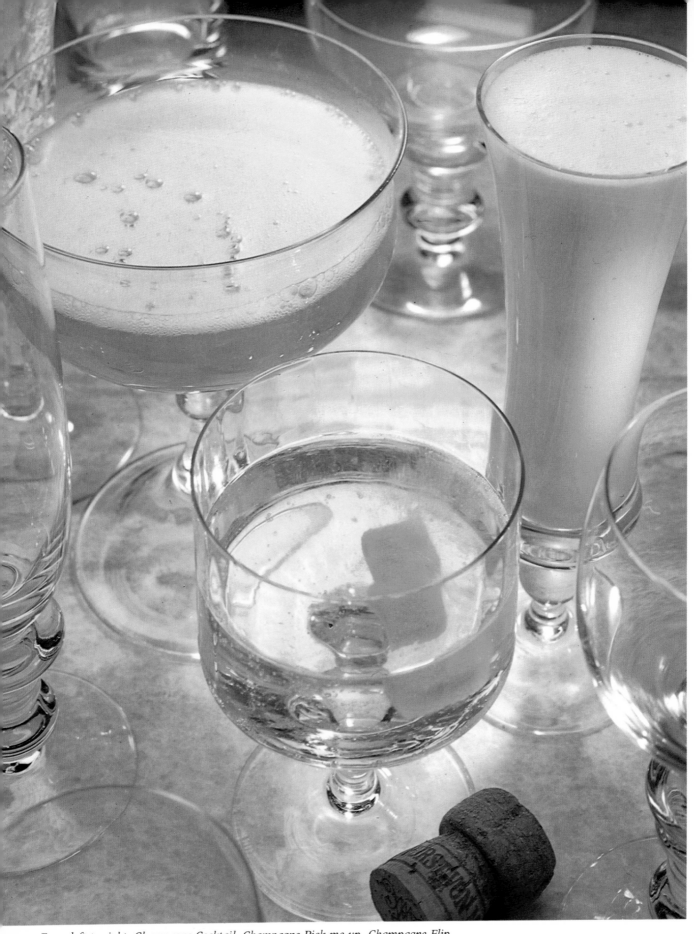

From left to right: Champagne Cocktail, Champagne Pick-me-up, Champagne Flip

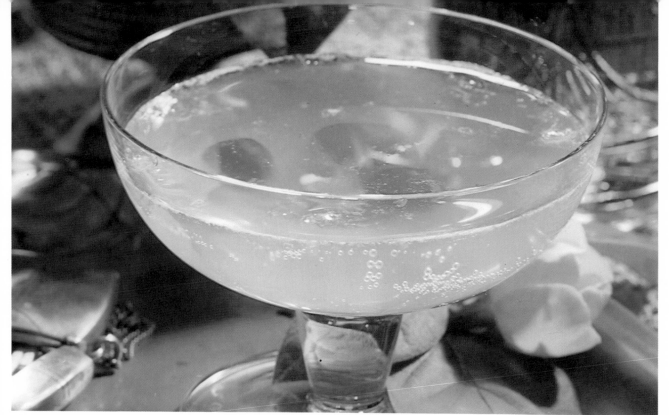

Chartreuse Daisy

Champagne Flip

2–3 ice cubes
1 egg yolk
2 teaspoons sugar syrup
50 ml/2 oz Rhine wine
champagne

Crack ice and put in a shaker with egg yolk, sugar syrup and wine. Shake very well and strain into a flip glass. Top up with champagne and serve with a straw.

Champagne Pick-me-up

2–3 ice cubes
15 ml/½ oz brandy
15 ml/½ oz dry vermouth
1 teaspoon sugar syrup
champagne

Put ice in a mixing glass with brandy, vermouth and sugar syrup. Stir and strain into a goblet. Top up with champagne.

Charleston

2–3 ice cubes
15 ml/½ oz gin
15 ml/½ oz dry vermouth
15 ml/½ oz bianco vermouth
2 teaspoons maraschino
1 teaspoon kirsch
1 teaspoon Cointreau
piece of lemon peel

Put ice in a mixing glass with gin, vermouths, maraschino, kirsch and Cointreau. Stir well and strain into a cocktail glass. Squeeze lemon peel over top.

Charlie Chaplin

2–3 ice cubes
25 ml/1 oz gin
20 ml/¾ oz lemon juice
15 ml/½ oz apricot brandy
1 cocktail cherry

Crack ice and put in a shaker with gin, lemon juice and apricot brandy. Shake well, strain into a cocktail glass. Decorate with cherry, serve with a cocktail stick.

Chartreuse Daisy

2–3 ice cubes
40 ml/1½ oz brandy
20 ml/¾ oz green Chartreuse
1 teaspoon lemon juice
soda water
3 cocktail cherries

Crack ice and put in a shaker with brandy, Chartreuse and lemon juice. Shake and strain into a shallow champagne glass. Top up with soda water and decorate with cherries. Serve with a cocktail stick.

Chartreuse Straight

40 ml/1½ oz yellow Chartreuse
20 ml/¾ oz green Chartreuse
1 ice cube

Put yellow and green Chartreuse in a cocktail glass. Stir, then add ice. Serve very cold.

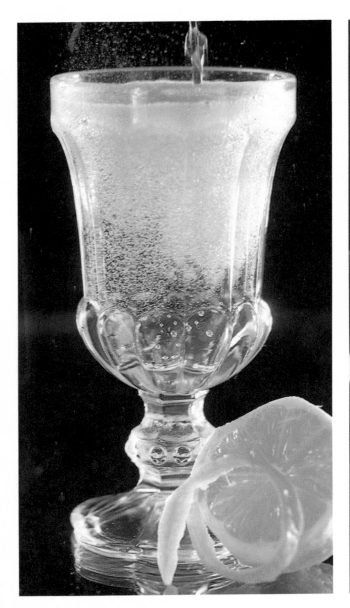

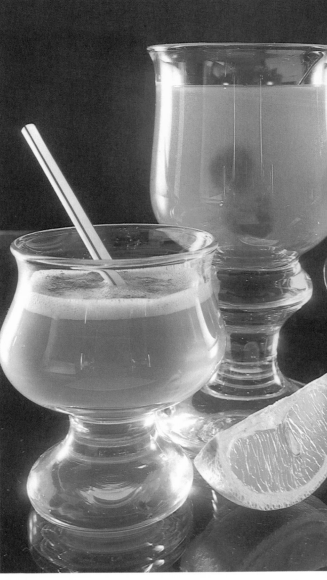

Chartreuse Temptation (above), Cherry Brandy Flip and Cherry Blossom (above right)

Chartreuse Temptation

25 ml/1 oz green Chartreuse
1 ice cube
1 teaspoon lemon juice
sparkling wine

Pour Chartreuse into a tall champagne glass. Add ice and lemon juice and top up with sparkling wine.

Cherry Blossom

2–3 ice cubes
25 ml/1 oz brandy
20 ml/¾ oz orange juice
15 ml/½ oz cherry brandy
3 dashes Cointreau
3 dashes grenadine
2–5 cocktail cherries

Crack ice and put in a shaker with all other ingredients except cherries. Shake well and strain into a cocktail glass. Decorate with cherries.

Cherry Brandy Flip

2–3 ice cubes
1 egg yolk
2 teaspoons sugar syrup
25 ml/1 oz cherry brandy
nutmeg

Crack ice and put in a shaker with egg yolk, sugar syrup and cherry brandy. Shake very well and strain into a cocktail glass. Grate a little nutmeg over top and serve with a straw.

Cherry Sour

2–3 ice cubes
40 ml/1½ oz cherry brandy
25 ml/1 oz lemon juice
1 teaspoon sugar syrup
soda water
3 cocktail cherries
1 lemon slice

Crack ice and put in a shaker with cherry brandy, lemon juice and sugar syrup. Shake well and strain into a tumbler. Top up with soda water, add cherries and fix lemon slice on rim of glass.

Chicago Cocktail

2 ice cubes
40 ml/1½ oz brandy
1 teaspoon Cointreau
1 dash Angostura bitters
sparkling wine

Put ice in a mixing glass with brandy, Cointreau and bitters. Stir well and strain into a shallow champagne glass. Top up with sparkling wine and serve with a straw.

Chicago Cooler

2–3 ice cubes
15 ml/½ oz red wine
2 teaspoons lemon juice
1 teaspoon sugar syrup
ginger ale
1 lemon slice
1 cocktail cherry

Put ice, wine, lemon juice and sugar syrup in a tumbler and stir. Top up with ginger ale. Decorate with lemon slice and cherry.

Cherry Sour (top right)
Chicago Cocktail (right)

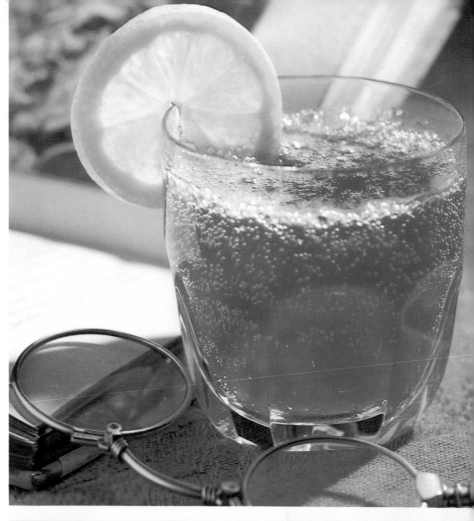

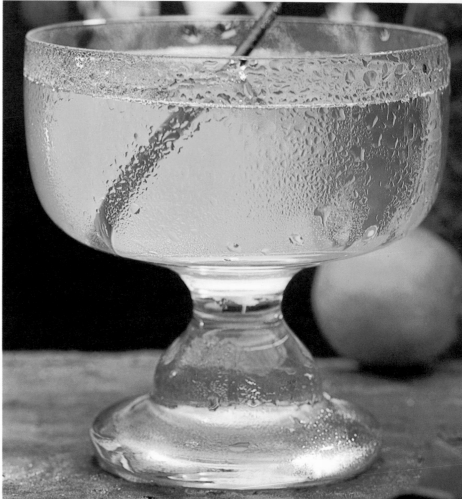

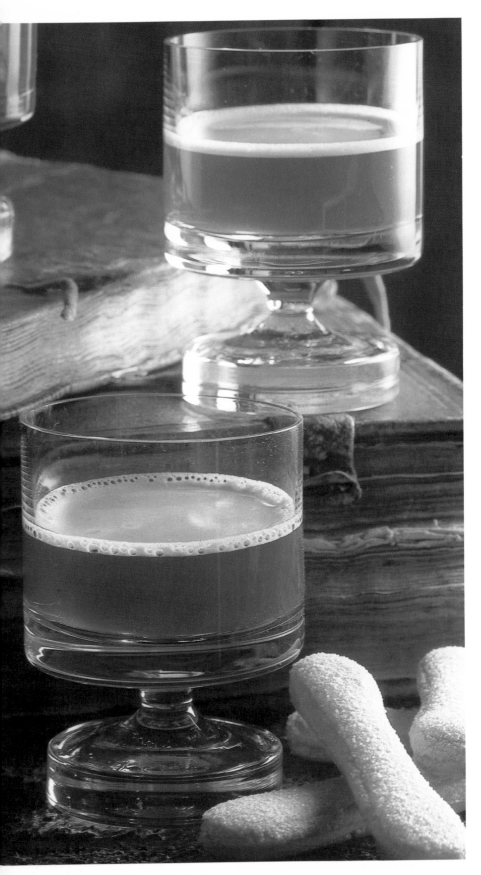

Chocolate Cocktail

2–3 ice cubes
40 ml/1½ oz port
2 teaspoons crème de cacao
2 teaspoons yellow Chartreuse
1 teaspoon grated bitter chocolate

Crack ice and put in a shaker with other ingredients. Shake well and strain into a cocktail glass.

Chocolate Soldier

2 ice cubes
25 ml/1 oz brandy
20 ml/¾ oz dry vermouth
2 teaspoons crème de cacao
1 dash orange bitters

Crack ice and put in an electric blender with other ingredients. Blend and pour into a shallow goblet.

Claret Fizz

2–3 ice cubes
40 ml/1½ oz claret
25 ml/1 oz lemon juice
soda water

Crack ice and put in a shaker with claret and lemon juice. Shake well and strain into a large tumbler. Top up with soda water and serve with a straw.

Claret Flip

2–3 ice cubes
1 egg yolk
2 teaspoons sugar syrup
50 ml/2 oz claret
nutmeg

Crack ice and put in a shaker with egg yolk, sugar syrup and claret. Shake very well and strain into a goblet. Grate a little nutmeg over top and serve with a straw.

Chocolate Soldier

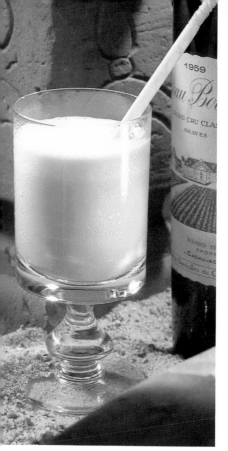

Claret Flip

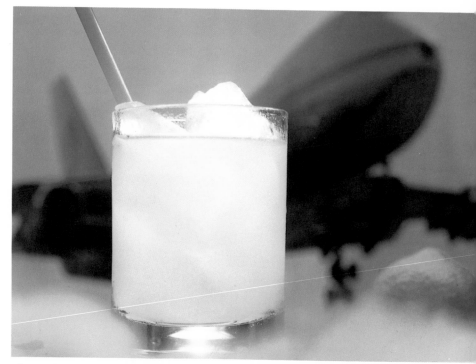

Clipper (above), Coffee Advocaat (below)

Claret Sour

1 ice cube
20 ml/¾ oz rum
15 ml/½ oz lemon juice
1 teaspoon castor sugar
claret
½ lemon slice

Crush ice and put in a shaker with rum, lemon juice and sugar. Shake well and pour into a goblet. Top up with claret and add lemon slice.

Clipper

25 ml/1 oz white rum
25 ml/1 oz lemon juice
15 ml/½ oz gin
½ teaspoon castor sugar
2–3 ice cubes

Put rum, lemon juice, gin and sugar in a mixing glass and stir well. Put ice in a small goblet, strain contents of mixing glass over ice and serve with a straw.

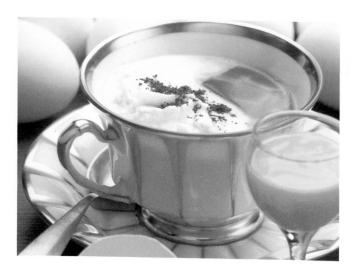

Clover Club

2–3 ice cubes
1 egg white
15 ml/½ oz lemon juice
40 ml/1½ oz gin
20 ml/¾ oz grenadine

Crack ice and put in a shaker with other ingredients. Shake very well and strain into a small goblet.

Coffee Advocaat

40 ml/1½ oz advocaat
hot coffee
25 ml/1 oz whipped cream
ground coffee

Pour advocaat into a warmed cup, top up with hot coffee, then add whipped cream. Sprinkle with a little ground coffee.

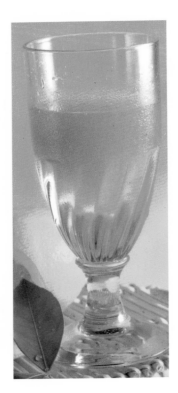

Coffee Cobbler

Coffee Cobbler

3–4 ice cubes
25 ml/1 oz brandy
strong cold sweetened coffee

Crush ice and put in a goblet. Add brandy and top up with coffee. Stir, and serve with a straw.

Colonel Collins

40 ml/1½ oz Bourbon whisky
25 ml/1 oz lemon juice
2 teaspoons castor sugar
4 ice cubes
soda water
1 lemon slice

Put whisky, lemon juice and sugar in a tall tumbler. Stir well. Crush ice and add to tumbler. Top up with soda water. Fix lemon slice on rim of glass and serve with a straw.

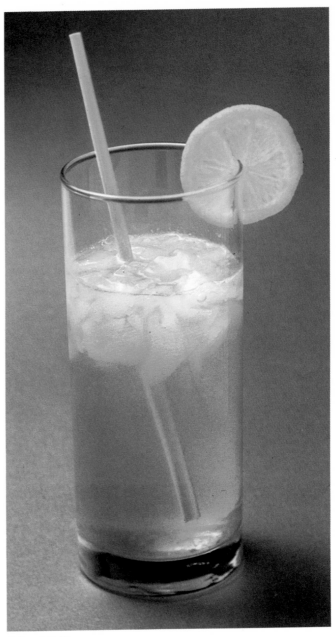

Colonel Collins

Colorado

2–3 ice cubes
20 ml/¾ oz cherry brandy
20 ml/¾ oz kirsch
20 ml/¾ oz cream

Crack ice and put in a shaker with other ingredients. Shake well, strain into a cocktail glass and serve with a straw.

Columbus

2–3 ice cubes
20 ml/¾ oz rum
20 ml/¾ oz apricot brandy
20 ml/¾ oz lime juice

Crack ice and put in a shaker with other ingredients. Shake well and strain into a cocktail glass.

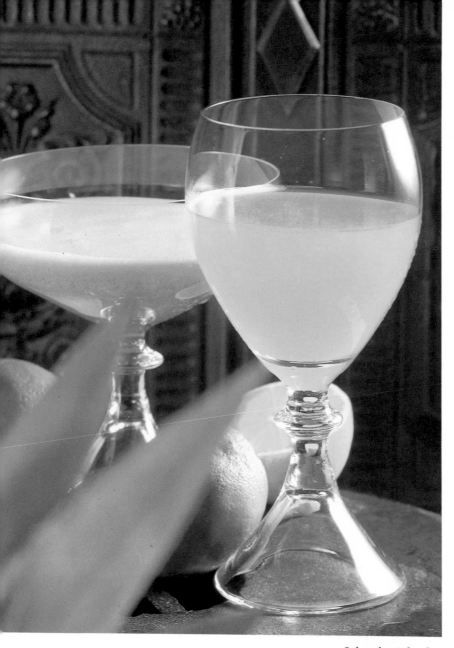

Colorado, Columbus

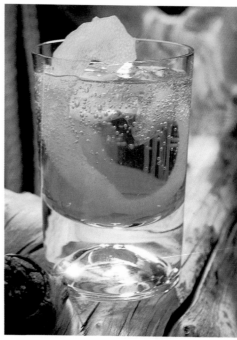

Country Club Highball

Continental

2—3 ice cubes
3 dashes dry vermouth
3 dashes red vermouth
2 dashes Cointreau
2 dashes orange bitters
2 dashes maraschino
sparkling wine
1 cocktail cherry

Put ice in a mixing glass with vermouths, Cointreau, bitters and maraschino. Stir well and strain into a shallow champagne glass. Top up with sparkling wine and decorate with cherry.

Cooperstown

2—3 ice cubes
25 ml/1 oz gin
15 ml/½ oz dry vermouth
15 ml/½ oz bianco vermouth
1 sprig of mint

Put ice in a mixing glass with gin and vermouths. Stir well and strain into a cocktail glass. Decorate with sprig of mint.

Copacabana

2—3 ice cubes
15 ml/½ oz brandy
25 ml/1 oz apricot brandy
15 ml/½ oz Cointreau
15 ml/½ oz lemon juice
1 orange slice

Crack ice and put in a shaker with brandy, apricot brandy, Cointreau and lemon juice. Shake well and strain into a large cocktail glass. Decorate with orange slice and serve with a straw.

Country Club Highball

2—3 ice cubes
80 ml/3 oz dry vermouth
25 ml/1 oz grenadine
soda water
spiral of lemon peel

Put ice in a large tumbler with vermouth and grenadine. Stir, then top up with soda water. Decorate with spiral of lemon peel.

39

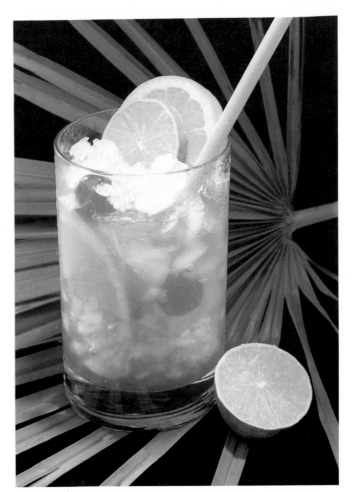

Creole Punch

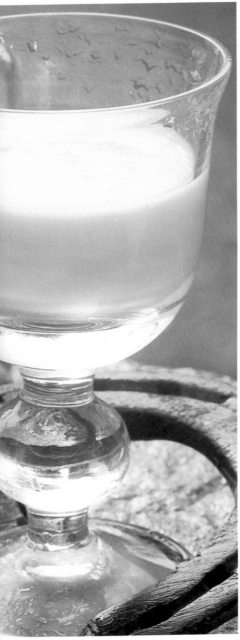

Cowboy

Cowboy

4 ice cubes
40 ml/1½ oz whisky
25 ml/1 oz cream

Crush ice and put in a shaker with whisky and cream. Shake and strain into a small goblet. Serve with a straw.

Creole Punch

4–6 ice cubes
50 ml/2 oz port
15 ml/½ oz lemon juice
2 teaspoons sugar syrup
1 teaspoon brandy
1 lemon slice
1 lime slice
½ orange slice
2 cocktail cherries

Crush ice and put half in a mixing glass with port, lemon juice, sugar syrup and brandy. Stir well. Put remaining crushed ice in a tumbler, strain contents of mixing glass over it and stir. Decorate with lemon, lime and orange slices and with cherries. Serve with a straw.

Crustino

15 ml/½ oz lemon juice
1 tablespoon castor sugar
50 ml/2 oz port
2 teaspoons grenadine
sparkling wine
spiral of lemon peel

Dip rim of a goblet first in lemon juice, shaking off excess, then in sugar. Allow frosting to dry. Put port, grenadine and remaining lemon juice in a mixing glass and stir. Pour into goblet and top up with sparkling wine. Spear lemon peel on a cocktail stick and use to decorate.

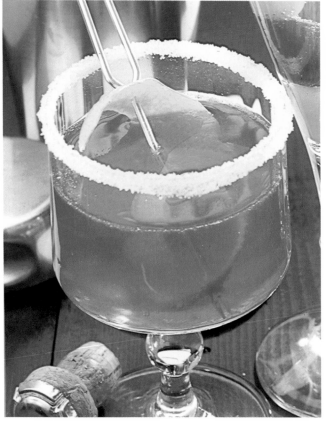
Crustino

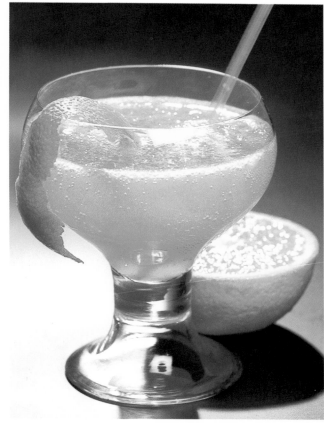
Crystal Highball

Crystal Highball

1–2 ice cubes
20 ml/¾ oz bianco vermouth
20 ml/¾ oz red vermouth
20 ml/¾ oz orange juice
soda water
spiral of orange peel

Put ice in a large cocktail glass. Add vermouths and orange juice and stir. Top up with soda water and decorate with spiral of orange peel. Serve with a straw.

Cuba Crusta

15 ml/½ oz lemon juice
1 tablespoon castor sugar
2–3 ice cubes
40 ml/1½ oz white rum
2 teaspoons pineapple juice
1 teaspoon Cointreau
spiral of lemon peel

Dip rim of a goblet first in lemon juice, shaking off excess, then in sugar. Allow frosting to dry. Crack ice and put in a shaker with rum, pineapple juice, Cointreau and remaining lemon juice. Shake and strain into glass. Decorate with spiral of lemon peel.

Cuba Libre

2–3 ice cubes
50 ml/2 oz white rum
15 ml/½ oz lemon juice
Coca-Cola
1 lemon slice

Put ice in a tall tumbler with rum and lemon juice. Top up with Coca-Cola and stir. Fix lemon slice on rim of glass and serve with a straw.

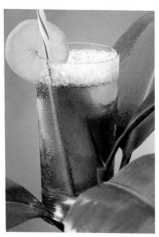
Cuba Libre

41

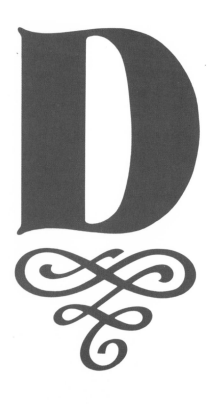

Daiquiri American-style

5–6 ice cubes
50 ml/1 oz white rum
25 ml/1 oz lime juice
1 teaspoon Cointreau
1 teaspoon sugar syrup
1 lemon or lime slice
1 cocktail cherry

Crack two ice cubes and put in an electric blender with rum, lime juice, Cointreau and sugar syrup. Blend. Crush remaining ice and put in a goblet. Strain contents of blender over crushed ice. Decorate with lemon or lime slice and cherry, and serve with a straw.

Daiquiri on the Rocks

6–7 ice cubes
50 ml/2 oz white rum
25 ml/1 oz lime juice
15 ml/½ oz sugar syrup

Crack two ice cubes and put in a shaker with rum, lime juice and sugar syrup. Shake very well. Put remaining ice in a tumbler, and strain in contents of shaker. Serve with a straw.

Dandy

2–3 ice cubes
20 ml/¾ oz Canadian whisky
20 ml/¾ oz Cointreau
20 ml/¾ oz orange juice

Crack ice and put in a shaker with other ingredients. Shake well and strain into a cocktail glass.

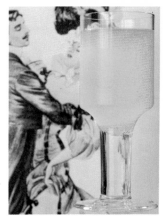

Dandy

Darling

25 ml/1 oz cherry brandy
25 ml/1 oz condensed milk
2 tablespoons vanilla ice cream
soda water
2 tablespoons raspberry ice cream
4 pineapple chunks or
   6 raspberries
25 ml/1 oz whipped cream

Pour cherry brandy into a tall glass, then add condensed milk and vanilla ice cream. Add soda water to about half way up glass, then add raspberry ice cream. Decorate with pineapple chunks or raspberries, and with whipped cream. Serve with a straw and a spoon.

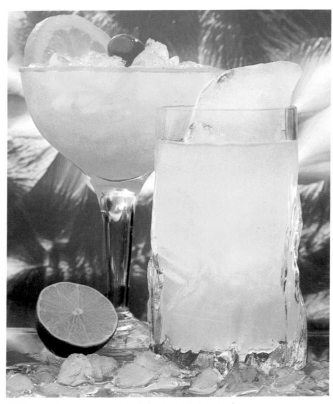

Daiquiri American-style, Daiquiri on the Rocks

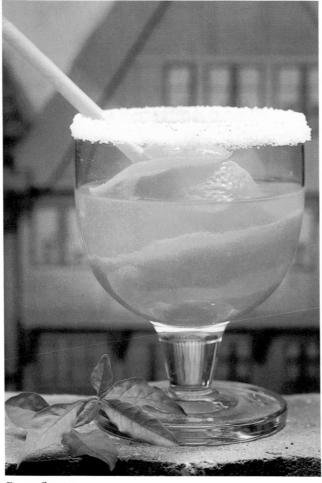

Dawn Crusta

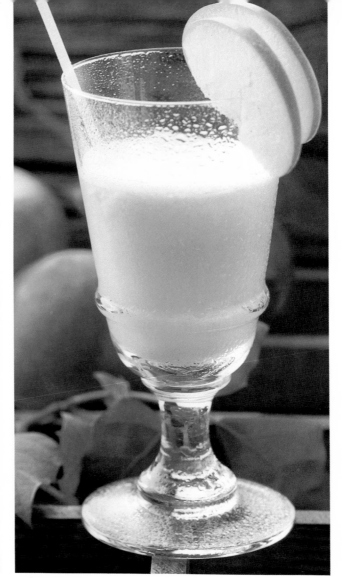

Delicious Sour

Dawn Crusta

15 ml/$\frac{1}{2}$ oz lemon juice
1 tablespoon castor sugar
2–3 ice cubes
40 ml/1$\frac{1}{2}$ oz white rum
15 ml/$\frac{1}{2}$ oz orange juice
1 teaspoon apricot brandy
1 dash grenadine
spiral of orange peel

Dip rim of a cocktail glass first in lemon juice, shaking off excess, then in sugar. Allow frosting to dry. Crack ice and put in a shaker with rum, orange juice, apricot brandy and grenadine. Shake and strain into glass. Decorate with spiral of orange peel.

Delicious Sour

2–3 ice cubes
1 egg white
1 teaspoon sugar syrup
15 ml/$\frac{1}{2}$ oz lemon juice
25 ml/1 oz calvados
25 ml/1 oz apricot brandy
soda water
2 apple slices

Crack ice and put in a shaker with egg white, sugar syrup, lemon juice, calvados and apricot brandy. Shake very well and strain into a goblet. Top up with soda water and fix apple slices on rim of glass. Serve with a straw.

Derby

40 ml/1$\frac{1}{2}$ oz gin
15 ml/$\frac{1}{2}$ oz peach brandy
1 sprig of mint

Chill gin and peach brandy, then pour into a cocktail glass and stir. Decorate with sprig of mint.

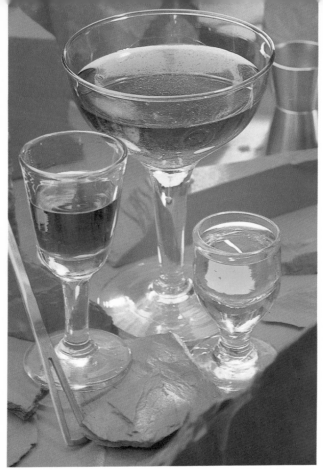

Devil's Own

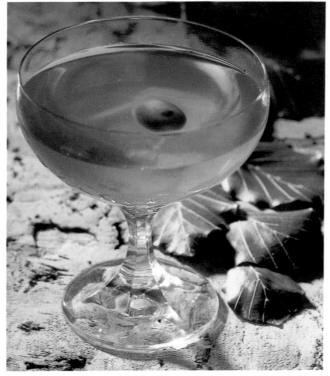

Douglas

Devil's Own

2–3 ice cubes
25 ml/1 oz brandy
25 ml/1 oz green crème de menthe
paprika

Crack ice and put in a shaker with brandy and crème de menthe. Shake well and strain into a cocktail glass. Sprinkle with paprika.

Dijon Fizz

2–3 ice cubes
50 ml/2 oz crème de cassis
40 ml/1½ oz kirsch
soda water
cluster of fresh blackcurrants
   (optional)

Crack ice and put in a shaker with crème de cassis and kirsch. Shake well and strain into a goblet. Top up with soda water and decorate with a cluster of fresh blackcurrants, if available.

Douglas

1 ice cube
20 ml/¾ oz whisky
20 ml/¾ oz gin
15 ml/½ oz grenadine
2 dashes Angostura bitters
1 olive

Put ice in a mixing glass with whisky, gin, grenadine and bitters. Stir and strain into a cocktail glass. Decorate with olive and serve with a cocktail stick.

Dubonnet Cocktail

2–3 ice cubes
40 ml/1½ oz gin
40 ml/1½ oz Dubonnet
piece of lemon peel

Put ice in mixing glass with gin and Dubonnet. Stir and strain into a large cocktail glass. Squeeze lemon peel over top.

Dubonnet Fizz

2–3 ice cubes
40 ml/1½ oz Dubonnet
25 ml/1 oz orange juice
15 ml/½ oz lemon juice
1 teaspoon cherry brandy
soda water

Crack ice and put in a shaker with Dubonnet, orange juice, lemon juice and cherry brandy. Shake well and strain into a large cocktail glass. Top up with soda water.

Duplex

2 tablespoons pineapple ice cream
25 ml/1 oz sherry
sparkling wine

Put pineapple ice cream in a tall champagne glass, add sherry and stir well. Top up with sparkling wine and serve with a straw.

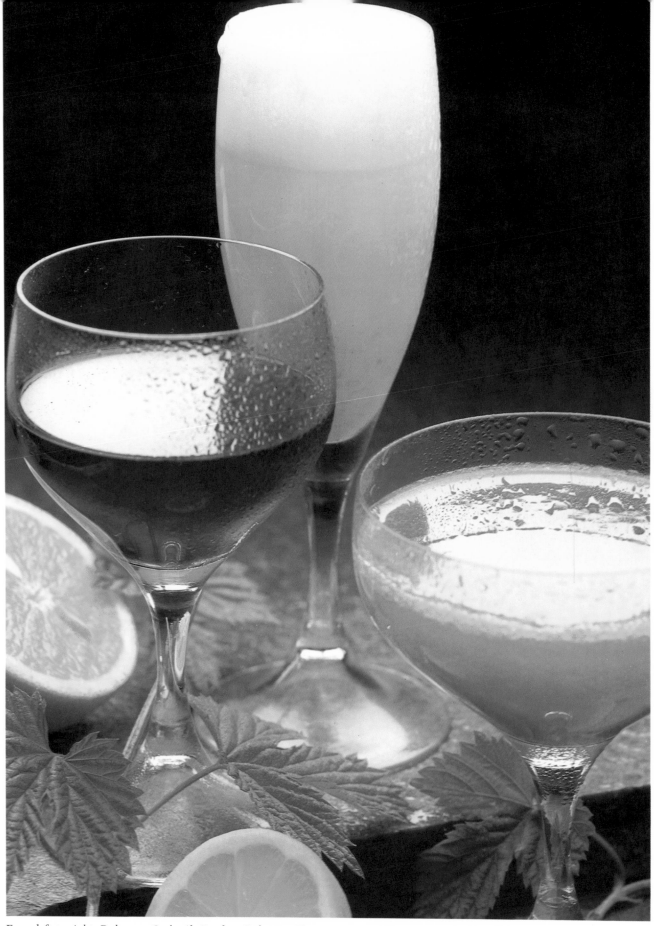

From left to right: Dubonnet Cocktail, Duplex, Dubonnet Fizz

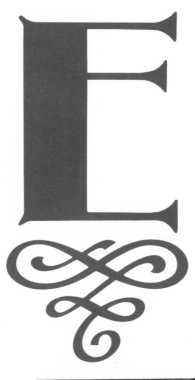

East India

2 ice cubes
40 ml/1½ oz white rum
1 teaspoon Cointreau
1 teaspoon pineapple juice
1 dash Angostura bitters
1 cocktail cherry

Crack ice and put in a shaker with rum, Cointreau, pineapple juice and bitters. Shake and strain into a cocktail glass. Decorate with cherry and serve with a cocktail stick.

East Wind

2–3 ice cubes
25 ml/1 oz vodka
15 ml/½ oz dry vermouth
15 ml/½ oz red vermouth
2–3 dashes rum

Crack ice and put in a shaker with other ingredients. Shake and strain into a cocktail glass.

Ecstasy

2–3 ice cubes
20 ml/¾ oz brandy
20 ml/¾ oz dry vermouth
20 ml/¾ oz Drambuie

Crack ice and put in a shaker with other ingredients. Shake well and strain into a cocktail glass.

East India (left)
El Dorado (below)

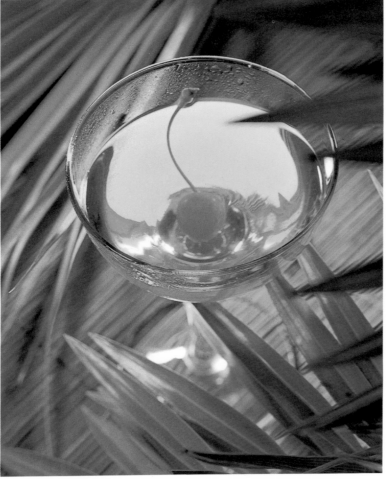

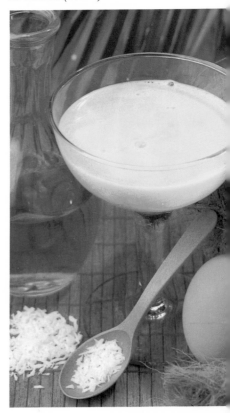

El Dorado   *El do Kroucher*

2–3 ice cubes
25 ml/1 oz white rum
25 ml/1 oz advocaat
25 ml/1 oz crème de cacao   *(Kummel)*
1 teaspoon grated coconut

Crack ice and put in a shaker with other ingredients. Shake very well and strain into a large cocktail glass. Serve with a straw.

Empire

2–3 ice cubes
25 ml/1 oz gin
15 ml/$\frac{1}{2}$ oz calvados
15 ml/$\frac{1}{2}$ oz apricot brandy
2 cocktail cherries

Put ice in a mixing glass with gin, calvados and apricot brandy. Stir well and strain into a cocktail glass. Decorate with cherries and serve with a cocktail stick.

Eton Blazer

3–4 ice cubes
25 ml/1 oz gin
25 ml/1 oz kirsch
15 ml/$\frac{1}{2}$ oz lemon juice
2 teaspoons sugar syrup
soda water
2 cocktail cherries

Place ice, gin, kirsch, lemon juice and sugar syrup in a tumbler. Stir, then top up with soda water. Decorate with cherries.

Evening Sun

1 tablespoon castor sugar
1 ice cube
25 ml/1 oz gin
25 ml/1 oz red vermouth
1 teaspoon orange juice
1 teaspoon grenadine
1 orange slice

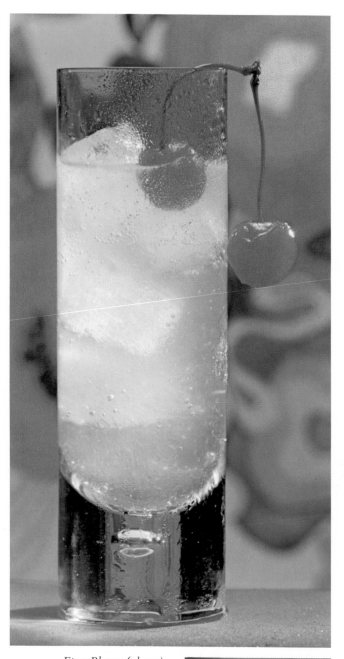

Eton Blazer (above)
Evening Sun (right)

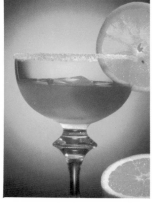

Dip rim of a cocktail glass first in water, shaking off excess, then in sugar. Allow frosting to dry. Put ice, gin, vermouth, orange juice and grenadine in a mixing glass and stir. Pour into cocktail glass. Fix orange slice on rim of glass.

F

Fanny Hill

15 ml/½ oz brandy
15 ml/½ oz Campari
15 ml/½ oz Cointreau
sparkling wine
1 lemon slice

Put brandy, Campari and Cointreau in a shallow champagne glass
and stir. Top up with sparkling
wine. Float lemon slice on top.

Favourite

25 ml/1 oz rum
25 ml/1 oz Cointreau
25 ml/1 oz condensed milk
2 teaspoons castor sugar
2 teaspoons instant coffee powder
1 egg yolk

Put all ingredients in an electric
blender and blend well. Pour into
a tumbler and serve with a straw.

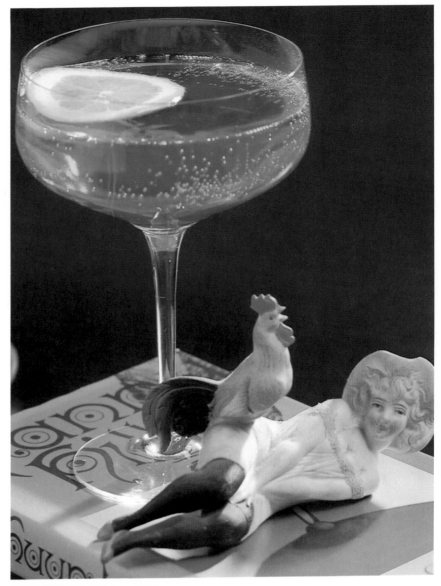

Fanny Hill

Feodora Cobbler

3 ice cubes
4–6 banana slices
15 ml/½ oz brandy
15 ml/½ oz rum
15 ml/½ oz Cointreau
soda water
1 orange slice

Crush ice and place in a shallow
glass. Smooth top of crushed ice
and lay banana slices on top. Add
brandy, rum and Cointreau. Top
up with soda water to taste. Fix
orange slice on rim of glass and
serve with a straw and a spoon.

Fire Extinguisher

100 ml/4 oz pale ale
100 ml/4 oz soda water
3–4 ice cubes

Put pale ale and soda water in a
tall glass and add ice.

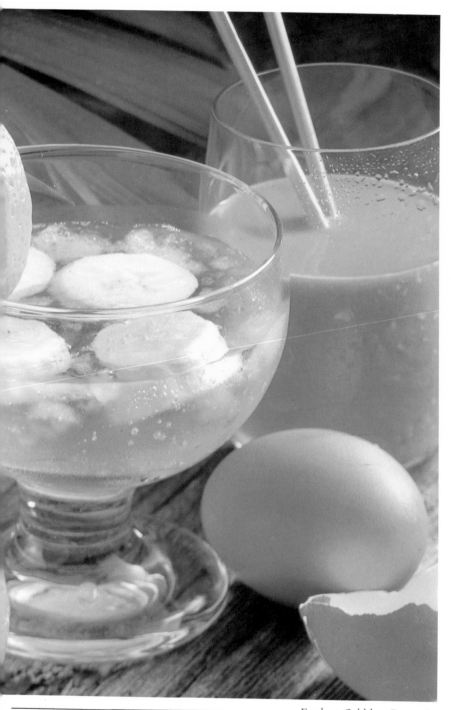

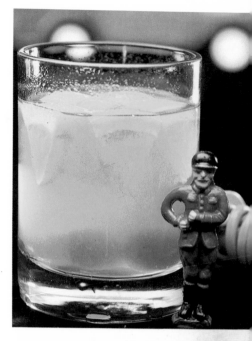

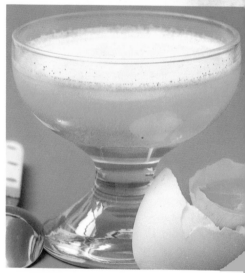

Fireman's Sour (top)
Flip Amore (above)

Feodora Cobbler, Favourite

Fireman's Sour

2–3 ice cubes
80 ml/3 oz white rum
15 ml/$\frac{1}{2}$ oz lemon juice
1 teaspoon grenadine
6 small triangles of lemon
3 cocktail cherries
soda water

Crack ice and put in a shaker with rum, lemon juice and grenadine. Shake well and strain into a tumbler. Decorate with small triangles of lemon and with cherries. Top up with a little soda water.

Flip Amore

2 ice cubes
1 egg yolk
20 ml/$\frac{3}{4}$ oz brandy
20 ml/$\frac{3}{4}$ oz crème de vanille
20 ml/$\frac{3}{4}$ oz maraschino

Crush ice and put in a shaker with other ingredients. Shake very well and pour into a large cocktail glass. Serve with a straw.

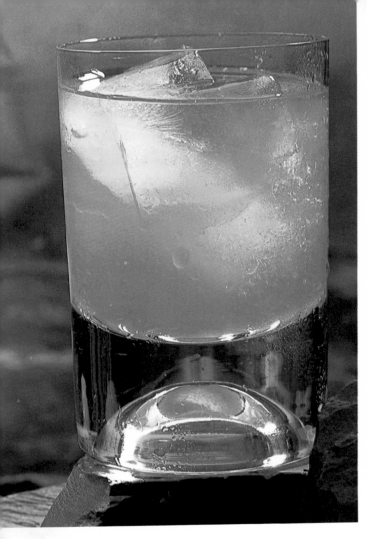
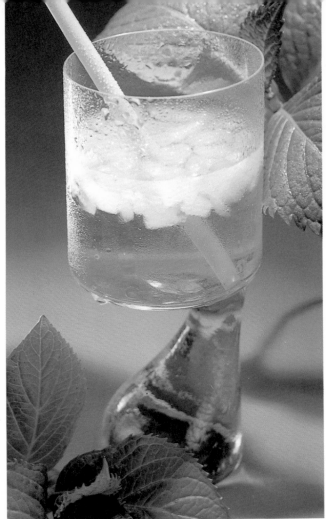

Flying Dutchman (above left)
Frozen Caruso (above)

Flying Dutchman

2–3 ice cubes
50 ml/2 oz gin
25 ml/1 oz grenadine
25 ml/1 oz lemon juice
mineral water

Put ice, gin, grenadine and lemon juice in a small tumbler and stir. Top up with mineral water.

French Cocktail

2–3 ice cubes
25 ml/1 oz gin
20 ml/¾ oz Pernod
1 teaspoon grenadine

Crack ice and put in a shaker with other ingredients. Shake and strain into a cocktail glass.

Fresco

3 sugar lumps
15 ml/½ oz lemon juice
sparkling wine
spiral of lemon peel

Put sugar lumps in a cocktail glass and soak with lemon juice. Top up with sparkling wine and decorate with spiral of lemon peel. Serve with a straw.

Frozen Caruso

4–5 ice cubes
20 ml/¾ oz gin
20 ml/¾ oz dry vermouth
20 ml/¾ oz green crème de menthe

Crack ice and put in a shaker with other ingredients. Shake well and pour into a small goblet. Serve with a straw.

Futurity

2–3 ice cubes
40 ml/1½ oz gin
20 ml/¾ oz red vermouth
2 dashes Angostura bitters

Crack ice and put in a shaker with other ingredients. Shake well and strain into a cocktail glass.

50

G

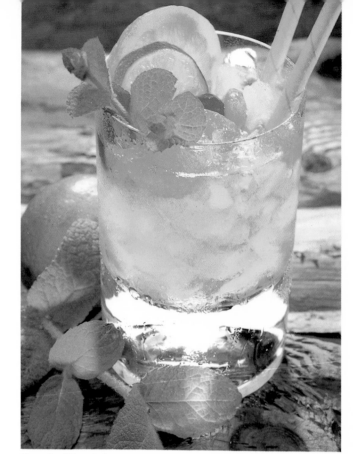

Georgia Mint Julep

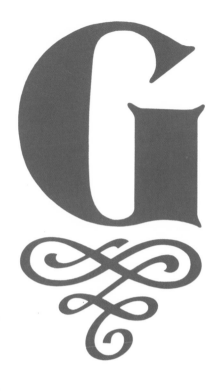

Geisha

15 ml/½ oz lemon juice
1 tablespoon castor sugar
2–3 ice cubes
20 ml/¾ oz gin
20 ml/¾ oz bianco vermouth
20 ml/¾ oz cherry brandy
1 pineapple chunk

Dip rim of a large cocktail glass first in lemon juice, shaking off excess, then in sugar. Allow frosting to dry. Crack ice and put in a shaker with gin, vermouth and cherry brandy. Shake and strain into glass. Decorate with pineapple chunk and serve with a cocktail stick.

Georgia Mint Julep

2 teaspoons castor sugar
65 ml/2½ oz water
4 sprigs of mint
3 ice cubes
25 ml/1 oz brandy
25 ml/1 oz apricot brandy

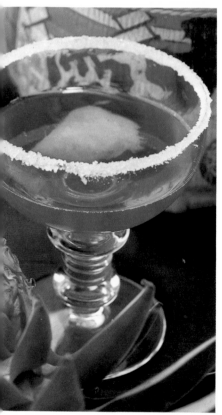

Geisha

4 apricot or peach slices
1 lemon slice
1 lime slice
1 cocktail cherry

Put sugar and water in a mixing glass, add three sprigs of mint and crush gently with a teaspoon. Remove mint. Crush ice and put in a tumbler. Add mint-flavoured sugar syrup, brandy and apricot brandy. Decorate with apricot or peach slices, lemon and lime slices, cherry and remaining sprig of mint. Serve with a straw and a spoon.

Gimlet

2–3 ice cubes
50 ml/2 oz gin
25 ml/1 oz lime juice cordial
soda water

Put ice in a mixing glass with gin and lime juice cordial. Stir well and strain into a large cocktail glass. Add a shot of soda water.

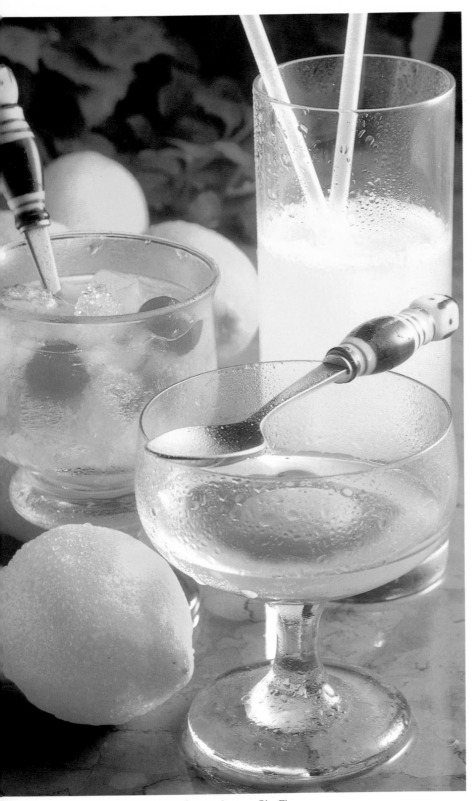

Gin Fizz

2–3 ice cubes
40 ml/1½ oz gin
25 ml/1 oz lemon juice
2 teaspoons sugar syrup
soda water

Crack ice and put in a shaker with gin, lemon juice and sugar syrup. Shake very well and strain into a tall glass. Top up with soda water to taste and serve with a straw.

Gin Oyster

1 teaspoon gin
1 egg yolk
2 teaspoons tomato ketchup
1 dash Worcestershire sauce
1 dash lemon juice
salt, pepper, paprika, nutmeg

Put gin in a shallow glass. Slide in egg yolk. Add tomato ketchup, Worcestershire sauce and lemon juice. Sprinkle with salt, pepper and paprika, and grate over a little nutmeg. Do not stir this drink, but swallow it in one gulp.

Gin Punch

3 ice cubes
40 ml/1½ oz gin
15 ml/½ oz lemon juice
2 teaspoons castor sugar
2 dashes maraschino
3–4 cocktail cherries
3–4 pineapple chunks

Crush ice and put in a shallow tumbler. Add gin, lemon juice, sugar and maraschino. Stir, then decorate with cherries and pineapple chunks. Serve with a straw and a spoon.

From left to right: Gin Punch, Gin Oyster, Gin Fizz

Gin Rickey

2–3 ice cubes
50 ml/2 oz gin
25 ml/1 oz lime or lemon juice
1 dash grenadine
soda water
spiral of lime or lemon peel

Put ice in a tall glass with gin, lime or lemon juice and grenadine. Stir and top up with soda water. Decorate with spiral of lime or lemon peel.

Ginger Daisy

1 piece preserved ginger
2–3 ice cubes
15 ml/½ oz brandy
15 ml/½ oz lemon juice
1 teaspoon orange syrup
1 teaspoon sugar syrup
ginger ale

Dice ginger and put in a shaker with ice, brandy, lemon juice, orange syrup and sugar syrup. Shake well, pour into a tumbler and top up with ginger ale.

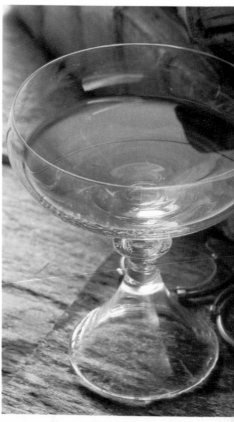

Gin Sling

2–3 ice cubes
40 ml/1½ oz gin
20 ml/¾ oz lemon juice
2 teaspoons castor sugar
1 dash Angostura bitters
mineral water

Put ice in a tumbler with gin, lemon juice, sugar and bitters. Stir and top up with mineral water.

Gipsy

2–3 ice cubes
25 ml/1 oz vodka
20 ml/¾ oz Bénédictine
1 dash Angostura bitters

Crack ice and put in a shaker with other ingredients. Shake and strain into a cocktail glass.

Golden Cocktail

2–3 ice cubes
20 ml/¾ oz gin
20 ml/¾ oz red vermouth
1 teaspoon Cointreau
1 teaspoon grenadine
1 cocktail cherry

Crack ice and put in a shaker with gin, vermouth, Cointreau and grenadine. Shake and strain into a cocktail glass. Spear cherry on a cocktail stick and use to decorate.

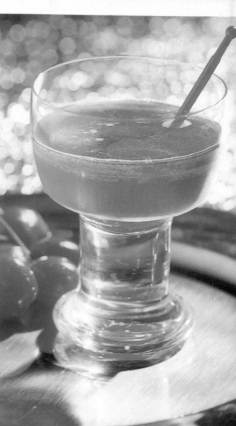

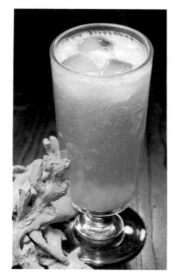

Ginger Daisy

Gipsy (top right)
Golden Cocktail (right)

53

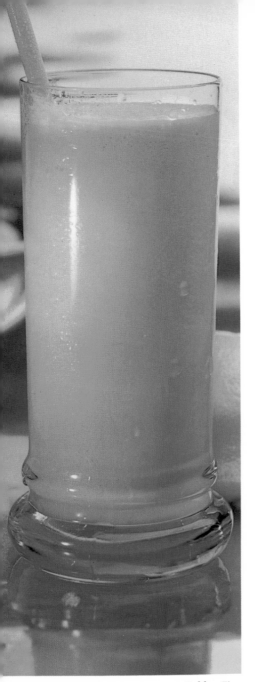

Golden Fizz

2–3 ice cubes
1 egg yolk
2 teaspoons castor sugar
50 ml/2 oz gin
25 ml/1 oz lemon juice
2 teaspoons grenadine
soda water

Crack ice and put in a shaker with egg yolk, sugar, gin, lemon juice and grenadine. Shake very well and strain into a tall tumbler. Top up with soda water and serve with a straw.

Golden Gate

2–3 ice cubes
40 ml/1½ oz orange juice
15 ml/½ oz Bourbon whisky
15 ml/½ oz Cointreau
1 teaspoon mandarin orange
    liqueur
sparkling wine
3 mandarin orange segments

Crack ice and put in a shaker with orange juice, whisky, Cointreau and mandarin orange liqueur. Shake very well, then strain into a champagne glass. Top up with sparkling wine and decorate with mandarin orange segments. Serve with a straw and a spoon.

Golden Fizz

Grapefruit Highball

Good Morning

2–3 ice cubes
1 egg white
1 teaspoon sugar syrup
15 ml/½ oz lemon juice
20 ml/¾ oz rum
20 ml/¾ oz port

Crack ice and put in a shaker with other ingredients. Shake very well and strain into a small tumbler. Serve with a straw.

Golden Daisy

2–3 ice cubes
40 ml/1½ oz whisky
25 ml/1 oz lemon juice
15 ml/½ oz Cointreau
2 teaspoons sugar syrup
soda water

Crack ice and put in a shaker with whisky, lemon juice, Cointreau and sugar syrup. Shake and strain into a large cocktail glass. Top up with soda water.

Golden Lady

2–3 ice cubes
15 ml/½ oz brandy
15 ml/½ oz Cointreau
15 ml/½ oz orange juice
sparkling wine

Crack ice and put in a shaker with brandy, Cointreau and orange juice. Shake and strain into a shallow champagne glass. Top up with sparkling wine.

Grapefruit Highball

2–3 ice cubes
80 ml/3 oz grapefruit juice
25 ml/1 oz grenadine
soda water or ginger ale

Put ice in a tall tumbler with grapefruit juice and grenadine. Top up with soda water or ginger ale, stir and serve with a straw. This highball may also be served in a hollowed-out grapefruit half.

54

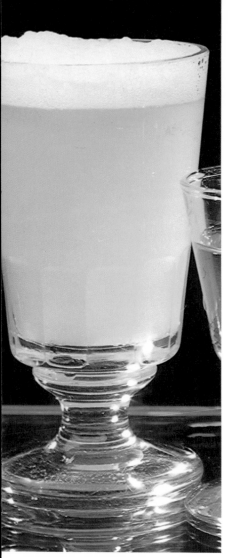

Green Fizz

Grasshopper

25 ml/1 oz crème de cacao
25 ml/1 oz green crème de menthe

Pour crème de cacao into a pousse-café glass. Add crème de menthe, pouring it gently over back of a spoon so that it floats on surface. Serve with a straw.

Green Dragon

2–3 ice cubes
40 ml/1½ oz vodka
40 ml/1½ oz green crème de menthe

Crack ice and put in a shaker with vodka and crème de menthe. Shake and strain into a small goblet.

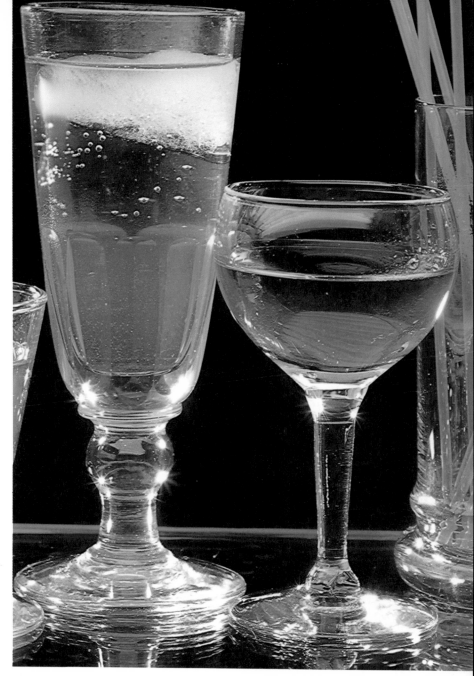

Green Hat, Green Sea

Green Fizz

4–5 ice cubes
1 egg white
2 teaspoons sugar syrup
25 ml/1 oz lemon juice
50 ml/2 oz gin
1 teaspoon green crème de menthe
soda water

Crack ice and put in a shaker with egg white, sugar syrup, lemon juice, gin and crème de menthe. Shake very well and strain into a tall glass. Top up with soda water and serve with a straw.

Green Hat

2–3 ice cubes
25 ml/1 oz gin
25 ml/1 oz green crème de menthe
soda water

Put ice in a large goblet or tumbler with gin and crème de menthe. Stir and top up with soda water. Serve with a straw.

55

Green Sea

(picture on page 55)

2–3 ice cubes
25 ml/1 oz vodka
20ml/¾ oz dry vermouth
20 ml/¾ oz green crème de menthe

Crack ice and put in a shaker with other ingredients. Shake and strain into a small goblet.

Greenhorn

50 ml/2 oz green crème de menthe
20 ml/¾ oz lemon juice
2–3 ice cubes
mineral water

Put crème de menthe and lemon juice in a shaker and shake well. Put ice in a tumbler, pour in contents of shaker and top up to taste with mineral water.

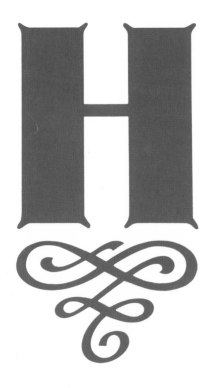

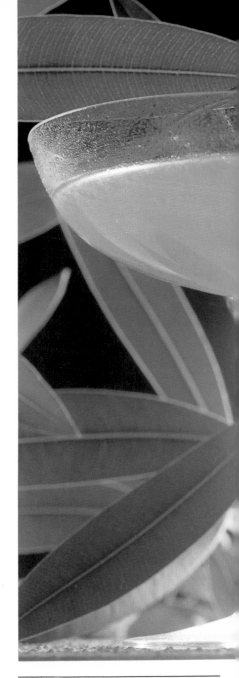

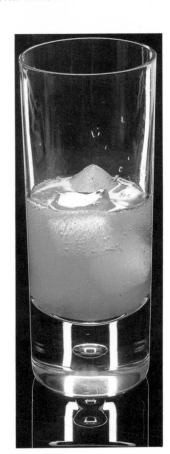

Greenhorn

Half and Half

2–3 ice cubes
25 ml/1 oz bianco vermouth
25 ml/1 oz grapefruit juice
1 teaspoon Campari

Crack ice and put in a shaker with other ingredients. Shake and strain into a cocktail glass.

Harvard Cooler

3 ice cubes
40 ml/1½ oz calvados
40 ml/1½ oz orange juice
1 teaspoon maple syrup
ginger ale
spiral of lemon peel

Crush ice and put in a shaker with calvados, orange juice and maple syrup. Shake well and pour into a tall glass. Top up with ginger ale and decorate with spiral of lemon peel. Serve with a straw.

Harvey Wallbanger

4 ice cubes
50 ml/2 oz vodka
25 ml/1 oz Galliano
25 ml/1 oz orange juice
½ teaspoon castor sugar
1 orange slice

Crack two ice cubes and put in a shaker with vodka, Galliano, orange juice and sugar. Shake and strain into a tumbler. Add remaining ice and decorate with orange slice.

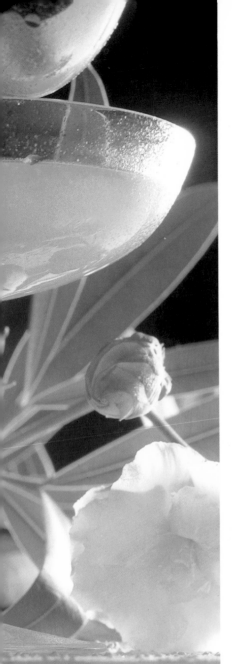

Hawaii Kiss

Serves 2
1 pineapple
25 ml/1 oz gin
2 ice cubes
sparkling wine

Scoop out flesh from pineapple, press juice out of flesh and return juice to hollowed-out shell. Add gin and ice and top up with sparkling wine. Serve with straws.

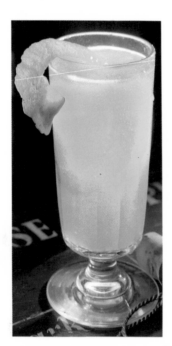

Hemingway

2–3 ice cubes
40 ml/1½ oz white rum
40 ml/1½ oz Cointreau
40 ml/1½ oz grapefruit juice
sparkling wine

Crack ice and put in a shaker with rum, Cointreau and grapefruit juice. Shake very well and strain into a champagne glass. Top up with sparkling wine and serve with a straw.

Honeymoon

2–3 ice cubes
25 ml/1 oz calvados
15 ml/½ oz Bénédictine
2 teaspoons orange juice
3 dashes Cointreau

Crack ice and put in a shaker with other ingredients. Shake and strain into a cocktail glass.

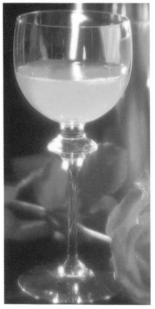

Honeymoon

Half and Half (above)
Harvard Cooler (above right)
Havana Club (below right)

Havana Club

2–3 ice cubes
40 ml/1½ oz white rum
20 ml/¾ oz red vermouth
1 cocktail cherry

Crack ice and put in a shaker with rum and vermouth. Shake well and strain into a cocktail glass. Spear cherry on a cocktail stick and use to decorate.

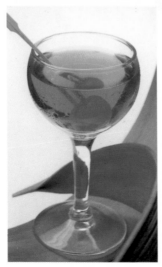

Horse Guards

2–3 ice cubes
1 egg yolk
20 ml/$\frac{3}{4}$ oz rum
20 ml/$\frac{3}{4}$ oz Cointreau
sparkling wine
spiral of lemon peel

Crack ice and put in a shaker with egg yolk, rum and Cointreau. Shake very well and strain into a tumbler. Top up with sparkling wine and decorate with spiral of lemon peel. Serve with a straw.

Hot Italy

4–5 ice cubes
40 ml/$1\frac{1}{2}$ oz whisky
red vermouth
1 dash Angostura bitters
piece of lemon peel

Crush ice and put in a tall tumbler. Add whisky and top up to taste with vermouth. Add bitters and squeeze lemon peel over top. Serve with a straw.

Imperial Crusta

15 ml/$\frac{1}{2}$ oz orange juice
1 tablespoon castor sugar
2–3 ice cubes
50 ml/2 oz kirsch
25 ml/1 oz mandarin orange juice
1 teaspoon sugar syrup
spiral of orange peel

Dip rim of a champagne glass first in orange juice, shaking off excess, then in sugar. Allow frosting to dry. Crack ice and put in a shaker with kirsch, mandarin orange juice and sugar syrup. Shake well and strain into glass. Decorate with spiral of orange peel.

Imperial Crusta

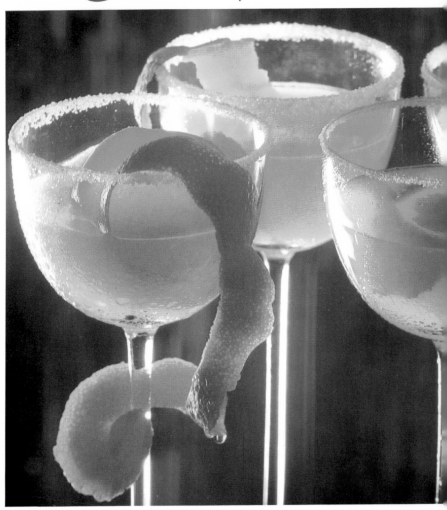

International

2–3 ice cubes
20 ml/$\frac{3}{4}$ oz brandy
20 ml/$\frac{3}{4}$ oz green Chartreuse
15 ml/$\frac{1}{2}$ oz pineapple juice
1 lemon wedge

Crack ice and put in a shaker with brandy, Chartreuse and pineapple juice. Shake very well and strain into a cocktail glass. Add lemon wedge and serve with a straw.

Intimate

2 ice cubes
20 ml/$\frac{3}{4}$ oz vodka
20 ml/$\frac{3}{4}$ oz apricot brandy
20 ml/$\frac{3}{4}$ oz dry vermouth
2 dashes orange bitters
1 black olive
piece of lemon peel

Put ice in a mixing glass with vodka, apricot brandy, vermouth and bitters. Stir and strain into a cocktail glass. Decorate with olive and lemon peel, and serve with a cocktail stick.

Irish Coffee

2 teaspoons castor sugar
40 ml/$1\frac{1}{2}$ oz Irish whisky
strong hot coffee
15 ml/$\frac{1}{2}$ oz cream

Put sugar in a goblet and add whisky. Top up with coffee and stir. Add cream, pouring it gently over back of a spoon so that it floats on surface.

Island Dream

3–4 ice cubes
2 teaspoons Cointreau
2 teaspoons grenadine
2 teaspoons orange juice
2 teaspoons lemon juice
white rum
1 cocktail cherry
1 lemon slice

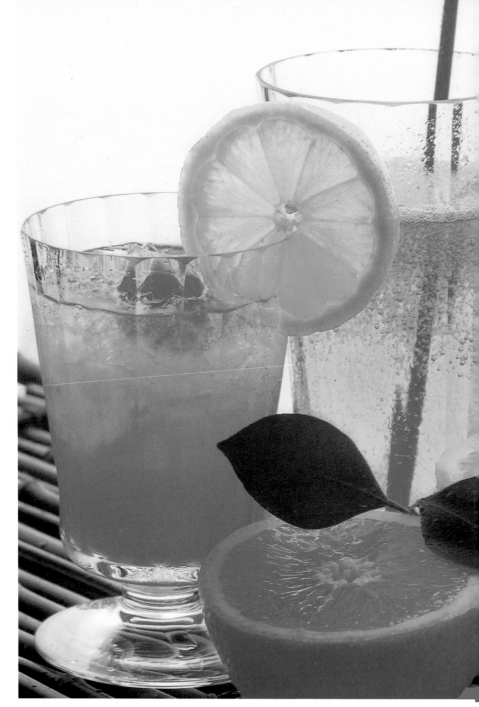

Island Dream, Island Highball

Crush ice and put in a tumbler with Cointreau, grenadine, orange juice and lemon juice. Top up with rum to taste and stir well. Add cherry and fix lemon slice on rim of glass. Serve with a straw.

Island Highball

2 ice cubes
15 ml/$\frac{1}{2}$ oz brandy
15 ml/$\frac{1}{2}$ oz gin
15 ml/$\frac{1}{2}$ oz red vermouth
1 dash orange bitters
soda water

Put ice in a tumbler with brandy, gin, vermouth and bitters. Stir and top up to taste with soda water. Serve with a straw.

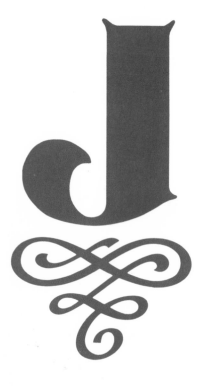

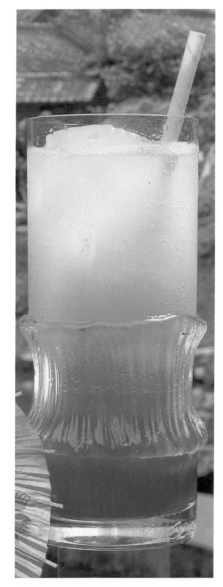

Japonaise

2–3 ice cubes
25 ml/1 oz advocaat
15 ml/½ oz kirsch
2 teaspoons grenadine
soda water

Put ice in a tall tumbler with advocaat, kirsch and grenadine. Stir well and top up to taste with soda water. Serve with a straw.

Japonaise

Kangaroo

2–3 ice cubes
40 ml/1½ oz vodka
15 ml/½ oz dry vermouth
piece of lemon peel

Put ice in a mixing glass with vodka and vermouth. Stir well and strain into a cocktail glass. Squeeze lemon peel over top.

Jeune Homme

2–3 ice cubes
25 ml/1 oz dry vermouth
15 ml/½ oz gin
15 ml/½ oz Cointreau
15 ml/½ oz Bénédictine
1 dash Angostura bitters

Crack ice and put in a shaker with other ingredients. Shake and strain into a large cocktail glass.

John Collins

2–3 ice cubes
25 ml/1 oz gin
15 ml/½ oz lemon juice
2 teaspoons castor sugar
soda water

Put ice in a tumbler with gin, lemon juice and sugar. Top up with soda water and stir.

Kiku Kiku

2 ice cubes
65 ml/2½ oz rice wine
40 ml/1½ oz pineapple juice
15 ml/½ oz gin

Crush ice and put in a shallow champagne glass. Add other ingredients and stir. Serve with a straw.

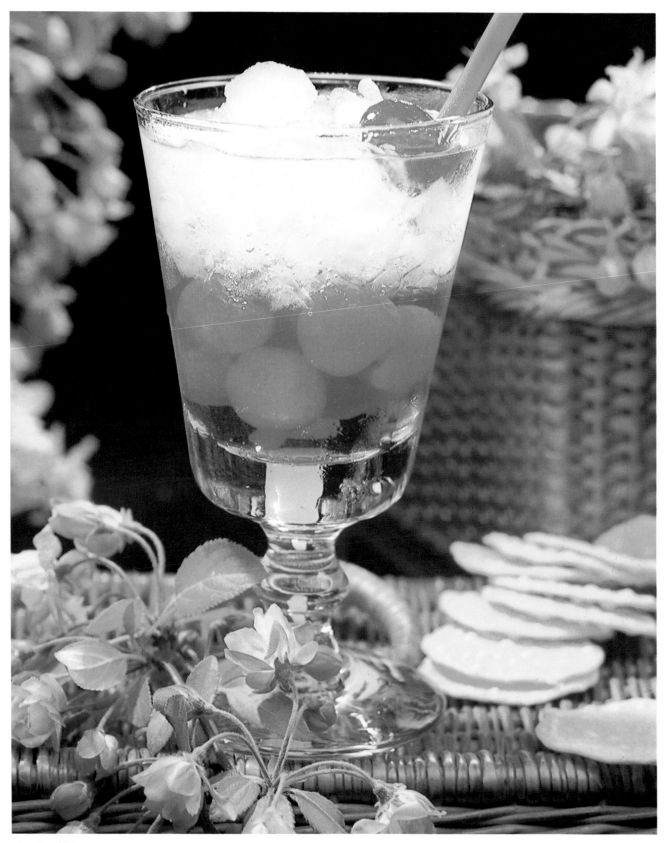

Kirsch Cobbler

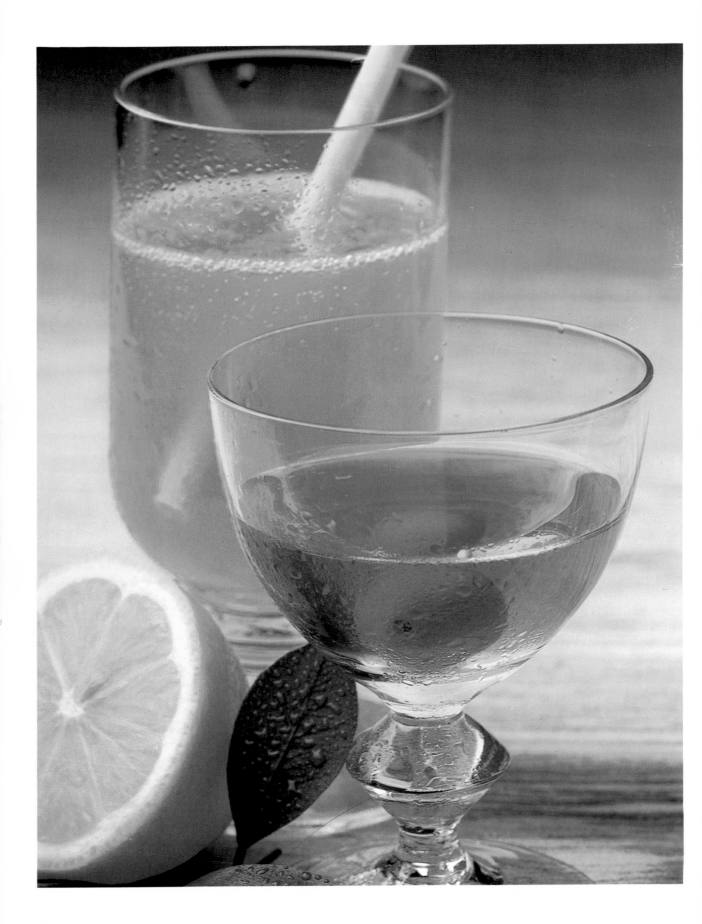

Kirsch Cobbler

(picture on page 61)

4 ice cubes
40 ml/1½ oz kirsch
40 ml/1½ oz maraschino
6–8 cocktail cherries
soda water

Crush ice and put in a goblet. Add
kirsch, maraschino and cherries.
Stir and top up with soda water.
Serve with a straw and spoon.

Klondyke Cocktail

3 ice cubes
40 ml/1½ oz calvados
15 ml/½ oz dry vermouth
1 dash Angostura bitters
1 olive
piece of lemon peel

Put ice in a mixing glass with
calvados, vermouth and bitters.
Stir well and strain into a cocktail
glass. Decorate with olive and
squeeze lemon peel over top.
Serve with a cocktail stick.

Klondyke Cooler

2–3 ice cubes
25 ml/1 oz dry vermouth
25 ml/1 oz red vermouth
25 ml/1 oz lemon juice
2 teaspoons castor sugar
ginger ale

Crack ice and put in a shaker with
vermouths, lemon juice and sugar.
Shake very well and strain into a
tumbler. Top up with ginger ale
and serve with a straw.

Klondyke Cooler, Klondyke Cocktail

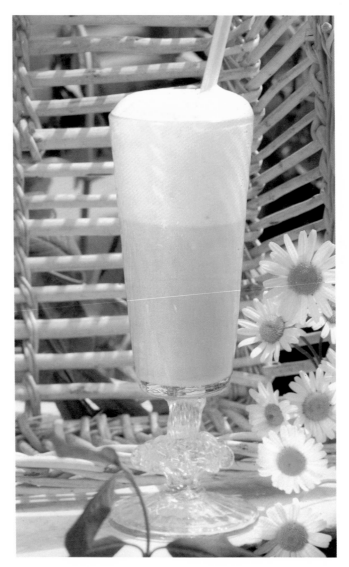

Knockout

Knockout

2–3 ice cubes
1 egg yolk
2 teaspoons sugar syrup
25 ml/1 oz Scotch whisky
sparkling wine

Crack ice and put in a shaker. Add
egg yolk, sugar syrup and whisky.
Shake well and strain into a tall
glass. Top up with sparkling wine
and serve with a straw.

Lady Brown

2–3 ice cubes
40 ml/1½ oz gin
20 ml/¾ oz Grand Marnier
20 ml/¾ oz mandarin orange juice
15 ml/½ oz lemon juice
2 mandarin orange segments

Crack ice and put in a shaker with gin, Grand Marnier, mandarin orange juice and lemon juice. Shake very well. Place mandarin orange segments in a large cocktail glass, strain in contents of shaker and serve with a straw.

Lady's Crusta

50 ml/2 oz orange juice
1 tablespoon castor sugar
2–3 ice cubes
50 ml/2 oz port
1 teaspoon sugar syrup
spiral of orange peel

Dip rim of a goblet first in orange juice, shaking off excess, then in sugar. Allow frosting to dry. Crack ice and put in a shaker with port, sugar syrup and remaining orange juice. Shake and strain into glass. Decorate with spiral of orange peel.

Leo's Special

2–3 ice cubes
25 ml/1 oz brandy
25 ml/1 oz Cointreau
2 teaspoons orange juice
2 teaspoons grapefruit juice
sparkling wine
1 cocktail cherry

Crack ice and put in a shaker with brandy, Cointreau, orange juice and grapefruit juice. Shake and strain into a shallow champagne glass. Top up with sparkling wine. Decorate with cherry and serve with a cocktail stick.

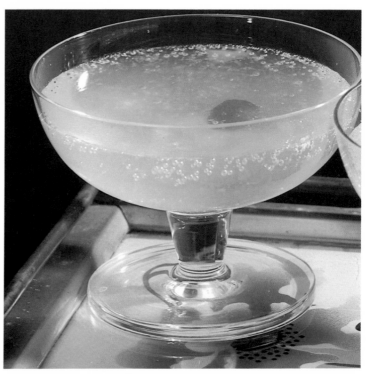

Lady's Crusta   *Leo's Special*

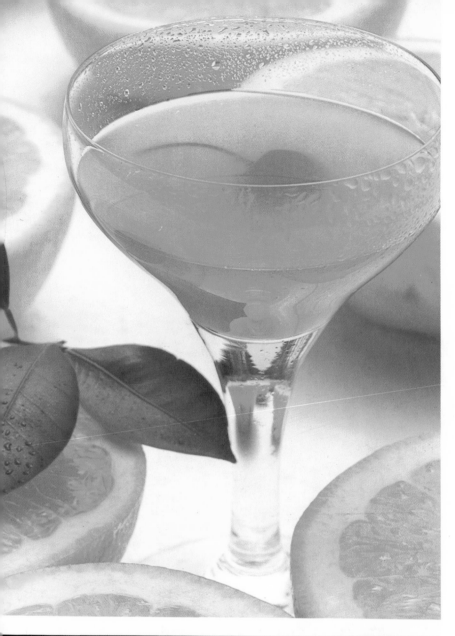

Lieutenant

2–3 ice cubes
25 ml/1 oz Bourbon whisky
15 ml/½ oz apricot brandy
15 ml/½ oz grapefruit juice
1 teaspoon sugar syrup
1 cocktail cherry

Crack ice and put in a shaker with whisky, apricot brandy, grapefruit juice and sugar syrup. Shake and strain into a cocktail glass. Decorate with cherry and serve with a cocktail stick.

Lightning Punch

Serves 2
15 ml/½ oz lemon juice
2 teaspoons castor sugar
100 ml/4 oz whisky
boiling water
2 teaspoons plum brandy

Put lemon juice and sugar in a mixing glass and stir. Add whisky and pour into warmed punch glasses. Top up with boiling water. Add plum brandy and stir well.

Little Prince

3 ice cubes
25 ml/1 oz gin
20 ml/¾ oz bianco vermouth
20 ml/¾ oz kirsch
bitter lemon
1 apple slice
1 banana slice
1 cocktail cherry
piece of cucumber peel
1 lemon slice

Put ice in a tumbler with gin, vermouth and kirsch. Stir and top up with bitter lemon. Add apple slice, banana slice, cherry and cucumber peel. Fix lemon slice on rim of glass.

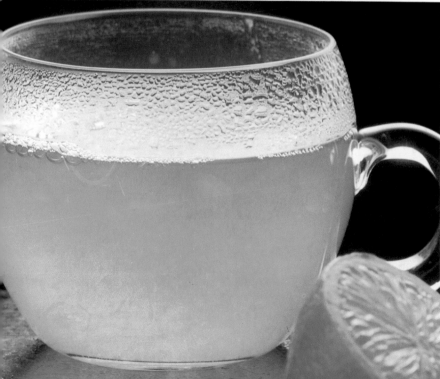

Lieutenant (top left)
Lightning Punch (left)

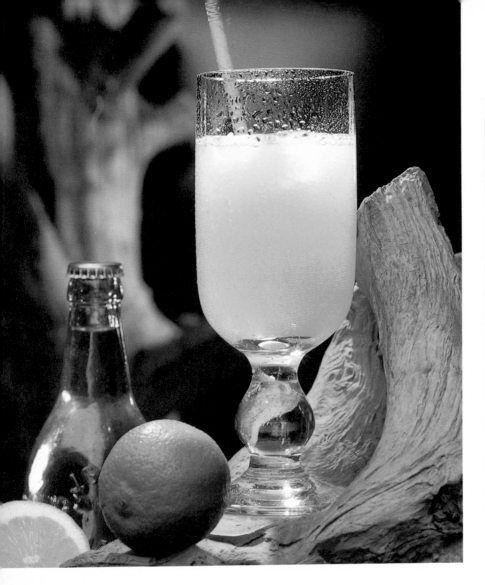

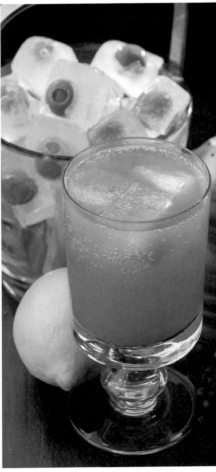

Lone Tree Cooler (above left)
Louisa (above)

Lone Tree Cooler

2–3 ice cubes
40 ml/1½ oz apricot brandy
25 ml/1 oz lemon juice
20 ml/¾ oz lime juice
1 dash grenadine
1 dash Angostura bitters
soda water

Crush ice and put in a shaker with all other ingredients except soda water. Shake and pour into a tall stemmed glass. Top up with soda water and serve with a straw.

Louisa

3 ice cubes, each containing a
    stuffed olive
40 ml/1½ oz vodka
65 ml/2½ oz tomato juice
1 teaspoon lemon juice
4 dashes Worcestershire sauce
salt, pepper
soda water

To prepare frozen stuffed olives, run a little water into the compartments of an ice tray, freeze, then add a stuffed olive to each compartment; fill up with water and freeze till hard. Place three frozen stuffed olives in a goblet. Add vodka, tomato juice, lemon juice, Worcestershire sauce, salt and pepper. Stir. Top up with soda water.

Lychee Cocktail

1 lychee
2–3 ice cubes
40 ml/1½ oz lychee juice
20 ml/¾ oz gin
20 ml/¾ oz white rum
1 teaspoon lemon juice

Put lychee in a large cocktail glass. Crack ice and put in a shaker with other ingredients. Shake very well and strain into glass.

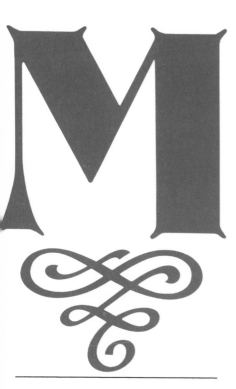

Madeira Cobbler

4 ice cubes
2 peach slices
2 grapes
2 cocktail cherries
3 pineapple chunks
2 teaspoons grenadine
1 dash kirsch
1 dash Cointreau
1 dash maraschino
Madeira

Crush ice and put in a goblet. Add fruits, then grenadine, kirsch, Cointreau and maraschino. Top up with Madeira and serve with a straw and a spoon.

Madeira Flip

2–3 ice cubes
1 egg yolk
2 teaspoons sugar syrup
50 ml/2 oz Madeira
nutmeg

Crack ice and put in a shaker with egg yolk, sugar syrup and Madeira. Shake well, strain into a tumbler. Grate a little nutmeg over top and serve with a straw.

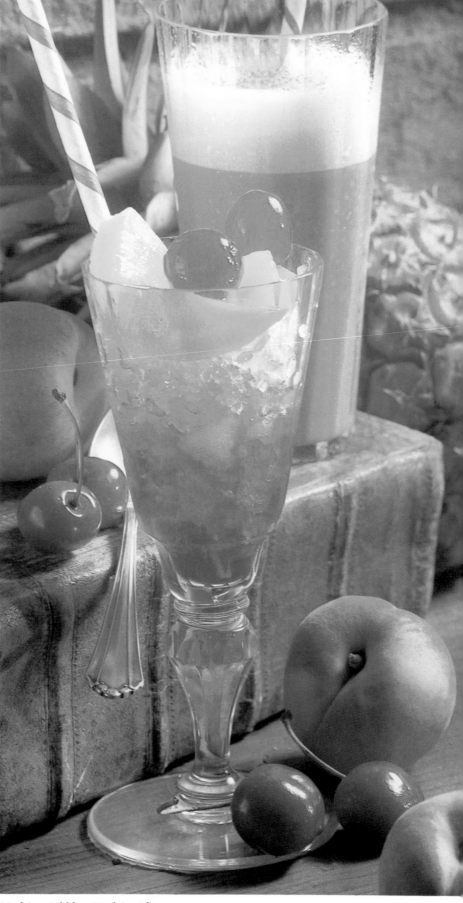

Madeira Cobbler, Madeira Flip

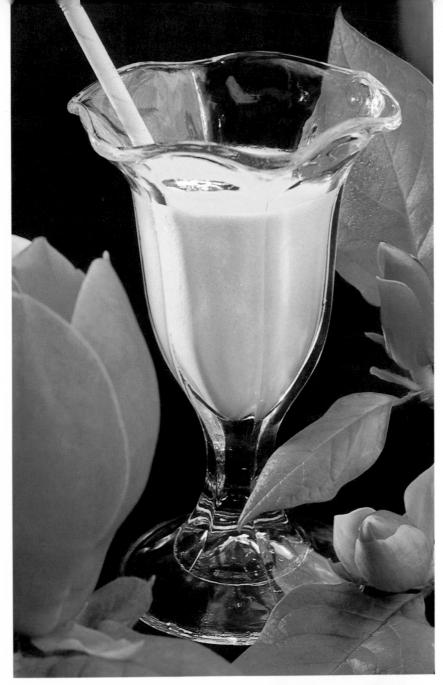

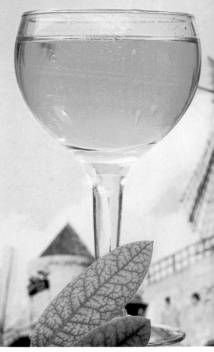

Mallorca

Mai Tai

50 ml/2 oz white rum
25 ml/1 oz orange juice
25 ml/1 oz lime juice
3 ice cubes
3 cocktail cherries
3 pineapple chunks
2 orange slices

Put rum, orange juice and lime juice in a small goblet and stir well. Crush ice and add to glass. Decorate with cherries, pineapple chunks and orange slices. Serve with a straw and a spoon.

Magnolia Blossom (above)
Mai Tai (right)

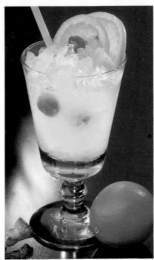

Magnolia Blossom

2–3 ice cubes
25 ml/1 oz gin
15 ml/$\frac{1}{2}$ oz cream
2 teaspoons lemon juice
2 dashes grenadine

Crack ice and put in a shaker with other ingredients. Shake and strain into a cocktail glass. Serve with a straw.

Maiden

2–3 ice cubes
25 ml/1 oz orange juice
20 ml/$\frac{3}{4}$ oz gin
20 ml/$\frac{3}{4}$ oz Cointreau
15 ml/$\frac{1}{2}$ oz lemon juice

Crack ice and put in a shaker with other ingredients. Shake well and strain into a large cocktail glass.

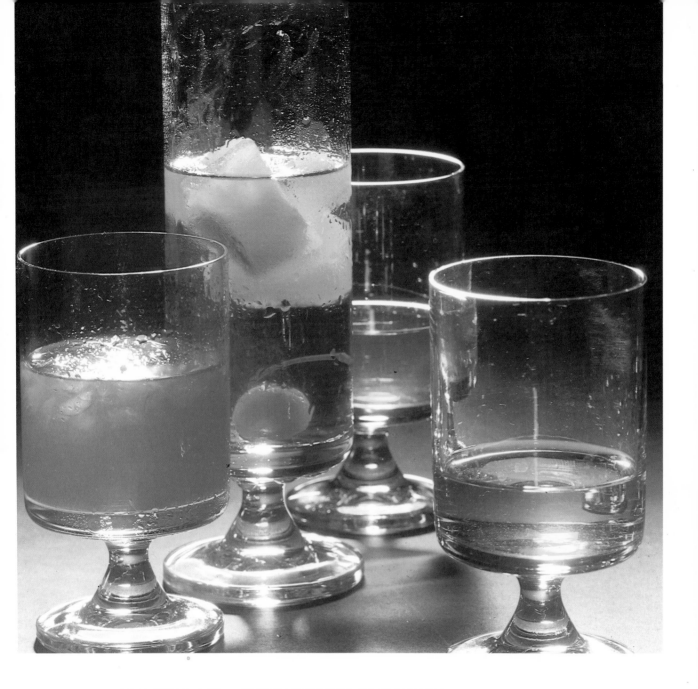

Mallorca

3 ice cubes
25 ml/1 oz rum
2 teaspoons Drambuie
2 teaspoons dry vermouth
2 teaspoons banana liqueur
piece of lemon peel

Put ice in a mixing glass with rum, Drambuie, vermouth and banana liqueur. Stir well and strain into a cocktail glass. Squeeze lemon peel over top.

Manhattan Cooler

4 ice cubes
80 ml/3 oz claret
15 ml/$\frac{1}{2}$ oz lemon juice
3 dashes rum
2 teaspoons castor sugar
ginger ale
1 cocktail cherry

Crack two ice cubes and put in a shaker with claret, lemon juice, rum and sugar. Shake very well and strain into a tall goblet. Top up to taste with ginger ale. Add cherry and remaining ice.

From left to right: Manhattan Latin, Manhattan Cooler, Manhattan Sweet, Manhattan Dry

Manhattan Dry

2–3 ice cubes
40 ml/1$\frac{1}{2}$ oz Bourbon whisky
15 ml/$\frac{1}{2}$ oz dry vermouth
1 dash Angostura bitters

Put ice in a mixing glass with whisky, vermouth and bitters. Stir well and strain into a goblet.

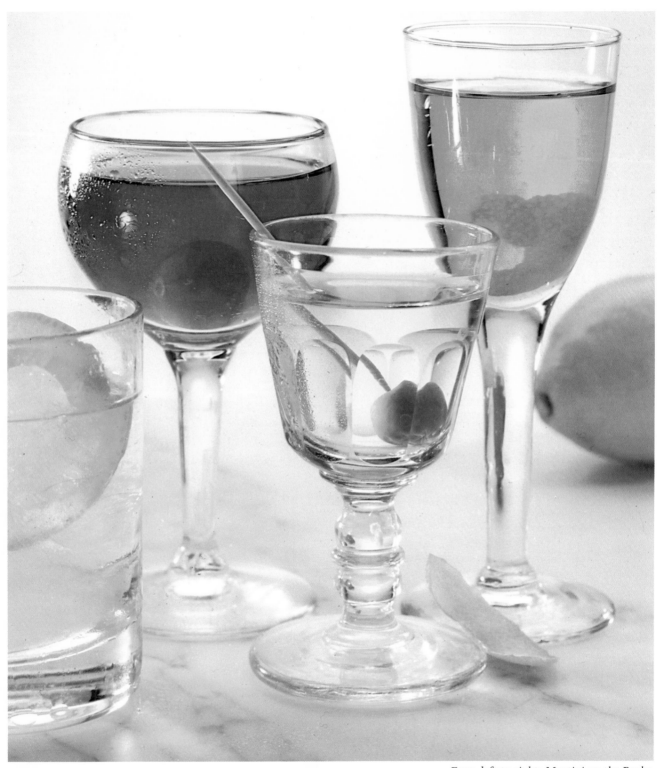

From left to right: Martini on the Rocks,
Martini Sweet, Martini Dry, Martini Medium

Manhattan Latin

(picture on page 69)

2−3 ice cubes
40 ml/1½ oz white rum
20 ml/¾ oz red vermouth

Crush ice and put in a mixing glass with rum and vermouth. Stir well and pour into a goblet. Serve with a straw.

Manhattan Sweet

(picture on page 69)

2−3 ice cubes
25 ml/1 oz Bourbon whisky
25 ml/1 oz bianco vermouth
1 dash Angostura bitters

Put ice in a mixing glass with whisky, vermouth and bitters. Stir well and strain into a goblet.

Margarita

salt
2−3 ice cubes
25 ml/1 oz tequila
15 ml/½ oz Cointreau
15 ml/½ oz lime or lemon juice

Dip rim of a cocktail glass first in water, shaking off excess, then in salt. Allow frosting to dry. Crack ice and put in a shaker with other ingredients. Shake and strain into glass.

Martini Dry

2−3 ice cubes
50 ml/2 oz gin
2 teaspoons dry vermouth
piece of lemon peel
1 olive (optional)

Put ice in a mixing glass with gin and vermouth and stir well. Strain into a cocktail glass and squeeze lemon peel over top. If liked, spear olive on a cocktail stick and use to decorate.

Martini Limone

2−3 ice cubes
50 ml/2 oz bianco vermouth
25 ml/1 oz lemon juice
soda water

Put ice in a mixing glass with vermouth and lemon juice. Stir well and pour into a tumbler. Top up with soda water and serve with a straw.

Martini Medium

2−3 ice cubes
40 ml/1½ oz gin
2 teaspoons dry vermouth
2 teaspoons red vermouth
piece of orange peel

Put ice in a mixing glass with gin and vermouths. Stir well and strain into a cocktail glass. Decorate with orange peel.

Martini on the Rocks

2−3 ice cubes
50 ml/2 oz gin
1 teaspoon dry vermouth
1 lemon slice

Put ice in a small tumbler with gin and vermouth. Stir, then decorate with lemon slice.

Martini Sweet

2−3 ice cubes
40 ml/1½ oz gin
15 ml/½ oz red vermouth
1 teaspoon sugar syrup or
   grenadine
1 cocktail cherry

Put ice in a mixing glass with gin, vermouth and sugar syrup or grenadine. Stir well and strain into a cocktail glass. Decorate with cherry and serve with a cocktail stick.

Mary Queen of Scots

15 ml/½ oz lemon juice
1 tablespoon castor sugar
2−3 ice cubes
25 ml/1 oz Scotch whisky
15 ml/½ oz Drambuie
15 ml/½ oz green Chartreuse
1 cocktail cherry

Dip rim of a cocktail glass first in lemon juice, shaking off excess, then in sugar. Allow frosting to dry. Crack ice and put in a shaker with whisky, Drambuie and Chartreuse. Shake and strain into glass. Spear cherry on a cocktail stick and use to decorate.

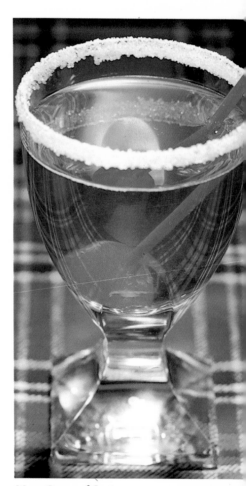

Mary Queen of Scots

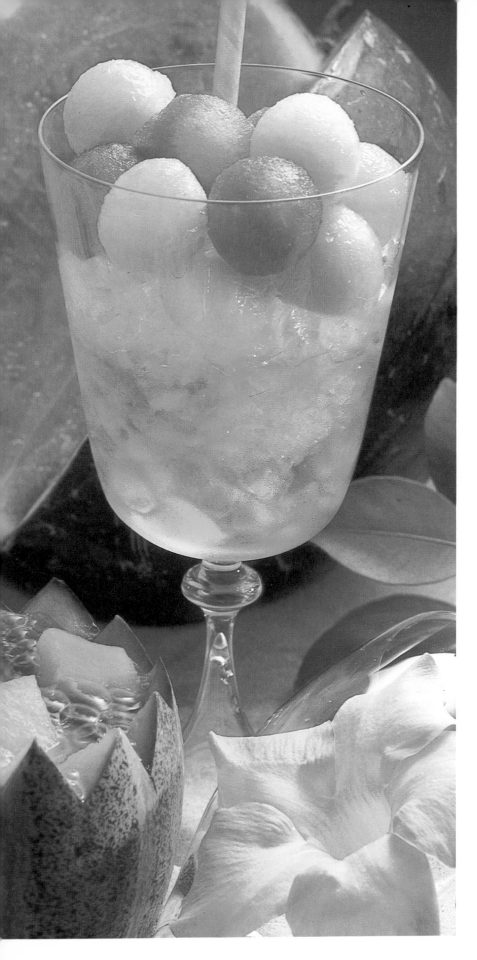

Melon Cobbler

4 ice cubes
4–6 balls cantaloupe melon
4–6 balls water melon
2 dashes brandy
2 dashes Cointreau
champagne

Crush ice and put in a goblet. Add melon, then brandy and Cointreau. Top up with champagne. Serve with a straw and a spoon.

Mississippi

2–3 ice cubes
25 ml/1 oz rye whisky
25 ml/1 oz rum
25 ml/1 oz lemon juice
2 dashes sugar syrup
spiral of lemon peel

Crack ice and put in a shaker with whisky, rum, lemon juice and sugar syrup. Shake and strain into a small goblet. To decorate, wind lemon peel round a wooden skewer or spear it on a cocktail stick.

Mona Lisa

15 ml/½ oz lemon juice
1 tablespoon castor sugar
2–3 ice cubes
40 ml/1½ oz crème de cacao
15 ml/½ oz dry vermouth
1 cocktail cherry

Dip rim of a cocktail glass first in lemon juice, shaking off excess, then in sugar. Allow frosting to dry. Crack ice and put in a shaker with crème de cacao and vermouth. Shake and strain into glass. Decorate with cherry and serve with a cocktail stick.

Melon Cobbler

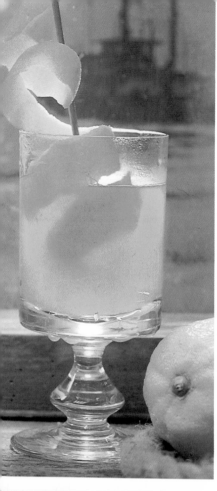

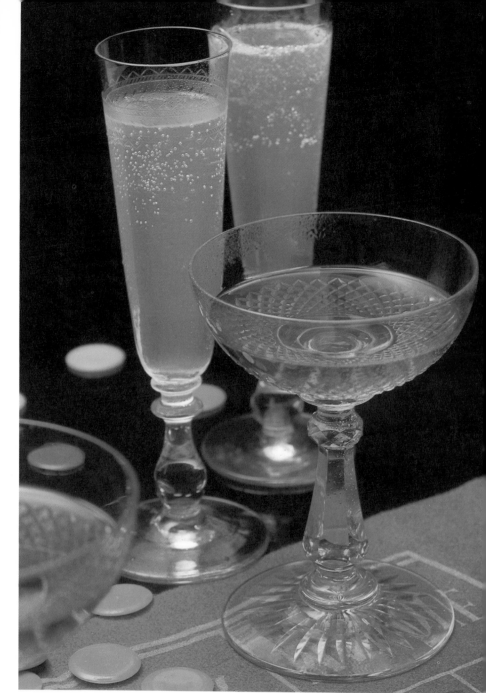

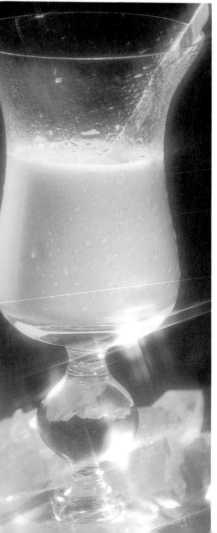

Mississippi (top left), Mont Blanc (below left)

Monte Carlo Imperial and Monte Carlo Cocktail (above)

Mont Blanc

2–3 ice cubes
20 ml/¾ oz gin
20 ml/¾ oz Cointreau
20 ml/¾ oz cream
2 teaspoons castor sugar

Crack ice and put in a shaker with other ingredients. Shake and strain into a cocktail glass. Serve with a straw.

Monte Carlo Cocktail

2–3 ice cubes
40 ml/1½ oz Canadian whisky
15 ml/½ oz Bénédictine
2 dashes Angostura bitters

Crack ice and put in a shaker with other ingredients. Shake and strain into a cocktail glass.

73

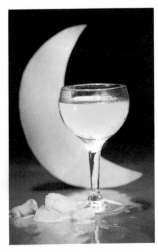

Moonlight

Monte Carlo Imperial

(picture on page 73)

2–3 ice cubes
25 ml/1 oz gin
15 ml/½ oz white crème de menthe
2 teaspoons lime juice
champagne

Crack ice and put in a shaker with gin, crème de menthe and lime juice. Shake and strain into a tall champagne glass. Top up with champagne.

Moonlight

3–4 ice cubes
40 ml/1½ oz bianco vermouth
15 ml/½ oz pear brandy

Put ice in a mixing glass with vermouth and pear brandy. Stir well and strain into a cocktail glass.

Morning Glory

2–3 ice cubes
20 ml/¾ oz brandy
20 ml/¾ oz Bourbon whisky
2 teaspoons sugar syrup
2 dashes Cointreau
1 dash Pernod
soda water
spiral of lemon peel

Put ice in a mixing glass with brandy, whisky, sugar syrup, Cointreau and Pernod. Stir well and strain into a small tumbler or balloon glass. Top up with soda water and stir. Decorate with spiral of lemon peel.

Morning Glory Fizz

2–3 ice cubes
1 egg white
2 teaspoons castor sugar
25 ml/1 oz lemon juice
50 ml/2 oz Bourbon whisky
1 teaspoon Pernod
soda water

Crush ice and put in a shaker with egg white, sugar, lemon juice, whisky and Pernod. Shake very well and strain into a tumbler or balloon glass. Top up with soda water and serve with a straw.

Morning Glory, Morning Glory Fizz

Moulin Rouge

2–3 ice cubes
25 ml/1 oz gin
20 ml/¾ oz apricot brandy
20 ml/¾ oz lemon juice
1 teaspoon grenadine
sparkling wine
1 orange slice

Crack ice and put in a shaker with gin, apricot brandy, lemon juice and grenadine. Shake and strain into a shallow champagne glass. Top up with sparkling wine and decorate with orange slice. Serve with a straw.

Moulin Rouge (below)
Mule's Hind Leg (top right)
Myra (below right)

Mule's Hind Leg

2–3 ice cubes
15 ml/½ oz gin
15 ml/½ oz calvados
15 ml/½ oz Bénédictine
15 ml/½ oz apricot brandy
2 teaspoons maple syrup

Put ice in a mixing glass with other ingredients. Stir well and strain into a cocktail glass.

Myra

2–3 ice cubes
25 ml/1 oz red wine
15 ml/½ oz vodka
15 ml/½ oz dry vermouth

Put ice in a mixing glass with other ingredients. Stir well and strain into a cocktail glass.

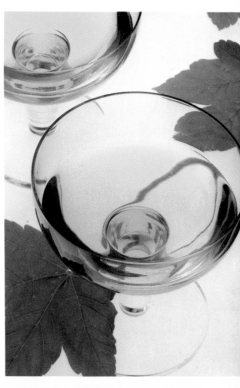

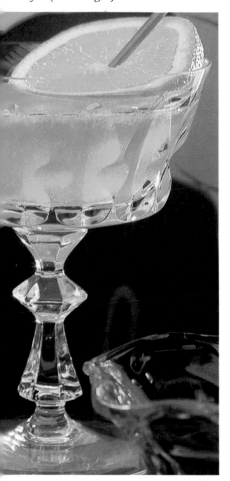

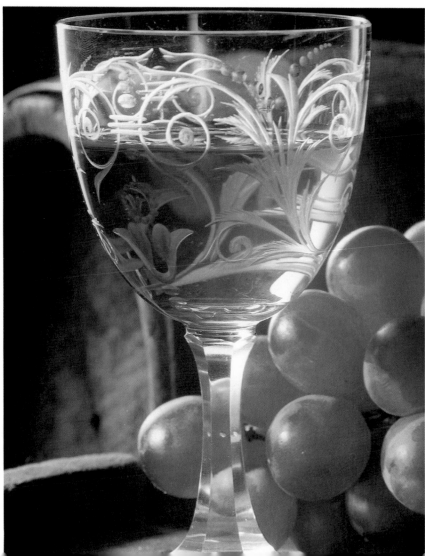

Napoleon

2–3 ice cubes
25 ml/1 oz whisky
25 ml/1 oz gin
1 teaspoon sugar syrup
1 teaspoon lemon juice
spiral of lemon peel

Put ice in a mixing glass with whisky, gin, sugar syrup and lemon juice. Stir and strain into a cocktail glass. Decorate with spiral of lemon peel.

Natasha

2–3 ice cubes
15 ml/½ oz apricot brandy
15 ml/½ oz pear brandy
15 ml/½ oz red vermouth
1 dash orange bitters
1 cocktail cherry

Put ice in a mixing glass with apricot brandy, pear brandy, vermouth and bitters. Stir and strain into a cocktail glass. Decorate with cherry.

Negroni

3 ice cubes
25 ml/1 oz gin
15 ml/½ oz Campari
15 ml/½ oz red vermouth
soda water
1 orange slice

Put ice in a tall tumbler. Add gin, Campari and vermouth and top up with soda water. Decorate with orange slice and serve with a straw.

New Orleans Fizz

2–3 ice cubes
1 egg white
2 teaspoons sugar syrup
25 ml/1 oz lemon juice
40 ml/1½ oz gin
40 ml/1½ oz Cointreau
25 ml/1 oz cream
soda water

Crack ice and put in a shaker with egg white, sugar syrup, lemon juice, gin, Cointreau and cream. Shake very well and strain into a goblet. Top up with soda water and serve with a straw.

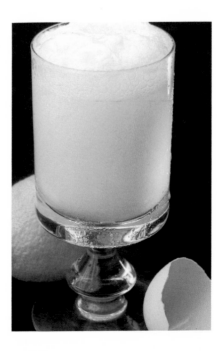

New Yorker

2–3 ice cubes
40 ml/1½ oz Bourbon whisky
15 ml/½ oz lemon juice
1 teaspoon grenadine
piece of orange peel

Crack ice and put in a shaker with whisky, lemon juice and grenadine. Shake and strain into a cocktail glass. Squeeze orange peel over top.

Noddy

2–3 ice cubes
25 ml/1 oz gin
15 ml/½ oz Bourbon whisky
2 teaspoons Pernod

Crack ice and put in a shaker with other ingredients. Shake and strain into a cocktail glass.

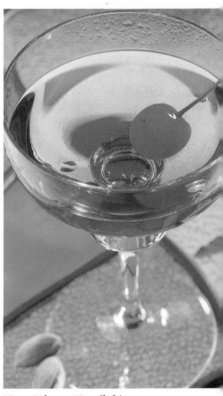

New Orleans Fizz (left)
Natasha (above)
Negroni (right)

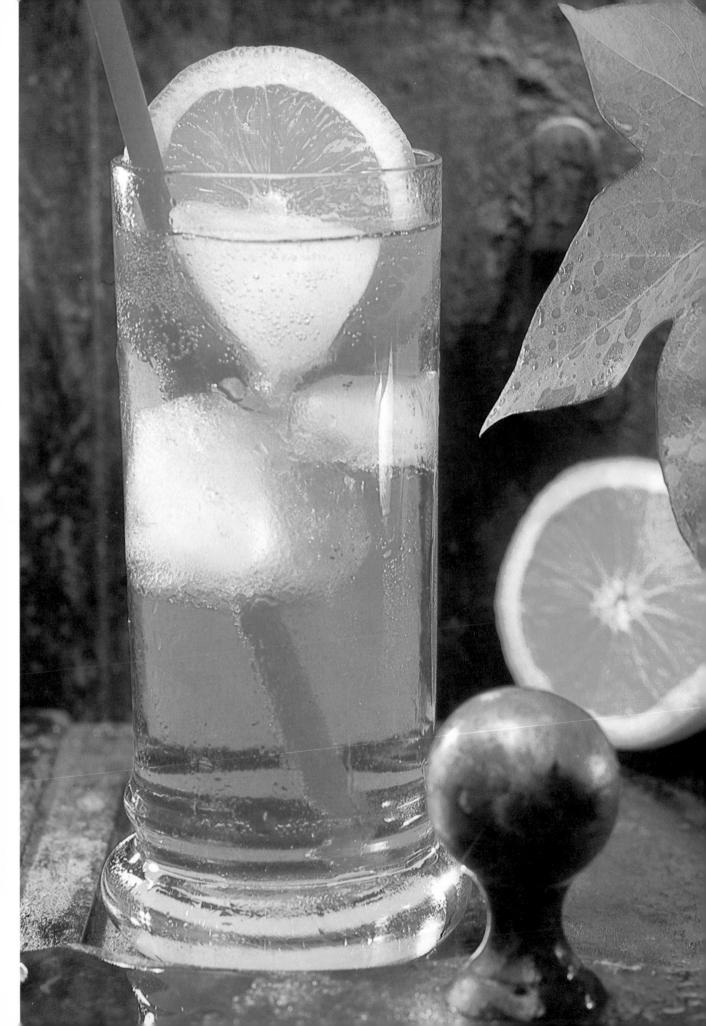

Old-fashioned

1 teaspoon castor sugar
1 teaspoon water
2 dashes Angostura bitters
2–3 ice cubes
50 ml/2 oz Bourbon whisky
1 orange slice
1 cocktail cherry

Put sugar, water and bitters in a small tumbler and stir well. Add ice and whisky. Stir again. Decorate with orange slice and cherry.

Old Pale

2–3 ice cubes
25 ml/1 oz Bourbon whisky
15 ml/$\frac{1}{2}$ oz dry vermouth
15 ml/$\frac{1}{2}$ oz Campari
piece of lemon peel

Put ice in a mixing glass with whisky, vermouth and Campari. Stir well and strain into a cocktail glass. Add lemon peel.

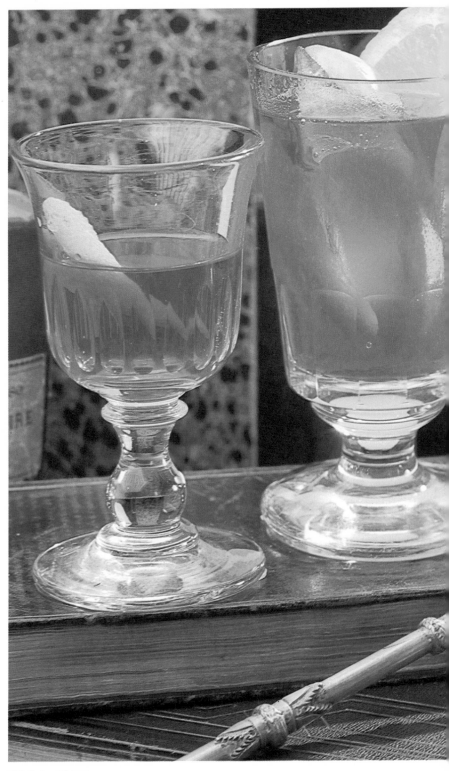

Old Pale, Old Time

Old Time

2–3 ice cubes
25 ml/1 oz Bourbon whisky
25 ml/1 oz Dubonnet
2 dashes Cointreau
2 dashes Pernod
1 dash Angostura bitters
2 orange slices
2 pineapple chunks
piece of lemon peel

Put ice in a tall goblet with whisky, Dubonnet, Cointreau, Pernod and bitters. Stir well and add orange slices, pineapple chunks and lemon peel. Serve with a straw and a spoon.

Opera

2–3 ice cubes
25 ml/1 oz gin
15 ml/$\frac{1}{2}$ oz Dubonnet
15 ml/$\frac{1}{2}$ oz maraschino
piece of orange peel

Crack ice and put in a shaker with gin, Dubonnet and maraschino. Shake well and strain into a cocktail glass. Squeeze orange peel over top.

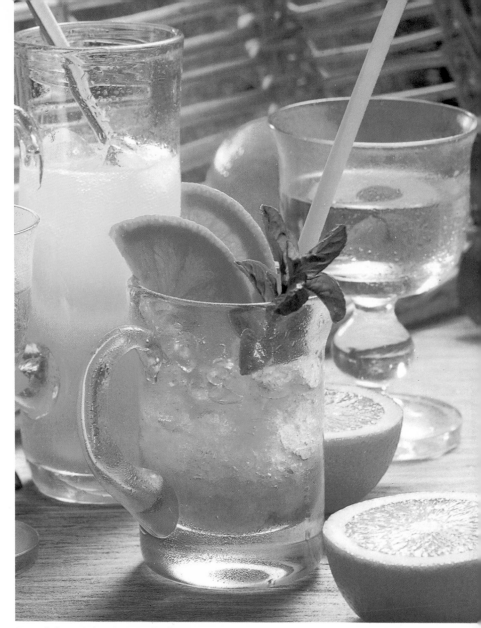

From left to right: Orange Cooler, Orange County Julep, Orange Bloom

Orange Bloom

2–3 ice cubes
25 ml/1 oz gin
15 ml/$\frac{1}{2}$ oz bianco vermouth
15 ml/$\frac{1}{2}$ oz Cointreau
1 cocktail cherry

Put ice in a mixing glass with gin, vermouth and Cointreau. Stir well and strain into a cocktail glass. Decorate with cherry.

Orange Cooler

3–4 ice cubes
2 teaspoons castor sugar
100 ml/4 oz orange juice
ginger ale

Put ice in a large tumbler with sugar and orange juice. Stir and top up with ginger ale. Serve with a straw.

Orange County Julep

3 ice cubes
50 ml/2 oz Cointreau
1 teaspoon lemon or grapefruit juice
2 dashes grenadine
1 orange slice
1 sprig of mint

Crush ice and put in a tumbler. Add Cointreau, lemon or grapefruit juice, and grenadine. Stir well. Decorate with halved orange slice and with sprig of mint. Serve with a straw.

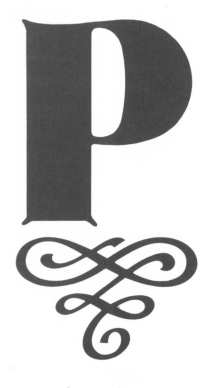

P

Panther's Sweat

2−3 ice cubes
25 ml/1 oz gin
25 ml/1 oz dry vermouth
1 teaspoon Cointreau
1 teaspoon lemon juice
1 dash Angostura bitters

Crack ice and put in a shaker with other ingredients. Shake well and strain into a cocktail glass.

Paprika Cocktail

2−3 ice cubes
25 ml/1 oz Cointreau
15 ml/½ oz Grand Marnier
15 ml/½ oz brandy
paprika

Crack ice and put in a shaker with Cointreau, Grand Marnier and brandy. Shake well and strain into a cocktail glass. Sprinkle a little paprika over top.

Pernod Fizz

2−3 ice cubes
1 egg white
1 teaspoon grenadine
15 ml/½ oz lemon juice
40 ml/1½ oz Pernod
soda water

Crack ice and put in a shaker with egg white, grenadine, lemon juice and Pernod. Shake very well and strain into a tumbler. Top up with soda water and serve with a straw.

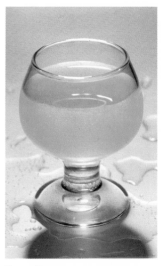

Peter Pan

Peter Pan

2−3 ice cubes
20 ml/¾ oz gin
20 ml/¾ oz dry vermouth
15 ml/½ oz orange juice
2 teaspoons peach bitters

Crack ice and put in a shaker with other ingredients. Shake and strain into a cocktail glass.

Peter Tower

2−3 ice cubes
40 ml/1½ oz brandy
15 ml/½ oz white rum
2 teaspoons grenadine
2 teaspoons Cointreau
2 teaspoons lemon juice

Put ice in a mixing glass with other ingredients. Stir well and strain into a cocktail glass.

Paddy

2−3 ice cubes
25 ml/1 oz Irish whisky
25 ml/1 oz red vermouth
1 dash Angostura bitters

Put ice in a mixing glass with other ingredients. Stir and strain into a cocktail glass.

Page Court

2−3 ice cubes
50 ml/2 oz orange juice
15 ml/½ oz Canadian whisky
15 ml/½ oz gin
15 ml/½ oz white rum
1 dash peach bitters

Crack ice and put in a shaker with other ingredients. Shake well and strain into a large cocktail glass.

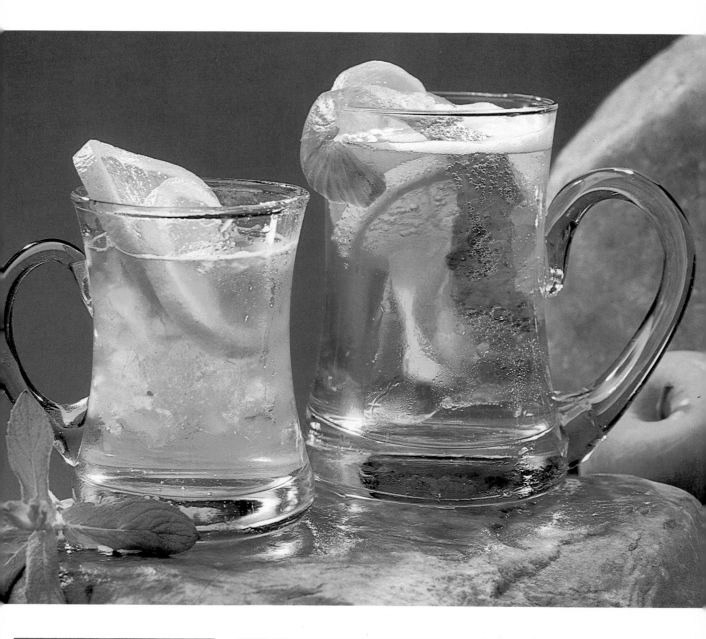

Pimlet, Pimm's

Pimlet

3–4 ice cubes
25 ml/1 oz Pimm's No 1
ginger ale
1 orange slice
1 lemon slice

Crush ice and put in a small tumbler. Add Pimm's and top up with ginger ale. Decorate with orange and lemon slices and serve with a straw.

Pimm's

2–3 ice cubes
40 ml/1½ oz Pimm's No 1
2 orange slices
1 lemon slice
lemonade
spiral of cucumber peel or sprig of
    mint

Put ice in a tall tumbler. Add Pimm's and orange and lemon slices. Top up with lemonade and decorate with spiral of cucumber peel or sprig of mint.

Pinky

2–3 ice cubes
½ egg white
2 teaspoons grenadine
40 ml/1½ oz gin

Crack ice and put in a shaker with other ingredients. Shake very well and strain into a cocktail glass.

Planter's Cocktail

2–3 ice cubes
40 ml/1½ oz rum
20 ml/¾ oz orange juice
20 ml/¾ oz lemon juice
2 dashes Angostura bitters
1 teaspoon castor sugar
3 pineapple chunks
1 cocktail cherry

Crack ice and put in a shaker with rum, orange juice, lemon juice, bitters and sugar. Shake very well and strain into a large cocktail glass. Decorate with pineapple chunks and cherry and serve with a cocktail stick.

Planter's Punch

4–6 ice cubes
50 ml/2 oz white rum
15 ml/½ oz lemon juice
2 teaspoons sugar syrup
1 orange slice
1 cocktail cherry
1 strawberry
2 raspberries

Crack half ice and put in a shaker with rum, lemon juice and sugar syrup. Shake well. Crush remaining ice and put in a tall tumbler. Pour in contents of shaker and stir. Decorate with orange slice, cherry, strawberry and raspberries. Serve with a straw and a spoon.

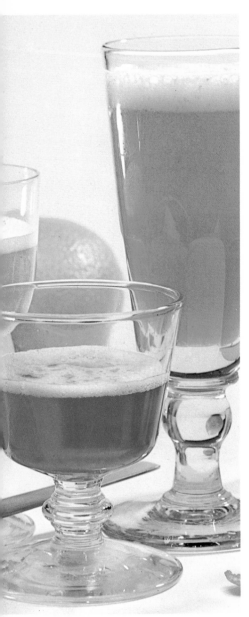
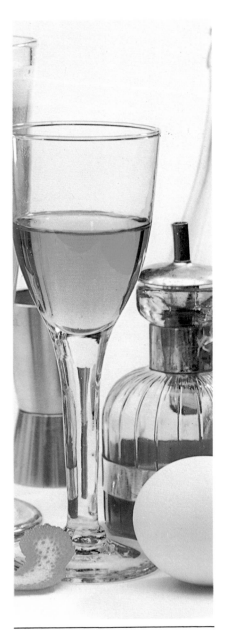

Pinky and Pink Lady Fizz (above)
Pink Gin (above right)

Pink Lady Fizz

2–3 ice cubes
1 egg white
2 teaspoons grenadine
25 ml/1 oz lemon juice
50 ml/2 oz gin
soda water

Crack ice and put in a shaker with egg white, grenadine, lemon juice and gin. Shake very well and strain into a goblet. Top up with soda water and serve with a straw.

Pink Gin

3–4 ice cubes
50 ml/2 oz gin
3 dashes Angostura bitters

Put ice in a mixing glass with gin and bitters. Stir and strain into a cocktail glass.

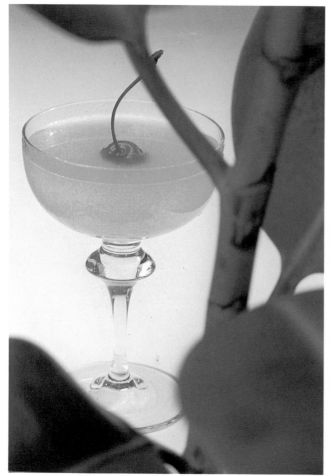

Planter's Cocktail

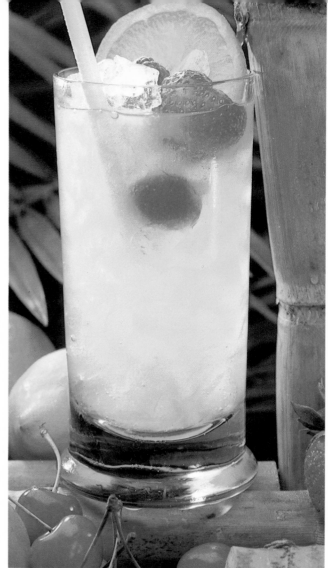

Planter's Punch

Port Cobbler

4 ice cubes
65 ml/2½ oz port
25 ml/1 oz Cointreau
1 teaspoon sugar syrup
soda water
5 pineapple chunks
1 cocktail cherry

Crush ice and put in a tall tumbler. Put port, Cointreau and sugar syrup in a shaker and shake well. Pour into tumbler, top up with soda water and decorate with pineapple chunks and cherry. Serve with a straw and a spoon.

Prairie Oyster

1 teaspoon Worcestershire sauce
1 egg yolk
2 teaspoons tomato ketchup
2 dashes lemon juice
2 dashes olive oil
salt, pepper, paprika

Put Worcestershire sauce in a shallow glass. Slide in egg yolk. Add tomato ketchup, lemon juice, olive oil, salt, pepper and paprika. Do not stir this drink, but swallow it in one gulp.

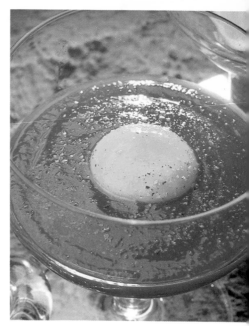

Prairie Oyster

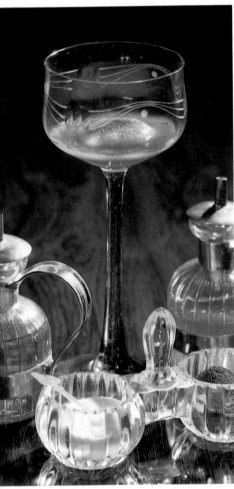

President Taft's Opossum

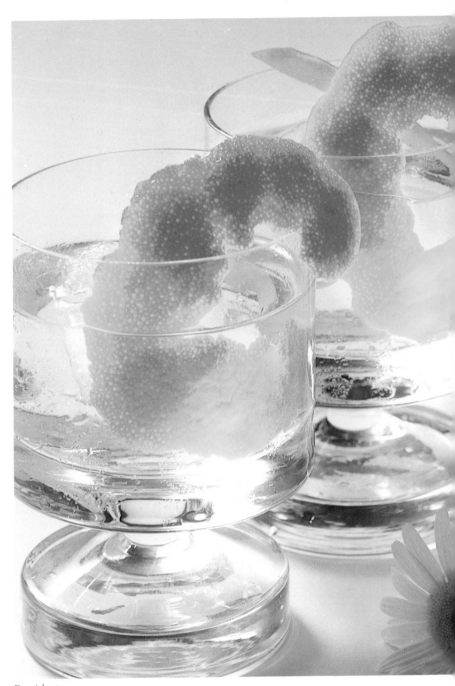

Presidente

President Taft's Opossum

1 teaspoon Angostura bitters
1 teaspoon vinegar
1 egg yolk
1 dash olive oil
1 dash Worcestershire sauce
1–2 teaspoons brandy
salt, paprika, cayenne pepper

Rinse out a shallow glass with bitters. Add vinegar and slide in egg yolk. Add olive oil, Worcestershire sauce, brandy, salt, paprika and cayenne. Do not stir this drink, but swallow it in one gulp.

Presidente

3–4 ice cubes
40 ml/1½ oz white rum
25 ml/1 oz dry vermouth
spiral of orange peel

Put ice in a mixing glass with rum and vermouth. Stir very well and pour into a small goblet. Decorate with spiral of orange peel.

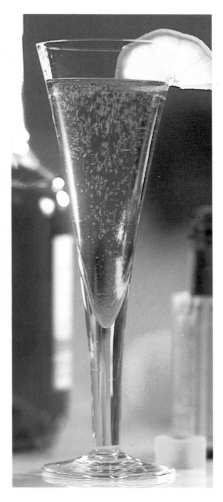

Prince of Wales

Prince of Wales

2–3 ice cubes
15 ml/½ oz brandy
15 ml/½ oz Cointreau
1 dash Angostura bitters
sparkling wine
½ lemon slice

Crack ice and put in a shaker with brandy, Cointreau and bitters. Shake well and strain into a tall champagne glass. Top up with sparkling wine and fix lemon slice on rim of glass.

Quarter Deck

2–3 ice cubes
40 ml/1½ oz dark rum
15 ml/½ oz sherry
2 teaspoons lime juice

Crack ice and put in a shaker with other ingredients. Shake very well and strain into a cocktail glass.

Queen Bee

(picture on page 86)

2–3 ice cubes
25 ml/1 oz sloe gin
25 ml/1 oz Cointreau
1 dash Pernod

Crack ice and put in a shaker with other ingredients. Shake well and strain into a cocktail glass.

Queen Elizabeth

(picture on page 86)

2–3 ice cubes
25 ml/1 oz gin
15 ml/½ oz Cointreau
15 ml/½ oz lemon juice
1 dash Pernod
1 cocktail cherry

Crack ice and put in a shaker with gin, Cointreau, lemon juice and Pernod. Shake well and strain into a cocktail glass. Decorate with cherry.

Queen Mary

(picture on page 86)

2–3 ice cubes
25 ml/1 oz brandy
25 ml/1 oz Cointreau
2 dashes strawberry syrup
1 dash Pernod
1 strawberry

Crack ice and put in a shaker with brandy, Cointreau, strawberry syrup and Pernod. Shake well and strain into a cocktail glass. Decorate with strawberry and serve with a cocktail stick.

Queen's Cocktail

(picture on page 86)

4 pineapple chunks
2–3 ice cubes
25 ml/1 oz gin
15 ml/½ oz bianco vermouth
15 ml/½ oz dry vermouth

Put pineapple chunks in a mixing glass and crush with a spoon. Add other ingredients and stir well. Strain into a cocktail glass.

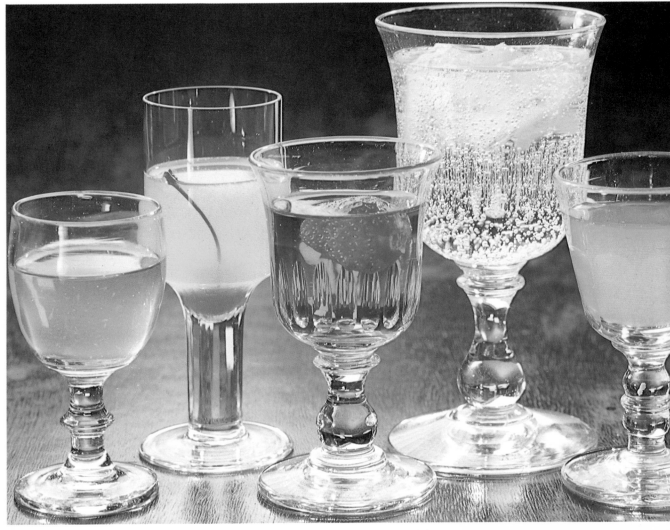

From left to right: Queen Bee,
Queen Elizabeth, Queen Mary,
Queen's Peg, Queen's Cocktail

Quo Vadis (right)

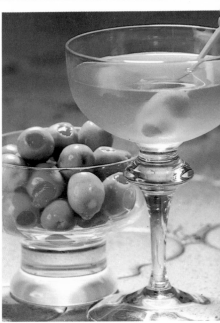

Queen's Peg

1 large ice cube
25 ml/1 oz gin
sparkling wine

Put ice in a goblet, add gin and
top up with sparkling wine.

Quo Vadis

2–3 ice cubes
25 ml/1 oz gin
25 ml/1 oz green Chartreuse
1 dash Bénédictine
1 dash Cointreau
1 olive

Crack ice and put in a shaker with
gin, Chartreuse, Bénédictine and
Cointreau. Shake and strain into a
cocktail glass. Spear olive on a
cocktail stick and use to decorate.

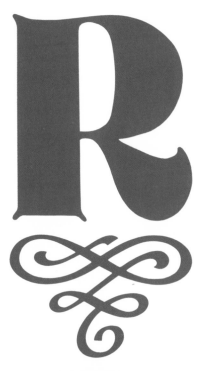

Rabbit's Revenge

2–3 ice cubes
40 ml/1½ oz Bourbon whisky
25 ml/1 oz pineapple juice
2–3 dashes grenadine
tonic water
1 orange slice

Put ice in a shaker with whisky, pineapple juice and grenadine. Shake well and pour into a tumbler. Top up with tonic water and fix orange slice on rim of glass. Serve with a straw.

Ramona Cocktail
(picture on page 88)

1 sprig of mint
2–3 ice cubes
25 ml/1 oz gin
25 ml/1 oz lemon juice
2 dashes grenadine

Coarsely chop mint. Crack ice and put in a shaker with mint and other ingredients. Shake well and strain into a cocktail glass.

Rabbit's Revenge

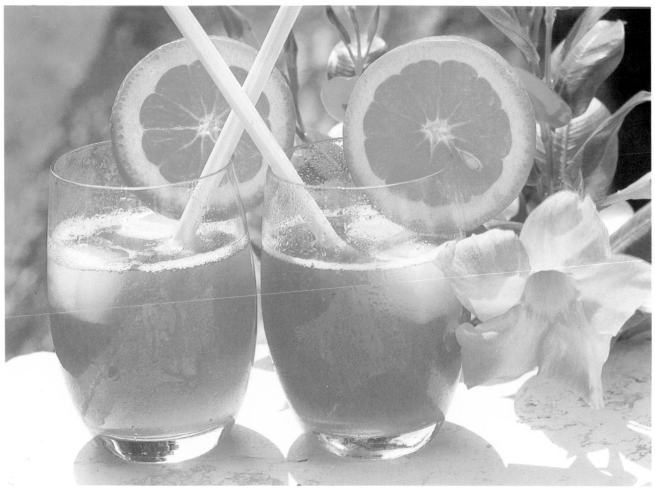

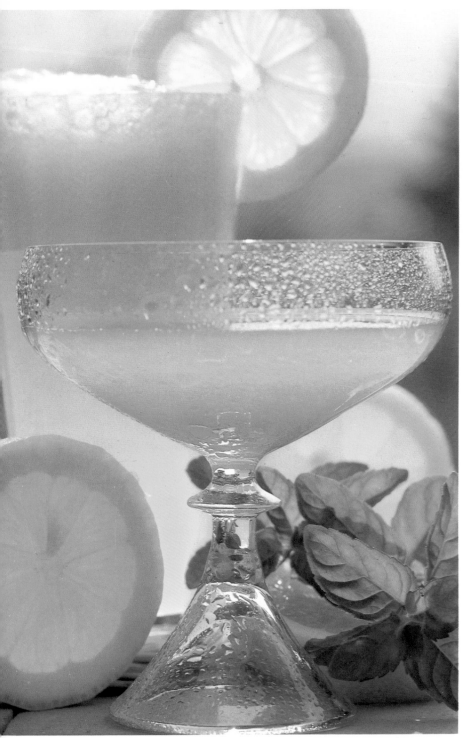
Ramona Fizz, Ramona Cocktail

Ramona Fizz

2–3 ice cubes
50 ml/2 oz white rum
50 ml/2 oz lemon juice
25 ml/1 oz Cointreau
2 teaspoons castor sugar
soda water
1 lemon slice

Crack ice and put in a shaker with rum, lemon juice, Cointreau and sugar. Shake very well and strain into a tall tumbler. Top up with soda water and fix lemon slice on rim of glass. Serve with a straw.

Ray Long

3 ice cubes
25 ml/1 oz bianco vermouth
20 ml/$\frac{3}{4}$ oz brandy
1 teaspoon Pernod
1 dash Angostura bitters

Put ice in a mixing glass with other ingredients. Stir well and strain into a cocktail glass.

Raymond Hitch Cocktail

3 ice cubes
80 ml/3 oz bianco vermouth
25 ml/1 oz orange juice
1 dash Angostura bitters
1 pineapple slice

Put ice in a mixing glass with vermouth, orange juice and bitters. Stir well and strain into a shallow glass. Decorate with pineapple slice and serve with a spoon.

Red Kiss

2–3 ice cubes
25 ml/1 oz dry vermouth
15 ml/½ oz gin
15 ml/½ oz cherry brandy
spiral of lemon peel

Put ice in a mixing glass with vermouth, gin and cherry brandy. Stir well and strain into a cocktail glass. Decorate with spiral of lemon peel.

Red Pearl

25 ml/1 oz blackberry liqueur
½ pineapple slice
sparkling wine

Put blackberry liqueur in a shallow champagne glass, add pineapple slice and top up with sparkling wine. Serve with a spoon.

Red Shadow

2–3 ice cubes
25 ml/1 oz whisky
15 ml/½ oz apricot brandy
15 ml/½ oz cherry brandy
1 teaspoon lemon juice

Crack ice and put in a shaker with other ingredients. Shake well and strain into a cocktail glass.

Red Tonic

25 ml/1 oz vodka
25 ml/1 oz grenadine
2 teaspoons lemon juice
1 ice cube
1 lemon slice
tonic water

Put vodka, grenadine and lemon juice in a mixing glass and stir well. Strain into a tall glass. Add ice and lemon slice and top up with tonic water. Serve with a straw.

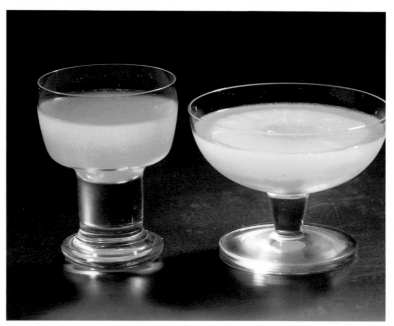

Ray Long, Raymond Hitch Cocktail

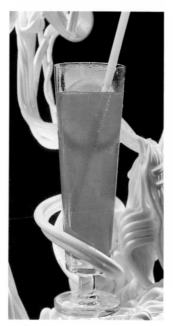

Red Tonic

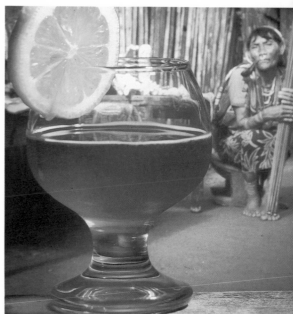

Redskin

Redskin

2–3 ice cubes
50 ml/2 oz white rum
2 teaspoons grenadine
pepper, cinnamon, nutmeg
1 lemon slice

Crack ice and put in a shaker with rum and grenadine. Add pepper, ground cinnamon and grated nutmeg. Shake and strain into a cocktail glass. Fix lemon slice on rim of glass to decorate.

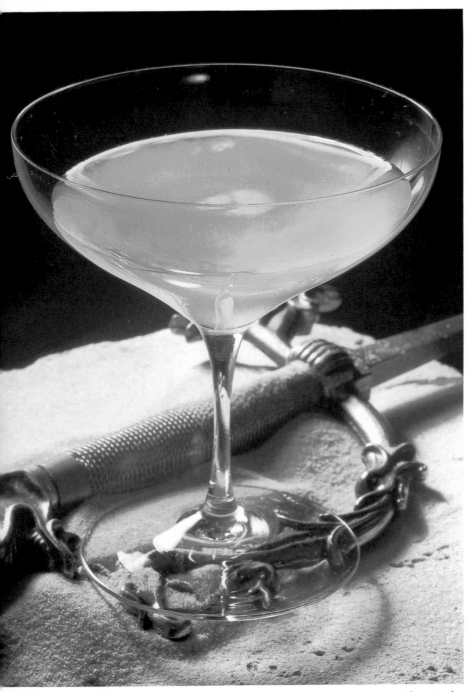

Rhett Butler

Rickey

1 small lemon
50 ml/2 oz whisky
soda water

Cut lemon in two and put in a
large tumbler. Press out juice with
a spoon and add whisky. Top up
with chilled soda water and serve
with spoon.

Ritz

2−3 ice cubes
25 ml/1 oz brandy
15 ml/½ oz Cointreau
15 ml/½ oz orange juice
champagne

Crack ice and put in a shaker with
brandy, Cointreau and orange
juice. Shake well and strain into a
tall champagne glass. Top up with
champagne.

Rob Roy

2−3 ice cubes
25 ml/1 oz Scotch whisky
25 ml/1 oz red vermouth
1 dash Angostura bitters
1 cocktail cherry

Put ice in a mixing glass with
whisky, vermouth and bitters.
Stir well and strain into a cocktail
glass. Decorate with cherry and
serve with a cocktail stick.

Rhett Butler

2−3 ice cubes
50 ml/2 oz Southern Comfort
15 ml/½ oz Cointreau
1 teaspoon lemon juice
1 teaspoon lime juice
1 teaspoon castor sugar

Crack ice and put in a shaker with
other ingredients. Shake well and
strain into a shallow champagne
glass.

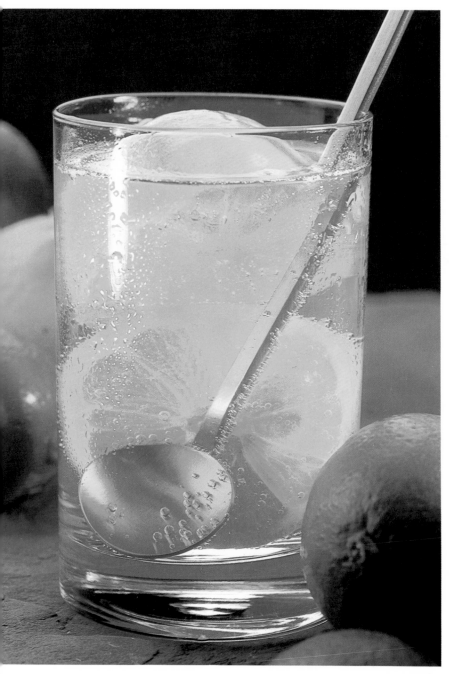

Rickey

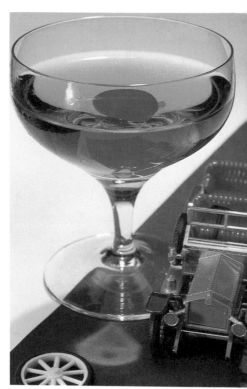

Rolls-Royce

Rolls-Royce

2–3 ice cubes
25 ml/1 oz gin
15 ml/$\frac{1}{2}$ oz dry vermouth
15 ml/$\frac{1}{2}$ oz bianco vermouth
1–2 dashes Bénédictine
1 cocktail cherry

Put ice in a mixing glass with gin, vermouths and Bénédictine. Stir well and strain into a cocktail glass. Decorate with cherry and serve with a cocktail stick.

Rocky Mountains Punch

2–3 ice cubes
25 ml/1 oz rum
15 ml/$\frac{1}{2}$ oz lemon juice
2 teaspoons maraschino
2–3 pineapple chunks
2–3 strawberries
1–2 cherries
sparkling wine

Crack ice and put in a shaker with rum, lemon juice and maraschino. Shake and strain into a goblet. Decorate with fruits and top up with sparkling wine. Serve with a straw and a spoon.

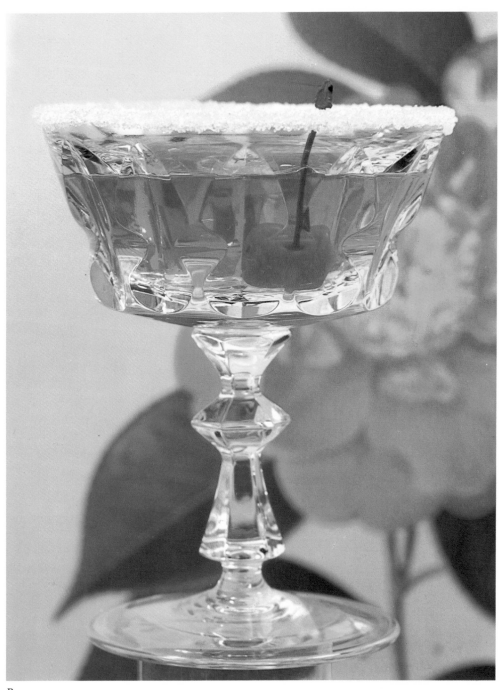

Rose

Rose

15 ml/$\frac{1}{2}$ oz lemon juice
1 tablespoon castor sugar
3 ice cubes
25 ml/1 oz gin
15 ml/$\frac{1}{2}$ oz apricot brandy
15 ml/$\frac{1}{2}$ oz dry vermouth
1 dash grenadine
1 cocktail cherry

Dip rim of a cocktail glass first in lemon juice, shaking off excess, then in sugar. Allow frosting to dry. Put ice in a mixing glass with gin, apricot brandy, vermouth, grenadine and a dash of remaining lemon juice. Stir and strain into cocktail glass. Decorate with cherry.

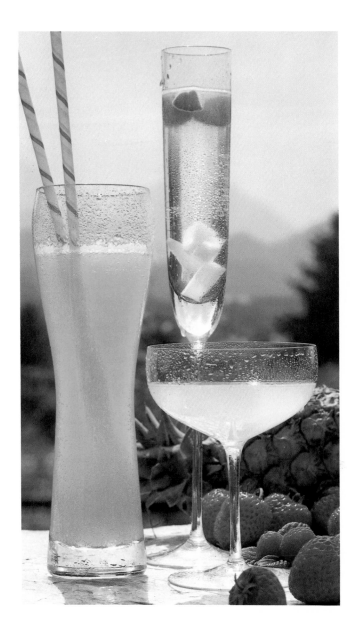

From left to right:
Royal Fizz, Royal Long,
Royal Bermuda

Royal Long

3–4 pineapple chunks
2–4 ice cubes
15 ml/$\frac{1}{2}$ oz Cointreau
15 ml/$\frac{1}{2}$ oz white wine
3–4 strawberries
sparkling wine

Put pineapple chunks in a tall narrow glass. Crush ice and add to glass with Cointreau and white wine. Stir, then add strawberries. Top up with sparkling wine and serve with a straw and a spoon.

Rum Alexander

2–3 ice cubes
25 ml/1 oz crème de cacao
15 ml/$\frac{1}{2}$ oz white rum
15 ml/$\frac{1}{2}$ oz cream

Crack ice and put in a shaker with other ingredients. Shake well and strain into a cocktail glass.

Rum Cobbler

3–4 ice cubes
1 teaspoon maraschino
1 teaspoon grenadine
1 orange slice
1 lime slice
2 cocktail cherries
3–4 pineapple chunks
1–2 strawberries
rum

Crush ice and put in a tall goblet. Add maraschino and grenadine. Decorate with fruits and top up with rum to taste. Serve with a straw and a spoon.

Royal Bermuda

2–3 ice cubes
40 ml/1$\frac{1}{2}$ oz white rum
15 ml/$\frac{1}{2}$ oz lemon juice
1 teaspoon Cointreau
1 teaspoon sugar syrup

Crack ice and put in a shaker with other ingredients. Shake and strain into a cocktail glass.

Royal Fizz

2–3 ice cubes
50 ml/2 oz orange juice
40 ml/1$\frac{1}{2}$ oz gin
40 ml/1$\frac{1}{2}$ oz raspberry brandy
40 ml/1$\frac{1}{2}$ oz lime juice
soda water

Crack ice and put in a shaker with orange juice, gin, raspberry brandy and lime juice. Shake and strain into a tall tumbler. Top up with soda water and serve with a straw.

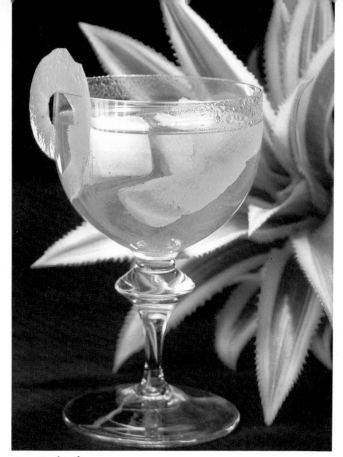

Rum Cocktail

Rum Cocktail

25 ml/1 oz white rum
1 dash Angostura bitters
1 teaspoon sugar syrup
2 ice cubes
spiral of orange peel
piece of orange peel

Put rum, bitters and sugar syrup in a cocktail glass and stir well. Add ice and decorate with spiral of orange peel. Squeeze remaining piece of orange peel over top.

Rum Flip

2–3 ice cubes
1 egg yolk
2 teaspoons sugar syrup
25 ml/1 oz rum
25 ml/1 oz strong cold tea
2 teaspoons Cointreau

Crack ice and put in a shaker with other ingredients. Shake very well and strain into a flip glass. Serve with a straw.

Rum Sour

2–3 ice cubes
40 ml/1½ oz white rum
15 ml/½ oz lemon juice
1 teaspoon sugar syrup
2 cocktail cherries
2 lemon segments
soda water

Crack ice and put in a shaker with rum, lemon juice and sugar syrup. Shake well and strain into a shallow champagne glass. Decorate with cherries and lemon segments and top up with soda water. Serve with a cocktail stick.

Rusty Nail

2–3 ice cubes
40 ml/1½ oz Scotch whisky
20 ml/¾ oz Drambuie
spiral of lemon peel

Put ice in a small tumbler. Add whisky and Drambuie and stir. Decorate with lemon peel.

Rye Cocktail

2–3 ice cubes
50 ml/2 oz rye whisky
2–3 dashes grenadine
2 dashes Angostura bitters
1 cocktail cherry

Put ice in a mixing glass with whisky, grenadine and bitters. Stir well and strain into a small goblet. Spear cherry on a cocktail stick and use to decorate.

Rye Daisy

3–4 ice cubes
40 ml/1½ oz rye whisky
20 ml/¾ oz yellow Chartreuse
2 teaspoons lemon juice
1 teaspoon sugar syrup
soda water
2 peach slices
2 strawberries

Crack ice and put in a shaker with whisky, Chartreuse, lemon juice and sugar syrup. Shake well and strain into a small goblet. Top up with soda water and decorate with peach slices and strawberries. Serve with a straw and a spoon.

Rye Punch

4–5 ice cubes
50 ml/2 oz rye whisky
2 teaspoons lemon juice
2 teaspoons castor sugar
1 orange slice

Crush ice and put in a shaker with whisky, lemon juice and sugar. Shake well and pour into a tall tumbler. Fix orange slice on rim of glass and serve with a straw.

From left to right: Rye Daisy, Rye Punch, Rye Cocktail

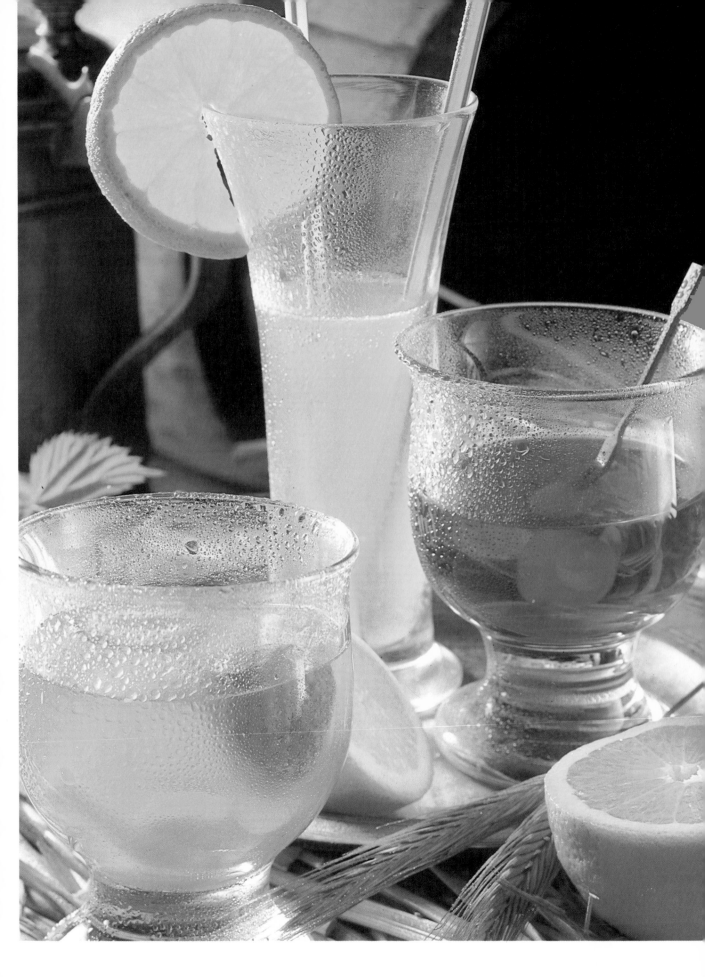

Sake Special

2–3 ice cubes
50 ml/2 oz gin
25 ml/1 oz sake
2 dashes Angostura bitters

Put ice in a mixing glass with other ingredients. Stir well and strain into a cocktail glass.

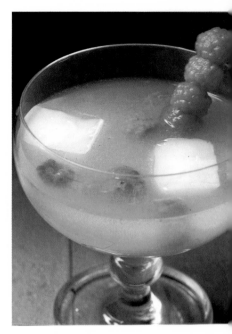

Santa Fé Express

Santa Fé Express

2–3 ice cubes
15 ml/½ oz Cointreau
1 teaspoon lemon juice
40 ml/1½ oz orange juice
soda water
10–12 frozen raspberries

Put ice, Cointreau and lemon juice in a large cocktail glass and stir. Top up with orange juice and soda water. Add raspberries, still frozen, spearing a few of them on a cocktail stick.

Saratoga Fizz

2–3 ice cubes
1 egg white
2 teaspoons castor sugar
15 ml/½ oz lemon juice
2 teaspoons lime juice
50 ml/2 oz Bourbon whisky
1 cocktail cherry
soda water

Crack ice and put in a shaker with egg white, sugar, lemon juice, lime juice and whisky. Shake very well and strain into a tall tumbler. Add cherry, top up with soda water and serve with a straw.

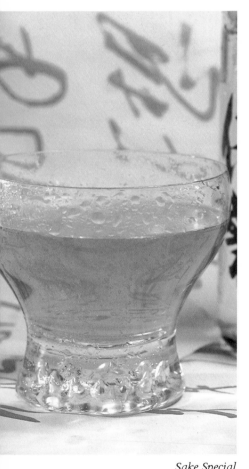

Sake Special

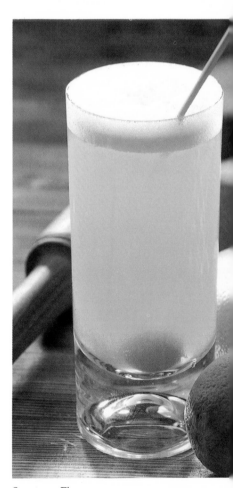

Saratoga Fizz

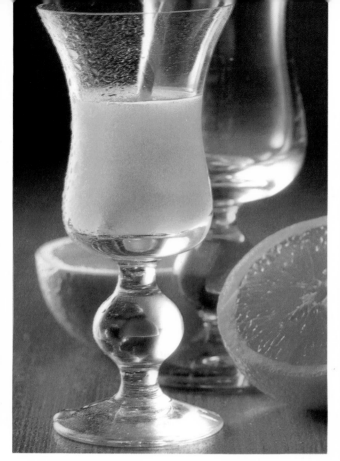

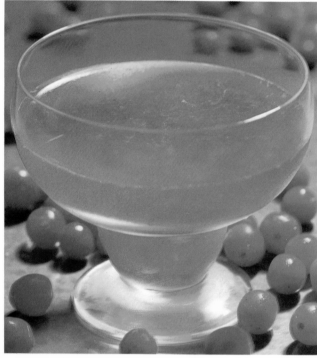

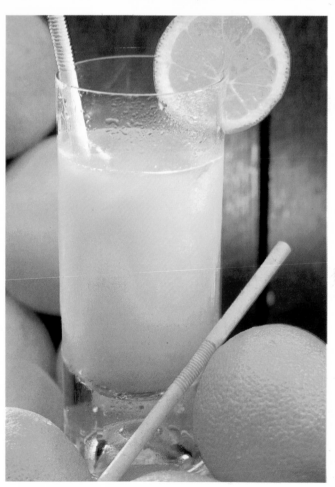

Satan's Whiskers (above)
Scarlett O'Hara (above right)
Screwdriver (right)

Satan's Whiskers

2–3 ice cubes
15 ml/½ oz gin
15 ml/½ oz dry vermouth
15 ml/½ oz bianco vermouth
15 ml/½ oz orange juice
1 teaspoon Cointreau
1 teaspoon orange bitters

Put ice in a mixing glass with other ingredients. Stir well and strain into a cocktail glass.

Scarlett O'Hara

2–3 ice cubes
40 ml/1½ oz Southern Comfort
40 ml/1½ oz cranberry juice
2–3 teaspoons lime juice

Crack ice and put in a shaker with other ingredients. Shake well and strain into a large cocktail glass.

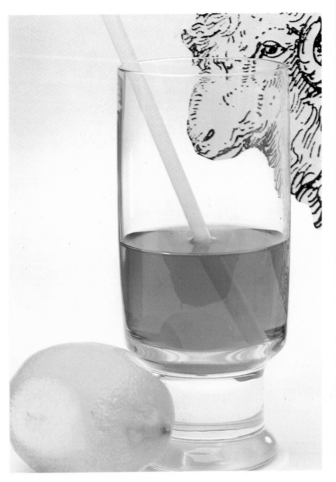
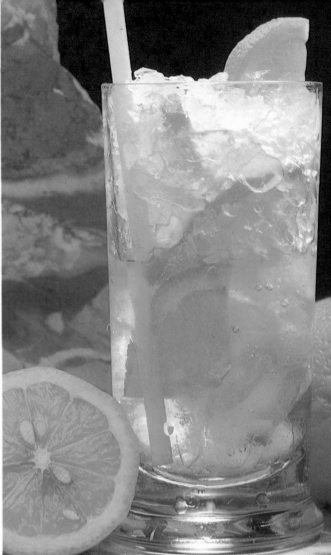

Sheep's Head (above left)
Sherry Cobbler (above)

Screwdriver

(picture on page 97)

2–3 ice cubes
80 ml/3 oz orange juice
25 ml/1 oz vodka
1 orange slice

Put ice in a mixing glass with orange juice and vodka. Stir very well and strain into a tumbler. Fix orange slice on rim of glass and serve with a straw.

Sheep's Head

3 ice cubes
40 ml/1½ oz Bourbon whisky
15 ml/½ oz red vermouth
1 teaspoon Bénédictine
piece of lemon peel
1 cocktail cherry

Put ice in a mixing glass with whisky, vermouth and Bénédictine. Stir and strain into a small tumbler. Squeeze lemon peel over top and decorate with cherry. Serve with a straw.

Sherry Cobbler

4 ice cubes
2 orange slices
1 lemon slice
65 ml/2½ oz sherry
15ml/½ oz sugar syrup

Crush ice and put in a tall tumbler or tall champagne glass. Halve orange and lemon slices and add to glass. Pour in sherry and sugar syrup. Stir, and serve with a straw.

Sidecar

2–3 ice cubes
25 ml/1 oz brandy
15 ml/½ oz Cointreau
15 ml/½ oz lemon juice
1 cocktail cherry

Crack ice and put in a shaker with brandy, Cointreau and lemon juice. Shake and strain into a cocktail glass. Spear cherry on a cocktail stick and use to decorate.

Silver Fizz

2–3 ice cubes
1 egg white
1 teaspoon castor sugar
25 ml/1 oz lemon juice
40 ml/1½ oz gin
soda water

Crack ice and put in a shaker with egg white, sugar, lemon juice and gin. Shake very well and strain into a tall tumbler. Top up with soda water, serve with a straw.

Singapore Gin Sling

2–3 ice cubes
50 ml/2 oz gin
25 ml/1 oz lemon juice
15 ml/½ oz cherry brandy
15 ml/½ oz Cointreau
2 teaspoons castor sugar
soda water
1 lemon slice

Put ice in a tall glass with gin, lemon juice, cherry brandy, Cointreau and sugar. Stir and top up with soda water. Decorate with lemon slice.

Sink or Swim

2–3 ice cubes
40 ml/1½ oz brandy
15 ml/½ oz bianco vermouth
1 dash Angostura bitters

Put ice in a mixing glass with other ingredients. Stir well and strain into a cocktail glass.

Sir Ridgeway Knight

2–3 ice cubes
25 ml/1 oz brandy
25 ml/1 oz Cointreau
25 ml/1 oz yellow Chartreuse
2 dashes Angostura bitters

Crack ice and put in a shaker with other ingredients. Shake well and strain into a large cocktail glass or balloon glass.

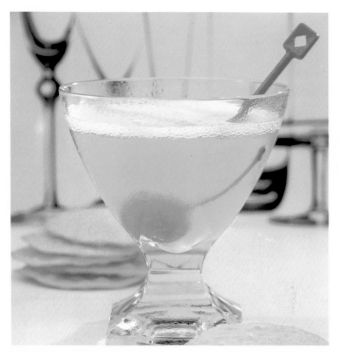

Sidecar

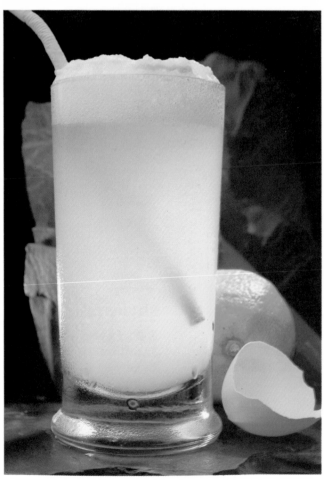

Silver Fizz

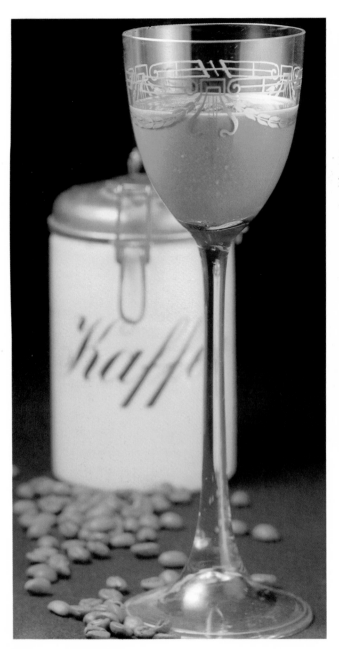

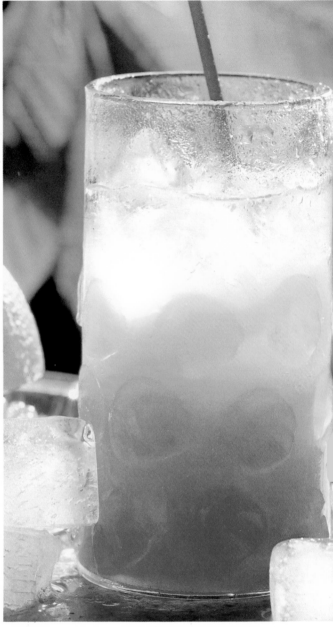

Slivovitz Cocktail (above)
Smiling Esther (above right)

Slivovitz Cocktail

2–3 ice cubes
25 ml/1 oz slivovitz
15 ml/$\frac{1}{2}$ oz strong cold coffee
15 ml/$\frac{1}{2}$ oz cream
instant coffee powder

Crack ice and put in a shaker with slivovitz, coffee and cream. Shake and strain into a cocktail glass. Sprinkle a little instant coffee powder over top.

Smiling Esther

4–6 ice cubes
25 ml/1 oz brandy
25 ml/1 oz Sabra
25 ml/1 oz orange juice

Crack half ice and put in a shaker with other ingredients. Shake well and strain into a tumbler. Add remaining ice and serve with a straw.

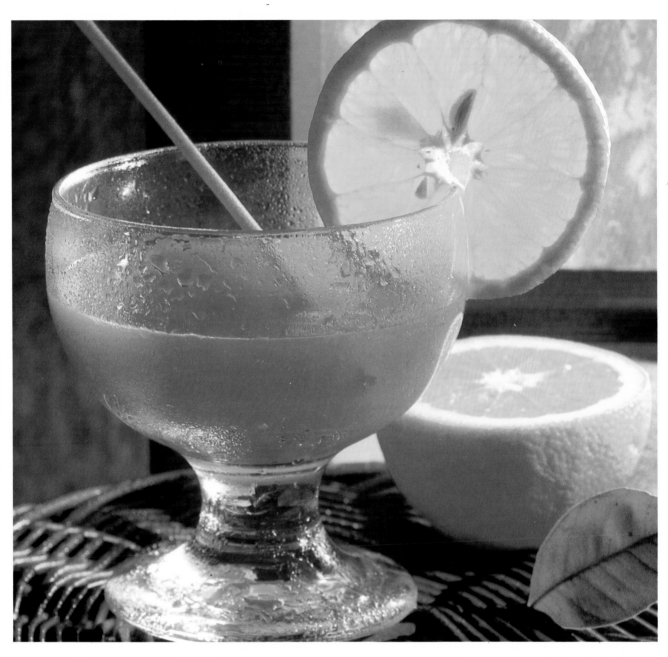

Soul Kiss

Soul Kiss

2−3 ice cubes
25 ml/1 oz Bourbon whisky
15 ml/½ oz dry vermouth
15 ml/½ oz Dubonnet
15 ml/½ oz orange juice
piece of orange peel
1 orange slice

Crack ice and put in a shaker with whisky, vermouth, Dubonnet and orange juice. Shake and strain into a large cocktail glass. Squeeze orange peel over top and fix orange slice on rim of glass. Serve with a straw.

Sparkling Grape Cocktail

4 white grapes
3 black grapes
sparkling wine

Spear grapes on wooden cocktail stick and stand stick in a tall champagne glass. Top up with sparkling wine.

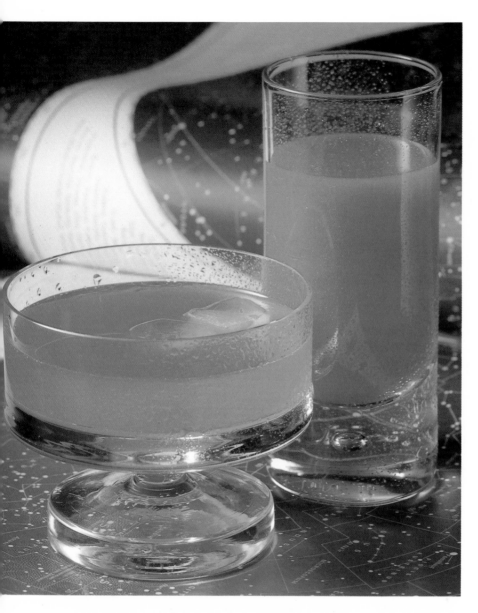

Star

2–3 ice cubes
25 ml/1 oz calvados
20 ml/¾ oz dry vermouth
1 dash Angostura bitters
piece of lemon peel
1 olive

Put ice in a mixing glass with calvados, vermouth and bitters. Stir very well and strain into a cocktail glass. Squeeze lemon peel over top. Spear olive on a cocktail stick and use to decorate.

Stinger

2–3 ice cubes
25 ml/1 oz brandy
25 ml/1 oz green crème de menthe

Crack ice and put in a shaker with brandy and crème de menthe. Shake and strain into a cocktail glass.

Stone Fence

2–3 ice cubes
50 ml/2 oz whisky
cider
spiral of apple peel

Put ice in a medium sized tumbler and add whisky. Top up with cider and decorate with spiral of apple peel.

Stonehammer

2–3 ice cubes
20 ml/¾ oz gin
20 ml/¾ oz red vermouth
15 ml/½ oz brandy
15 ml/½ oz lemon juice

Crack ice and put in a shaker with other ingredients. Shake and strain into a large cocktail glass.

Sputniks (1 and 2)

Sputnik (1)

4–6 ice cubes
65 ml/2½ oz vodka
25 ml/1 oz Fernet Branca
1 teaspoon lemon juice
½ teaspoon castor sugar

Crack half ice and put in a shaker with other ingredients. Shake well and strain into a large cocktail glass. Add remaining ice.

Sputnik (2)

2–3 ice cubes
25 ml/1 oz vodka
15 ml/½ oz brandy
15 ml/½ oz Bourbon whisky
sangrita
cayenne pepper

Crack ice and put in a shaker with vodka, brandy and whisky. Shake well and strain into a tumbler. Top up with sangrita. Sprinkle with cayenne pepper and stir well.

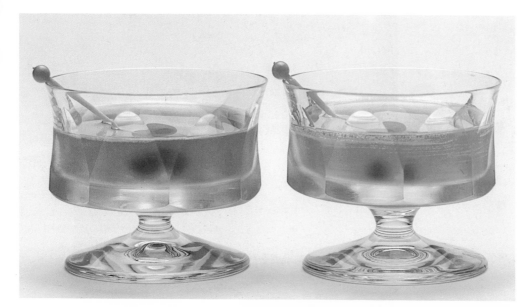

Star (left)
Stone Fence (below)

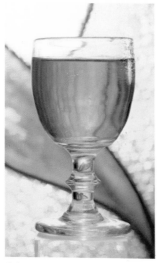

Stinger

Stromboli

3–4 ice cubes
50 ml/2 oz Bourbon whisky
1 teaspoon sugar syrup
3 dashes Angostura bitters
3 cocktail cherries
1 orange slice
1 lemon slice

Put ice in a small tumbler with whisky, sugar syrup and bitters. Stir well and decorate with cherries, orange slice and lemon slice.

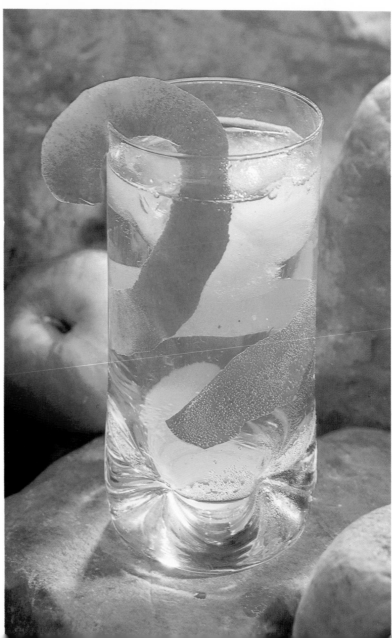

103

Summertime

3 ice cubes
25 ml/1 oz rum
25 ml/1 oz Cointreau
2 teaspoons grenadine
2 teaspoons orange juice
2 teaspoons lemon juice

Put ice in a mixing glass with other ingredients. Stir well and strain into a large cocktail glass.

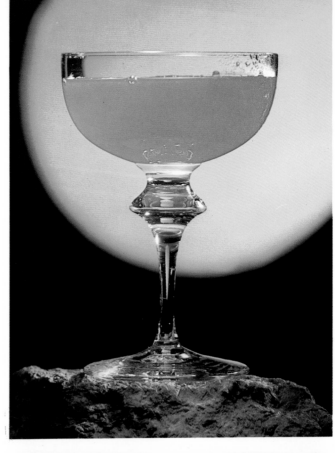

Swedish Fan

3 ice cubes
15 ml/$\frac{1}{2}$ oz gin
15 ml/$\frac{1}{2}$ oz brandy
15 ml/$\frac{1}{2}$ oz cherry brandy
1 dash orange bitters
piece of orange peel

Put ice in a mixing glass with gin, brandy, cherry brandy and bitters. Stir well and strain into a cocktail glass. Squeeze orange peel over top.

Sweet Girl

2–3 ice cubes
20 ml/$\frac{3}{4}$ oz gin
20 ml/$\frac{3}{4}$ oz apricot brandy
20 ml/$\frac{3}{4}$ oz cream

Crack ice and put in a shaker with other ingredients. Shake well and strain into a cocktail glass.

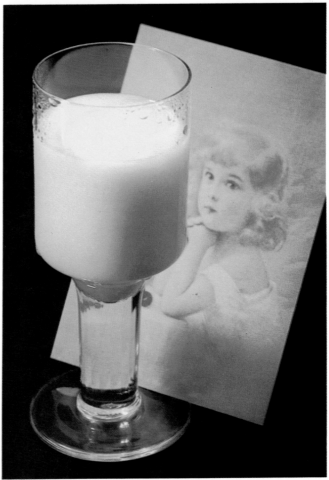

Summertime (top right)
Sweet Girl (right)

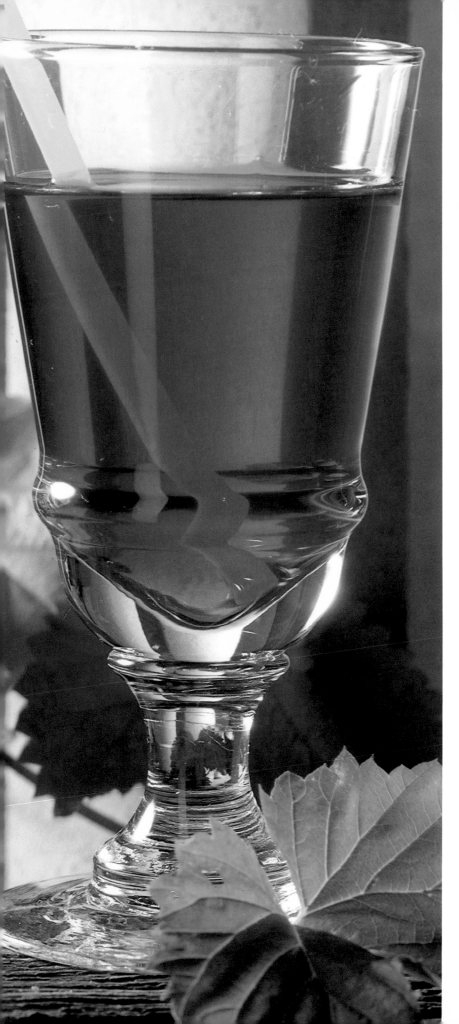

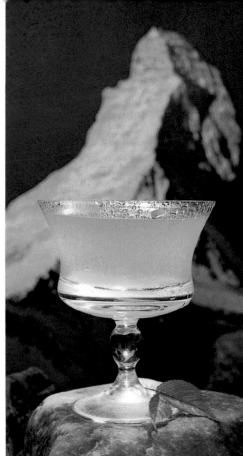

Swiss Sunset (above)
Sweet Lady (left)

Sweet Lady

2–3 ice cubes
25 ml/1 oz crème de cacao
15 ml/$\frac{1}{2}$ oz whisky
15 ml/$\frac{1}{2}$ oz peach brandy

Crack ice and put in a shaker with other ingredients. Shake well and strain into a cocktail glass.

Swiss Sunset

2–3 ice cubes
20 ml/$\frac{3}{4}$ oz brandy
20 ml/$\frac{3}{4}$ oz mandarin orange liqueur
2 teaspoons grapefruit juice
2 teaspoons lemon juice

Crack ice and put in a shaker with other ingredients. Shake and strain into a cocktail glass.

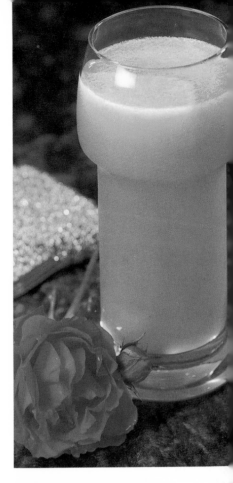

T

Take Two

2–3 ice cubes
25 ml/1 oz gin
15 ml/½ oz Cointreau
2 teaspoons Campari

Put ice in a mixing glass with other ingredients. Stir well and strain into a cocktail glass.

Tango

2–3 ice cubes
20 ml/¾ oz gin
20 ml/¾ oz red vermouth
15 ml/½ oz Cointreau
15 ml/½ oz orange juice
piece of orange peel

Crack ice and put in a shaker with gin, vermouth, Cointreau and orange juice. Shake and strain into a cocktail glass. Squeeze orange peel over top.

Tantalus

2–3 ice cubes
25 ml/1 oz Forbidden Fruit
    liqueur
15 ml/½ oz brandy
15 ml/½ oz lemon juice

Crack ice and put in a shaker with other ingredients. Shake and strain into a cocktail glass.

Taxi

2–3 ice cubes
25 ml/1 oz gin
25 ml/1 oz dry vermouth
2 teaspoons Pernod
2 teaspoons lime juice

Put ice in a mixing glass with other ingredients. Stir well and strain into a cocktail glass.

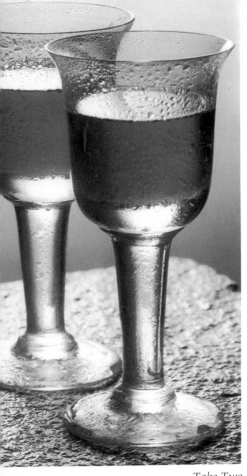

Take Two

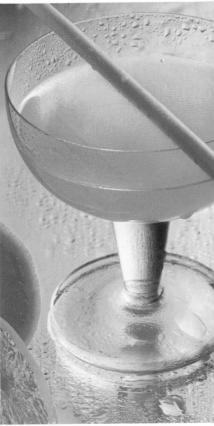

Tango (top)
Tantalus (above)

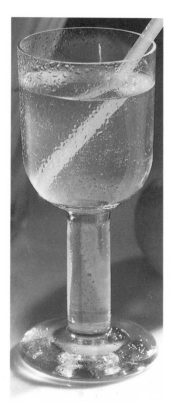

Taxi

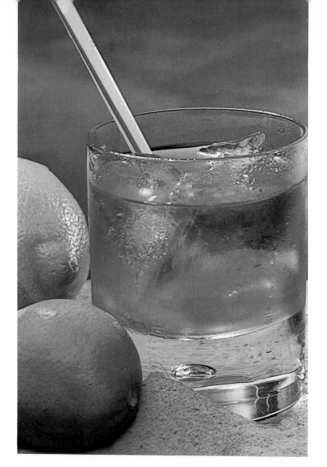

Tequila Caliente

2–3 ice cubes
40 ml/1½ oz tequila
15 ml/½ oz crème de cassis
15 ml/½ oz lime juice
2 dashes grenadine
soda water

Put ice in a small tumbler with tequila, crème de cassis, lime juice and grenadine. Stir well and add a shot of soda water. Serve with a straw.

Tequila Cocktail

2–3 ice cubes
25 ml/1 oz tequila
20 ml/¾ oz port
1 teaspoon lime juice
2 dashes Angostura bitters

Crack ice and put in a shaker with other ingredients. Shake and strain into a cocktail glass.

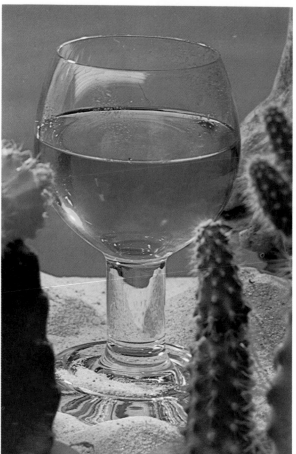

Tequila Caliente (top), Tequila Cocktail (above)

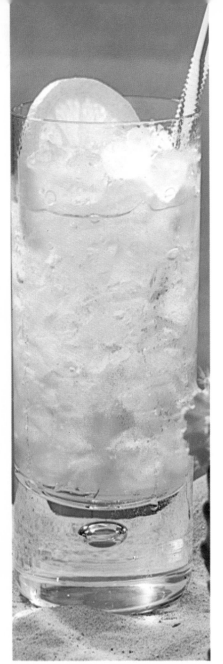

Tequila Fix

Tequila Sunrise

6–8 ice cubes
50 ml/2 oz tequila
25 ml/1 oz grenadine
25 ml/1 oz lemon juice
soda water
1 lime slice

Crack half ice and put in a shaker
with tequila, grenadine and lemon
juice. Shake and strain into a tumbler. Top up with soda water, add
remaining ice and fix lime slice on
rim of glass. Serve with a straw.

Third Rail

2–3 ice cubes
25 ml/1 oz rum
2 teaspoons dry vermouth
2 teaspoons red vermouth
2 teaspoons orange juice

Crack ice and put in a shaker with
other ingredients. Shake well and
strain into a cocktail glass.

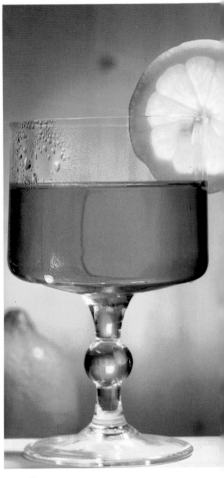

Tim Frazer

Tequila Fix

15 ml/½ oz lime juice
2 teaspoons honey
50 ml/2 oz tequila
2 dashes Cointreau
4–5 ice cubes
1 lemon slice

Put lime juice and honey in a tall
tumbler and stir well. Add tequila
and Cointreau. Crush ice and add
to glass. Stir well and decorate
with lemon slice. Serve with a
straw.

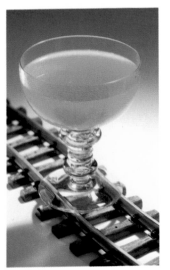

Third Rail

Tim Frazer

2–3 ice cubes
25 ml/1 oz whisky
25 ml/1 oz dry vermouth
15 ml/½ oz Campari
soda water
1 lemon slice

Crack ice and put in a shaker with
whisky, vermouth and Campari.
Shake well and strain into a large
cocktail glass. Add a shot of soda
water and fix lemon slice on rim
of glass.

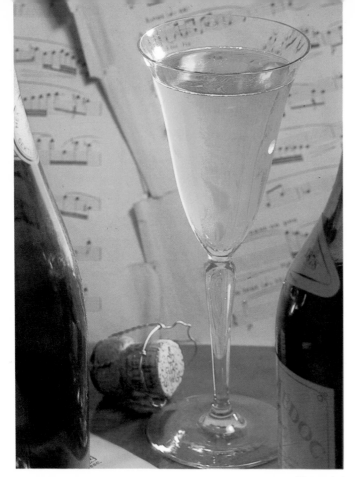

Toscanini

Tomato Cocktail

2–3 ice cubes
50 ml/2 oz tomato juice
2 dashes lemon juice
1 dash tomato ketchup
1 dash Worcestershire sauce
celery salt

Crack ice and put in a shaker with tomato juice, lemon juice, tomato ketchup, Worcestershire sauce and a little celery salt. Shake well and strain into a small goblet.

Tous les Garçons

2–3 ice cubes
20 ml/¾ oz brandy
20 ml/¾ oz dry vermouth
20 ml/¾ oz crème de cacao
1 dash orange bitters

Crack ice and put in a shaker with other ingredients. Shake well and strain into a cocktail glass.

Toscanini

3–4 ice cubes
25 ml/1 oz Cordial Médoc
15 ml/½ oz Cointreau
15 ml/½ oz brandy
champagne

Crack ice and put in a shaker with Cordial Médoc, Cointreau and brandy. Shake well and strain into a tall champagne glass. Top up with champagne.

Tovarich

8 ice cubes
50 ml/2 oz vodka
25 ml/1 oz kümmel
20 ml/¾ oz lime juice

Crack two ice cubes and put in a shaker with vodka, kümmel and lime juice. Shake well. Crush remaining ice and put in a tall, narrow goblet. Strain in contents of shaker and serve with a straw.

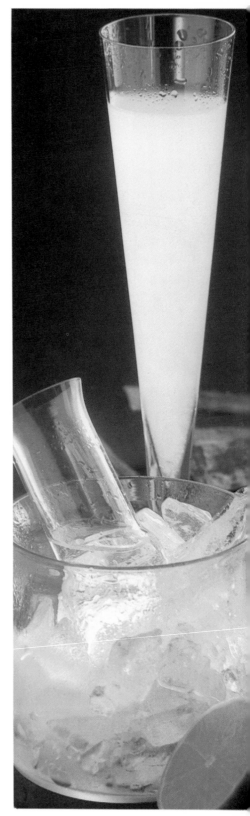

Tovarich

Ultimo

2–3 ice cubes
25 ml/1 oz gin
2 teaspoons whisky
2 teaspoons vodka
2 teaspoons dry vermouth
1 teaspoon Campari
1 olive

Crack ice and put in a shaker with gin, whisky, vodka, vermouth and Campari. Shake very well and strain into a cocktail glass. Spear olive on a cocktail stick and use to decorate.

Union Jack

2–3 ice cubes
40 ml/1½ oz gin
20 ml/¾ oz crème yvette

Crack ice and put in a shaker with gin and crème yvette. Shake and strain into a cocktail glass.

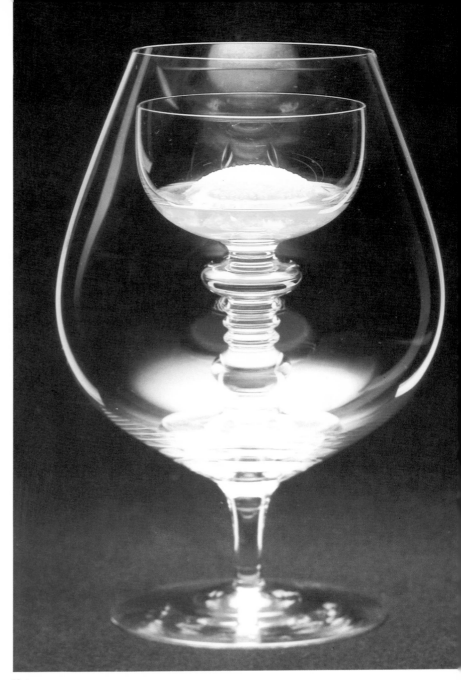

Upton

Up-to-date

2–3 ice cubes
25 ml/1 oz rye whisky
25 ml/1 oz sherry
2 dashes Grand Marnier
2 dashes Angostura bitters
piece of lemon peel

Put ice in a mixing glass with whisky, sherry, Grand Marnier and bitters. Stir well and strain into a cocktail glass. Squeeze lemon peel over top.

Upton

1 egg yolk
1 teaspoon castor sugar
50 ml/2 oz brandy

Slide egg yolk into a shallow glass. Sprinkle with sugar and add brandy. Do not stir this drink, but swallow it in one gulp.

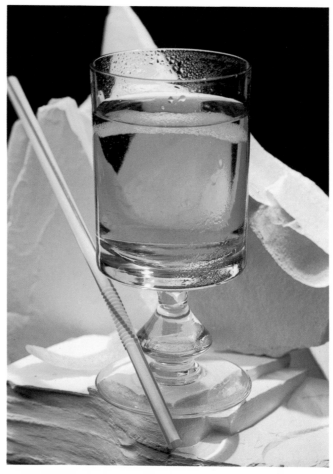

Vermouth Cassis

Vampire Killer

2–3 ice cubes
25 ml/1 oz gin
15 ml/½ oz Fernet Branca
15 ml/½ oz red vermouth

Crack ice and put in a shaker with other ingredients. Shake well and strain into a cocktail glass.

Vermouth Addington

2–3 ice cubes
25 ml/1 oz dry vermouth
25 ml/1 oz bianco vermouth
soda water
spiral of lemon peel

Crack ice and put in a shaker with vermouths. Shake and strain into a goblet. Top up with soda water and decorate with spiral of lemon peel. Serve with a straw.

Vermouth Cassis

2–3 ice cubes
80 ml/3 oz dry vermouth
40 ml/1½ oz crème de cassis
soda water
piece of lemon peel

Put ice in a goblet with vermouth and crème de cassis. Stir and top up with soda water. Decorate with piece of lemon peel and serve with a straw.

Vermouth Flip

2–3 ice cubes
1 egg yolk
1 teaspoon castor sugar
65 ml/2½ oz vermouth
nutmeg

Crack ice and put in a shaker with egg yolk, sugar and vermouth. Shake very well and strain into a flip glass. Grate a little nutmeg over top and serve with a straw.

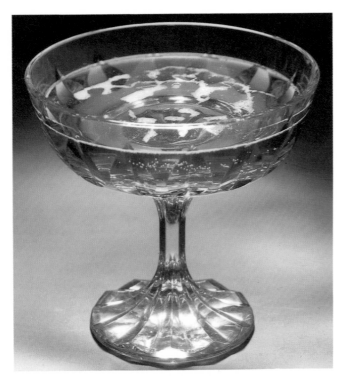

Vie - en-rose

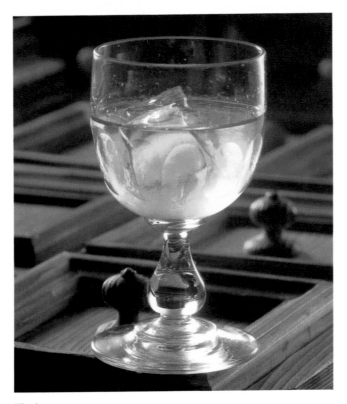

Virgin

Vie-en-rose

2–3 ice cubes
15 ml/½ oz plum brandy
15 ml/½ oz cherry brandy
15 ml/½ oz raspberry syrup
sparkling wine

Crack ice and put in a shaker with plum brandy, cherry brandy and raspberry syrup. Shake well and strain into a shallow champagne glass. Top up with sparkling wine.

Virgin

2 ice cubes
20 ml/¾ oz gin
20 ml/¾ oz Forbidden Fruit
   liqueur
2 teaspoons crème de menthe

Put ice in a shaker with other ingredients. Shake and pour into a cocktail glass.

Vodka Crusta

15 ml/½ oz orange juice
1 tablespoon castor sugar
4–5 ice cubes
40 ml/1½ oz vodka
15 ml/½ oz brandy
15 ml/½ oz red vermouth
1 dash orange bitters
1 dash Angostura bitters
spiral of lemon peel

Dip rim of a goblet first in orange juice, shaking off excess, then in sugar. Allow frosting to dry. Crack ice and put in a shaker with vodka, brandy, vermouth, bitters and two teaspoons of remaining sugar. Shake well and strain into glass. Decorate with spiral of lemon peel.

Vodka Daisy

4–6 pineapple chunks
4–6 ice cubes
50 ml/2 oz vodka
2 teaspoons sugar syrup
1 teaspoon Bénédictine
1 dash maraschino
1 dash calvados
soda water

Put pineapple chunks in a tall champagne glass. Crack ice and put in a shaker with vodka, sugar syrup, Bénédictine, maraschino and calvados. Shake very well and strain into glass. Add a shot of soda water and serve with a straw and a spoon.

Vodka Fizz

3 ice cubes
50 ml/2 oz pineapple juice
40 ml/1½ oz vodka
1 teaspoon lemon juice
1 teaspoon sugar syrup
soda water

Crack two ice cubes and put in a shaker with pineapple juice, vodka, lemon juice and sugar syrup. Shake very well and strain into a tall goblet. Top up with soda water, add remaining ice cube and serve with a straw.

Vodka Gibson

2–3 ice cubes
40 ml/1½ oz vodka
15 ml/½ oz dry vermouth
2–3 pearl onions

Put ice in a mixing glass with vodka and vermouth. Stir well and strain into a cocktail glass. Decorate with pearl onions and serve with a cocktail stick.

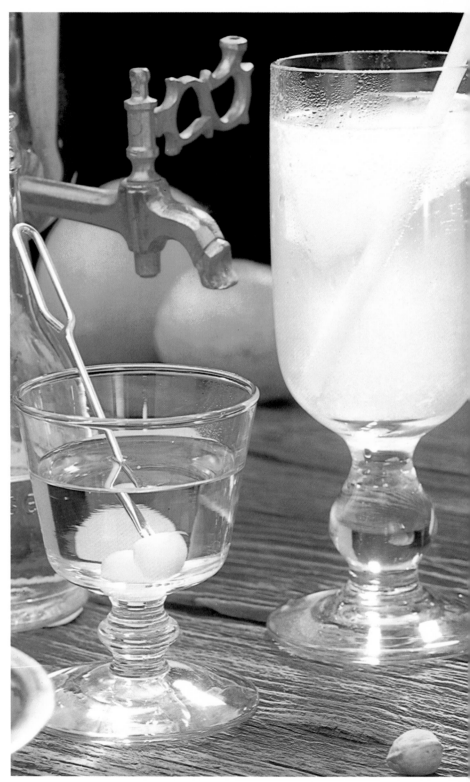

Vodka Gibson, Vodka Fizz

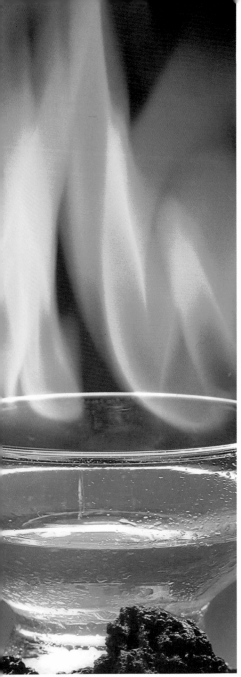

Vulcano

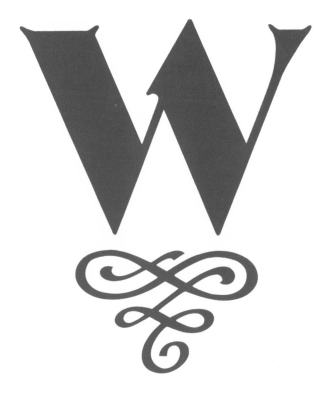

Vulcano

25 ml/1 oz green Chartreuse
25 ml/1 oz kirsch
1 dash Cointreau
1 dash blue curaçao
sparkling wine

Put Chartreuse, kirsch, Cointreau and blue curaçao in a shallow flameproof glass and stir. Stand glass on an asbestos mat and set light to contents. Put out flames with sparkling wine.

Wallflower

2–3 ice cubes
40 ml/1½ oz crème de cacao
25 ml/1 oz white rum
25 ml/1 oz orange juice
25 ml/1 oz cream
1 teaspoon grenadine
1 teaspoon castor sugar
½ teaspoon grated chocolate

Crack ice and put in a shaker with all other ingredients except grated chocolate. Shake very well and strain into a goblet. Sprinkle with grated chocolate.

Washington

2–3 ice cubes
40 ml/1½ oz brandy
15 ml/½ oz dry vermouth
1 teaspoon sugar syrup or
  grenadine
2 dashes Angostura bitters

Put ice in a mixing glass with other ingredients and stir well. Strain into a cocktail glass.

Wave of Sylt

1 tablespoon castor sugar
50 ml/2 oz boiling water
25 ml/1 oz rum
25 ml/1 oz red wine
1 clove
nutmeg
1 lemon slice

Put sugar in a warmed flameproof punch glass. Add boiling water and stir until sugar has dissolved. Put rum, red wine and clove in a pan, heat until just below boiling point, then pour into glass. Grate a little nutmeg over top and decorate with lemon slice.

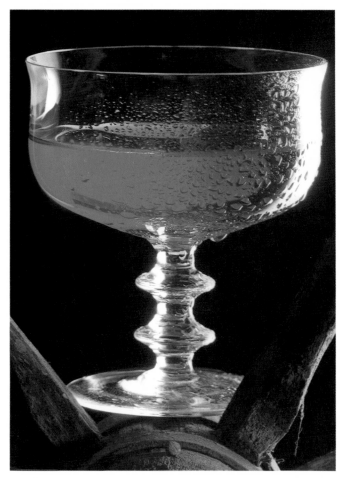
Washington

Whisky Sour

2–3 ice cubes
50 ml/2 oz Bourbon whisky
15 ml/½ oz orange juice
15 ml/½ oz lemon juice
2 teaspoons castor sugar
1 orange segment
1 lemon segment
3 cocktail cherries
soda water

Crack ice and put in a shaker with whisky, orange juice, lemon juice and sugar. Shake very well and strain into a tumbler. Add orange and lemon segments and cherries, and top up with soda water. Serve with a straw.

White Lady

2–3 ice cubes
½ egg white
2 teaspoons lemon juice
25 ml/1 oz gin
2 teaspoons Cointreau
1 cocktail cherry

Crack ice and put in a shaker with egg white, lemon juice, gin and Cointreau. Shake very well and strain into a cocktail glass. Spear cherry on a cocktail stick and use to decorate.

William's Favourite

20 ml/¾ oz pear brandy
20 ml/¾ oz dry vermouth
20 ml/¾ oz crème de cassis
1 pineapple chunk
sparkling wine
1 orange slice

Put pear brandy, vermouth and crème de cassis in a shallow champagne glass and stir. Add pineapple chunk and top up with chilled sparkling wine. Fix orange slice on rim of glass and serve with a cocktail stick.

Whisky Cocktail

2–3 ice cubes
50 ml/2 oz whisky
2 dashes Angostura bitters
2 dashes sugar syrup
1 cocktail cherry

Crack ice and put in a shaker with whisky, bitters and sugar syrup. Shake and strain into a cocktail glass. Decorate with cherry.

Whisky Cooler

4 ice cubes
50 ml/2 oz whisky
25 ml/1 oz lemon juice
1 teaspoon castor sugar
ginger ale

Crack two ice cubes and put in a shaker with whisky, lemon juice and sugar. Shake and strain into a tall tumbler. Top up with ginger ale and add remaining ice.

115

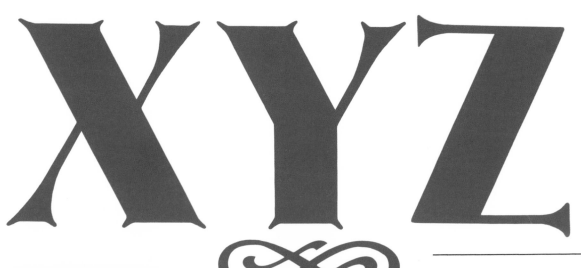

XYZ

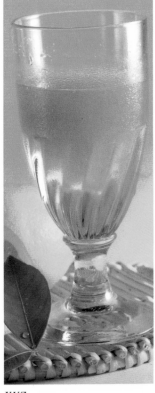

XYZ

XYZ

2–3 ice cubes
25 ml/1 oz dark rum
15 ml/½ oz Cointreau
15 ml/½ oz lemon juice

Crack ice and put in a shaker with other ingredients. Shake and strain into a cocktail glass.

Yankee Flip

2–3 ice cubes
1 egg yolk
1 teaspoon castor sugar
80 ml/3 oz red wine
40 ml/1½ oz pineapple juice
nutmeg

Crack ice and put in a shaker with egg yolk, sugar, wine and pineapple juice. Shake very well and strain into a flip glass. Grate a little nutmeg over top and serve with a straw.

Yellow Daisy

2–3 ice cubes
40 ml/1½ oz gin
40 ml/1½ oz dry vermouth
2 teaspoons Grand Marnier
1 cocktail cherry

Crack ice and put in a shaker with gin, vermouth and Grand Marnier. Shake well and strain into a large cocktail glass. Decorate with cherry and serve with a cocktail stick.

Yellow Parrot

2–3 ice cubes
25 ml/1 oz yellow Chartreuse
20 ml/¾ oz gin
20 ml/¾ oz Bénédictine
1 cocktail cherry

Crack ice and put in a shaker with Chartreuse, gin and Bénédictine. Shake and strain into a cocktail glass. Decorate with cherry and serve with a cocktail stick.

York

2–3 ice cubes
40 ml/1½ oz whisky
2 teaspoons red vermouth
2–3 dashes Angostura bitters
piece of lemon peel

Put ice in a mixing glass with whisky, vermouth and bitters. Stir well and strain into a cocktail glass. Squeeze lemon peel over top.

Zoom

2–3 ice cubes
40 ml/1½ oz brandy
20 ml/¾ oz cream
15 ml/½ oz honey

Crack ice and put in a shaker with other ingredients. Shake well and strain into a large cocktail glass.

Index

ADVOCAAT
Coffee Advocaat 37
El Dorado 47
Japonaise 60

ANISETTE
Anisette Cocktail 14

APRICOT BRANDY
Angel's Face 13
Angel's Kiss 14
Apricot Blossom 14
Apricot Brandy Daisy 14
Apricot Cooler 16
Bel Ami 18
Charlie Chaplin 33
Columbus 38
Copacabana 39
Dawn Crusta 43
Delicious Sour 43
Empire 47
Georgia Mint Julep 51
Intimate 59
Lieutenant 65
Lone Tree Cooler 66
Moulin Rouge 75
Mule's Hind Leg 75
Natasha 76
Red Shadow 89
Rose 92
Sweet Girl 104

BEER
Fire Extinguisher 48

BÉNÉDICTINE
ABC 10
Angel's Lips 14
April Shower 16
Bénédictine Frappé 18
Bénédictine Pick-me-up 18
Bourbon Cocktail 21
Calvados Smash 28
Cape Kennedy 29
Gipsy 53
Honeymoon 57
Jeune Homme 60
Monte Carlo Cocktail 73
Mule's Hind Leg 75
Rolls-Royce 91
Sheep's Head 98
Vodka Daisy 113
Yellow Parrot 116

BLUE CURACAO
Blue Day 20
Blue Lady 20

Blue Monday Nightcap (1) 20
Vulcano 114

BOURBON WHISKY
Bourbon Cocktail 21
Bourbon Highball 21
Colonel Collins 38
Golden Gate 54
Lieutenant 65
Manhattan Dry 69
Manhattan Sweet 71
Morning glory 74
Morning Glory Fizz 74
New Yorker 76
Noddy 76
Old-fashioned 78
Old Pale 78
Old Time 79
Rabbit's Revenge 87   2
Saratoga Fizz 96
Sheep's Head 98
Soul Kiss 101
Sputnik (2) 102
Stromboli 103
Whisky Sour 115

BRANDY
Adam and Eve 11
Afterwards 11
Alexander 13
American Beauty 13
April Shower 16
Bazooka 18
Bel Ami 18
Betsy Ross 19
Between the Sheets 19
Brandy Cocktail 23
Brandy Cooler 23
Brandy Crusta 23
Brandy Daisy 23
Brandy Fix 23
Brandy Flip 23
Brandy Highball 25
Brandy Pick-me-up 25
Brandy Rickey 25
Brandy Smash 25
Brandy Tea Punch 25
Butterfly Flip 27
Capri 30
Champagne Pick-me-up 33
Chartreuse Daisy 33
Cherry Blossom 34
Chicago Cocktail 35   5/4
Chocolate Soldier 36
Coffee Cobbler 38
Copacabana 39

Creole Punch 40
Devile's Own 44
Ecstasy 46
Fanny Hill 48   4
Feodora Cobbler 48
Georgia Mint Julep 51
Ginger Daisy 53
Golden Lady 54
International 59
Island Highball 59
Leo's Special 64
Melon Cobbler 72
Morning Glory 74
Paprika Cocktail 80
Peter Tower 80
President Taft's Opossum 84   3
Prince of Wales 85
Queen Mary 85
Ritz 90
Sidecar 98
Sink or Swim 99
Sir Ridgeway Knight 99
Smiling Esther 100
Sputnik (2) 102
Stinger 102
Stonehammer 102
Swedish Fan 104
Swiss Sunset 105
Tantalus 106
Toscanini 109
Tous les Garçons 109
Upton 110
Vodka Crusta 112
Wallflower 114
Zoom 116

CALVADOS
Applejack Rabbit 14
Calvados Cocktail 28
Calvados Smash 28
Delicious Sour 43
Empire 47
Harvard Cooler 56
Honeymoon 57
Klondyke Cocktail 63
Mule's Hind Leg 75
Star 102   1
Vodka Daisy 113

CAMPARI
Americano 13
Campari and Soda 29
Campino 29
Capri 30
Fanny Hill 48

Half and Half 56
Negroni 76
Old Pale 78
Take Two 106
Tim Frazer 108
Ultimo 110

CHAMPAGNE
ABC 10
Brandy Pick-me-up 25
Buck's Fizz 26
Champagne Cobbler 31
Champagne Cocktail 31
Champagne Daisy 31
Champagne Flip 33
Champagne Pick-me-up 33
Melon Cobbler 72
Monte Carlo Imperial 74
Ritz 90
Toscanini 109

CHARTREUSE
Alaska 11
Bazooka 18
Bijou 19
C and S 28
Champagne Daisy 31
Chartreuse Daisy 33
Chartreuse Straight 33
Chartreuse Temptation 34
Chocolate Cocktail 36
International 59
Mary Queen of Scots 71
Rye Daisy 94
Sir Ridgeway Knight 99
Vulcano 114
Yellow Parrot 116

CHERRY BRANDY
Bazooka 18
Brandy Fix 23
Cherry Blossom 34
Cherry Brandy Flip 34
Cherry Sour 35
Colorado 38
Darling 42
Dubonnet Fizz 44
Geisha 51
Red Kiss 89
Red Shadow 89
Singapore Gin Sling 99
Swedish Fan 104
Vie-en-rose 112

CIDER
Stone Fence 102

COFFEE
Agadir 11
Black Russian 19
Cacao Frappé 28
Carioca 30
Coffee Advocaat 37
Coffee Cobbler 38
Favourite 48
Irish Coffee 59
Slivovitz Cocktail 100

COINTREAU
Adam and Eve 11
Amour Crusta 13
Bacardi Highball 16
Balalaika 16
Between the Sheets 19 (1 and 2)
Blue Monday Nightcaps 20
Boniface the Good 20
Bourbon Cocktail 21
Brandy Tea Punch 25
Calvados Cocktail 28
Champagne Cobbler 31
Charleston 33
Cherry Blossom 34
Chicago Cocktail 35
Continental 39
Copacabana 39
Cuba Crusta 41
Daiquiri American-style 42
Dandy 42
East India 46
Fanny Hill 48
Favourite 48
Feodora Cobbler 48
Golden Cocktail 53
Golden Daisy 54
Golden Gate 54
Golden Lady 54
Hemingway 57
Honeymoon 57
Horse Guards 58
Island Dream 59
Jeune Homme 60
Leo's Special 64
Madeira Cobbler 67
Maiden 68
Margarita 71
Melon Cobbler 72
Mont Blanc 73
Morning Glory 74
New Orleans Fizz 76
Old Time 79
Orange Bloom 79
Orange County Julep 79
Panther's Sweat 80
Paprika Cocktail 80
Peter Tower 80
Port Cobbler 83
Prince of Wales 85
Queen Bee 85
Queen Elizabeth 85
Queen Mary 85
Ramona Fizz 88
Rhett Butler 90

Ritz 90
Royal Bermuda 93
Royal Long 93
Rum Flip 94
Sante Fé Express 96
Satan's Whiskers 97
Sidecar 98
Singapore Gin Sling 99
Sir Ridgeway Knight 99
Summertime 104
Take Two 106
Tango 106
Tequila Fix 108
Toscanini 109
Vulcano 114
White Lady 115
XYZ 116

CRÈME DE CACAO
Alexander 13
Barbarians' Tracks 17
Butterfly Flip 27
Cacao Frappé 28
Chocolate Cocktail 36
Chocolate Soldier 36
El Dorado 47
Grasshopper 55
Mona Lisa 72
Rum Alexander 93
Sweet Lady 105
Tous les Garçons 109
Wallflower 114

CRÈME DE CASSIS
Acapulco 10
Dijon Fizz 44
Tequila Caliente 107
Vermouth Cassis 111
William's Favourite 115

CRÈME DE MENTHE
Afterwards 11
Calvados Smash 28
Devil's Own 44
Frozen Caruso 50
Grasshopper 55
Green Dragon 55
Green Fizz 55
Green Hat 55
Green Sea 56   3+
Greenhorn 56
Monte Carlo Imperial 74
Stinger 102
Virgin 112

CRÈME DE VANILLE
Flip Amore 49

DRAMBUIE
Ecstasy 46
Mallorca 69
Mary Queen of Scots 71
Rusty Nail 94

DUBONNET
Dubonnet Cocktail 44
Dubonnet Fizz 44

Old Time 79
Opera 79
Soul Kiss 101

FRUIT LIQUEURS (MISCELLANEOUS)
Bloodhound 19
Golden Gate 54
Mallorca 69
Red Pearl 89
Swiss Sunset 105
Tantalus 106
Virgin 112

GIN
Adam and Eve 11
Alaska 11
Angel's Face 13
Anisette Cocktail 14
Barbarians' Tracks 17
Barfly's Dream 17
Bazooka 18
Beau Rivage 18
Beautiful 18
Berlin 18
Bijou 19
Bloodhound 19
Blue Lady 20
Bronx 26
Campino 29
Charleston 33
Charlie Chaplin 33
Clipper 37
Clover Club 37
Cooperstown 39
Derby 43
Douglas 44
Dubonnet Cocktail 44
Dubonnet Fizz 44
Empire 47
Eton Blazer 47
Evening Sun 47
Flying Dutchman 50
French Cocktail 50   4+
Frozen Caruso 50
Futurity 50
Geisha 51
Gimlet 51
Gin Fizz 52
Gin Oyster 52
Gin Punch 52
Gin Rickey 53
Gin Sling 53
Golden Cocktail 53
Golden Fizz 54
Green Hat 55
Hawaii Kiss 57
Island Highball 59
Jeune Homme 60
John Collins 60
Kiku Kiku 60
Lady Brown 64
Little Prince 65
Lychee Cocktail 66

Magnolia Blossom 68
Maiden 68
Martini Dry 71
Martini Medium 71
Martini on the Rocks 71
Martini Sweet 71
Mont Blanc 73
Monte Carlo Imperial 74
Moulin Rouge 75
Mule's Hind Leg 75
Napoleon 76
Negroni 76
New Orleans Fizz 76
Noddy 76
Opera 79
Orange Bloom 79
Page Court 80
Panther's Sweat 80
Peter Pan 80
Pink Gin 82
Pink Lady Fizz 82
Pinky 82
Queen Elizabeth 85
Queen's Cocktail 85
Ramona Cocktail 87
Red Kiss 89
Rolls-Royce 91
Rose 92
Royal Fizz 93
Sake Special 96
Satan's Whiskers 97
Silver Fizz 99
Singapore Gin Sling 99
Stonehammer 102
Swedish Fan 104
Sweet Girl 104
Take Two 106
Tango 106
Taxi 106
Ultimo 110   3
Union Jack 110
Vampire Killer 111
Virgin 112
White Lady 115
Yellow Daisy 116
Yellow Parrot 116

GRAND MARNIER
Annabelle 14
Carioca 30
Lady Brown 64
Paprika Cocktail 80
Up-to-date 110
Yellow Daisy 116

GRENADINE
Afterwards 11
American Beauty 13
American Glory 13
Apricot Cooler 16
Beau Rivage 18
Beautiful 18
Champagne Daisy 31
Cherry Blossom 34
Clover Club 37

Country Club Highball 39
Crustino 40
Dawn Crusta 43
Douglas 44
Evening Sun 47
Fireman's Sour 49
Flying Dutchman 50
French Cocktail 50
Gin Rickey 53
Golden Cocktail 53
Golden Fizz 54
Grapefruit Highball 54
Island Dream 59
Japonaise 60
Lone Tree Cooler 66
Madeira Cobbler 67
Magnolia Blossom 68
Martini Sweet 71
Moulin Rouge 75
New Yorker 76
Orange County Julep 7
Pernod Fizz 80
Peter Tower 80
Pink Lady Fizz 82
Pinky 82
Rabbit's Revenge 87
Ramona Cocktail 87
Red Tonic 89
Redskin 89
Rose 92
Rum Cobbler 93
Rye Cocktail 94
Summertime 104
Tequila Caliente 107
Tequila Sunrise 108
Wallflower 114

KIRSCH
Afterwards 11
Annabelle 14
Charleston 33
Colorado 38
Dijon Fizz 44
Eton Blazer 47
Imperial Crusta 58
Japonaise 60
Kirsch Cobbler 63
Little Prince 65
Madeira Cobbler 67
Vulcano 114

MADEIRA
Berlin 18
Madeira Cobbler 67
Madeira Flip 67

MARASCHINO
Amour Crusta 13
Brandy Crusta 23
Brooklyn 26
Charleston 33
Continental 39
Flip Amore 49
Gin Punch 52
Kirsch Cobbler 63

Madeira Cobbler 67
Opera 79
Rocky Mountains Punch 91
Rum Cobbler 93
Vodka Daisy 113

PEACH BRANDY
Derby 43
Sweet Lady 105

PEAR BRANDY
Moonlight 74
Natasha 76
William's Favourite 115

PERNOD
Anisette Cocktail 14
French Cocktail 50
Morning Glory 74
Morning Glory Fizz 74
Noddy 76
Old Time 79
Pernod Fizz 80
Queen Bee 85
Queen Elizabeth 85
Queen Mary 85
Taxi 106
Je ne sais quoi - 1
PIMM'S
Pimlet 81
Pimm's 81

PLUM BRANDY
Apricot Blossom 14
Lightning Punch 65
Slivovitz Cocktail 100
Vie-en-rose 112

PORT
Amour Crusta 13
Betsy Ross 19
Chocolate Cocktail 36
Creole Punch 40
Crustino 40
Good Morning 54
Lady's Crusta 64
Port Cobbler 83
Tequila Cocktail 107

RASPBERRY BRANDY
Royal Fizz 93

RED WINE
American Cooler 13
Burnt Punch 27
Chicago Cocktail 35
Claret Fizz 36
Claret Flip 36
Claret Sour 37
Manhattan Cooler 69
Myra 75
Wave of Sylt 114
Yankee Flip 116

RUM
American Cooler 13
Bacardi Blossom 16
Bacardi Highball 16
Barbarians' Tracks 17

Barfly's Dream 17
Beau Rivage 18
Beautiful 18
Between the Sheets 19
Burnt Punch 27
Cape Kennedy 29
Caricoca 30
Claret Sour 37
Clipper 37
Columbus 38
Cuba Crusta 41
Cuba Libre 41
Daiquiri American-style 42 4
Daiquiri on the Rocks 42
Dawn Crusta 43
East India 46
East Wind 46
El Dorado 47
Favourite 48
Feodora Cobbler 48
Fireman's Sour 49
Good Morning 54
Havana Club 57
Hemingway 57
Horse Guards 58
Island Dream 59
Lychee Cocktail 66
Mai Tai 68
Mallorca 69
Manhattan Cooler 69
Manhattan Latin 71
Mississippi 72
Page Court 80
Peter Tower 80
Planter's Cocktail 82
Planter's Punch 82
Presidente 84
Quarter Deck 85
Ramona Fizz 88
Redskin 89
Rocky Mountains Punch 91
Royal Bermuda 93
Rum Alexander 93
Rum Cobbler 93
Rum Cocktail 94
Rum Flip 94
Rum Sour 94
Summertime 104
Third Rail 108
Wallflower 114
Wave of Sylt 114
XYZ 116

RYE WHISKY
Byrrh Cocktail 28
Mississippi 72
Rye Cocktail 94
Rye Daisy 94
Rye Punch 94
Up-to-date 110

SHERRY
Adonis 11
Bamboo 17
Butler's Good Morning Flip 27

Duplex 44
Quarter Deck 85
Sherry Cobbler 98
Up-to-date 110

SLOE GIN
Queen Bee 85

SPARKLING WINE
Agadir 11
American Glory 13
Apricot Brandy Daisy 14
Boniface the Good 20
Butler's Good Morning Flip 27
Chartreuse Temptation 34
Continental 39
Crustino 40
Fanny Hill 48
Fresco 50
Golden Gate 54
Golden Lady 54
Hawaii Kiss 57
Hemingway 57
Horse Guards 58
Knockout 63
Leo's Special 64
Moulin Rouge 75
Prince of Wales 85
Red Pearl 89
Rocky Mountains Punch 91
Royal Long 93
Sparkling Grape Cocktail 101
Vie-en-rose 112
Vulcano 114
William's Favourite 115

TEA
Brandy Tea Punch 25
Rum Flip 94

TEQUILA
Acapulco 10
Margarita 71
Tequila Caliente 107
Tequila Cocktail 107
Tequila Fix 108
Tequila Sunrise 108

VERMOUTH
Adonis 11
American Beauty 13
Americano 13
Bamboo 17
Beau Rivage 18
Beautiful 18
Bijou 19
Bloodhound 19
Brandy Cocktail 23
Bronx 26
Brooklyn 26
Byrrh Cocktail 28
Campino 29
Capri 30
Champagne Pick-me-up 33
Charleston 33
Chocolate Soldier 36
Continental 39

Cooperstown 39
Country Club Highball 39
Crystal Highball 41
East Wind 46
Ecstasy 46
Evening Sun 47
Frozen Caruso 50
Futurity 50
Geisha 51
Golden Cocktail 53
Green Sea 56
Half and Half 56
Havana Club 57
Hot Italy 58
Intimate 59
Island Highball 59
Jeune Homme 60
Kangaroo 60
Klondyke Cocktail 63
Klondyke Cooler 63
Little Prince 65
Mallorca 69
Manhattan Dry 69
Manhattan Latin 71
Manhattan Sweet 71
Martini Dry 71
Martini Limone 71
Martini Medium 71
Martini on the Rocks 71
Martini Sweet 71
Mona Lisa 72
Moonlight 74
Myra 75

Natasha 76
Negroni 76
Old Pale 78
Orange Bloom 79
Paddy 80
Panther's Sweat 80
Peter Pan 80
Presidente 84
Queen's Cocktail 85
Ray Long 88
Raymond Hitch Cocktail 88
Red Kiss 89
Rob Roy 90
Rolls-Royce 91
Rose 92
Satan's Whiskers 97
Sheep's Head 98
Sink or Swim 99
Soul Kiss 101
Star 102
Stonehammer 102
Tango 106
Taxi 106
Third Rail 108
Tim Frazer 108
Tous les Garçons 109
Ultimo 110
Vampire Killer 111
Vermouth Addington 111
Vermouth Cassis 111
Vermouth Flip 111
Vodka Crusta 112
Vodka Gibson 113

Washington 114
William's Favourite 115
Yellow Daisy 116
York 116

VODKA
Balalaika 16
Black Russian 19
Bloody Mary 20
Blue Day 20
Blue Monday Nightcaps
  (1 and 2) 20
Bullshot 26
East Wind 46
Gipsy 53
Green Dragon 55
Green Sea 56
Harvey Wallbanger 56
Intimate 59
Kangaroo 60
Louisa 66
Red Tonic 89
Screwdriver 98
Sputniks (1 and 2) 102
Tovarich 109
Ultimo 110
Vodka Crusta 112
Vodka Daisy 113
Vodka Fizz 113
Vodka Gibson 113

WHISKY
Admiral's Highball 11
Barbarians' Tracks 17

Brooklyn 26
C and S 28
Cablegram Cooler 28
Cape Kennedy 29
Cowboy 40
Dandy 42
Douglas 44
Golden Daisy 54
Hot Italy 58
Irish Coffee 59
Knockout 63
Lightning Punch 65
Mary Queen of Scots 71
Monte Carlo Cocktail 73
Napoleon 76
Paddy 80
Page Court 80
Red Shadow 89
Rhett Butler 90
Rickey 90
Rob Roy 90
Rusty Nail 94
Scarlett O'Hara 97
Stone Fence 102
Sweet Lady 105
Tim Frazer 108
Ultimo 110
Whisky Cocktail 115
Whisky Cooler 115
York 116

WHITE WINE
Champagne Flip 33
Royal Long 93